Oxford Casebook of Forensic Psychiatry

Oxford Casebook of Forensic Psychiatry

Nigel Eastman

Emeritus Professor of Law and Ethics in Psychiatry, St George's, University of London
Honorary Consultant Forensic Psychiatrist, South West London & St George's Mental Health NHS Trust, UK

Gwen Adshead

Consultant Forensic Psychiatrist and Psychotherapist, Broadmoor Hospital, UK

Simone Fox

Consultant Clinical and Forensic Psychologist, South London and Maudsley NHS Foundation Trust, UK

Richard Latham

Consultant Forensic Psychiatrist, East London NHS Foundation Trust, UK

Seán Whyte

Consultant Forensic Psychiatrist & Clinical Director, South-West London &
St George's Mental Health NHS Trust
Visiting Senior Lecturer, Institute of Psychiatry, Psychology & Neuroscience, UK

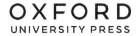

OXFORD
UNIVERSITY PRESS

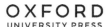

Great Clarendon Street, Oxford, OX2 6DP,
United Kingdom

Oxford University Press is a department of the University of Oxford.
It furthers the University's objective of excellence in research, scholarship,
and education by publishing worldwide. Oxford is a registered trade mark of
Oxford University Press in the UK and in certain other countries

© Oxford University Press 2023

The moral rights of the authors have been asserted

First Edition published in 2023

Published in the United States of America by Oxford University Press
198 Madison Avenue, New York, NY 10016, United States of America

British Library Cataloguing in Publication Data
Data available

Library of Congress Control Number is on file at the Library of Congress

ISBN 978-0-19-884205-7

DOI: 10.1093/med/9780198842057.001.0001

Printed in the UK by
Ashford Colour Press Ltd, Gosport, Hampshire

*The late Professor Gillian McGauley, Professor of Forensic Psychotherapy and
Medical Education, also Honorary Consultant Forensic Psychotherapist,
St George's, University of London, always a thoughtful, caring and inspirational teacher
at all levels of medical education.*

*Professor Nigel Eastman died unexpectedly in February 2022, while this work was still
in press. Prof. Eastman was a passionate and dedicated educator, and his publications are
a testimony to that passion, and the culmination of a lifetime of study, clinical practice
and research. This book would not exist without him and it is with both sadness and
respect that we, his co-authors and editors, dedicate this book to him, as a posthumous
thank you for the enthusiasm, intellect and generosity that made it possible.*

PREFACE

This *Oxford Casebook of Forensic Psychiatry* is a companion to the *Oxford Specialist Handbook of Forensic Psychiatry*. The handbook is written at the interface of law and psychiatry, covering not only the psychiatry of mental disorder and offending behaviour but also law in relation to all adult psychiatry. It is therefore not limited in its relevance to those who practise specialist forensic psychiatry but, we hope, is of value to all psychiatrists, and other mental health professionals, as well as to those lawyers, judges, police officers, and others who deal with branches of criminal and civil law where mental disorder is relevant. The handbook is a resource book which addresses both clinical forensic psychiatry and the developing practical and academic disciplines of psycho-legal studies, so that it offers exploration of the theory and practice of 'psychiatry and law'. The casebook is, as a companion volume, intended to supplement and complement the handbook in each of these domains.

As in all branches of both medicine and law, learning is greatly enhanced by the opportunity to put knowledge into practice, which in clinical forensic and clinico-legal practice includes the opportunity to think through not only the technical medical but also the legal and ethical aspects of real clinical and legal situations. The discursive and normative nature of this fact-based but heavily value-laden discipline makes such an approach crucial. For example, whereas in other branches of medicine a 'decision tree' approach to technical decision-making may occasionally be sufficient to guide practice, in forensic psychiatry the profound influence of both values and law renders this always inadequate as a sole approach. Hence the decision process must address not only technical clinical issues but also ethical and legal perspectives, constructs, and models, through recognition and exploration of the context and full range of consequences of alternative potential decisions.

The objective of the casebook is therefore to assist practitioners to improve the quality of their clinical, clinico-legal and ethical decision-making, including by enhancing comprehensive awareness of the substance of the decision at hand in any case they may confront in their practice.

Specifically as regards clinico-legal skills, the cases are written so as to be capable of being applied to practice in any common law jurisdiction. Although the law described within each case is that of one, usually all, of the UK & Irish jurisdictions which are dealt with in detail in the handbook, the division of each case into 'clinical', 'legal', and then 'clinico-legal' (then 'ethical') sections allows the reader from a jurisdiction not dealt with to insert for themselves the relevant law from that jurisdiction, and then to carry out 'clinico-legal' analysis based upon that law. Or the British or Irish reader might wish to test their clinico-legal skill by conducting analysis of the case using the law from one or more of the local jurisdictions that are not their own. Finally, we have included a pair of cases (criminal cases 16 and 17) written within other Commonwealth jurisdictions, which again require any reader from one of the UK or Irish jurisdictions to apply their clinical findings to an unfamiliar legal domain; further encouraging the development of generic clinico-legal skills that are not jurisdiction-specific, and which go beyond skills gained through working across the various jurisdictions. The casebook is therefore directly relevant to a wide range of clinicians working across Commonwealth jurisdictions.

The casebook offers explicit aids to decision-making both in positive, factual terms and in terms of norms and value judgments, based upon case scenarios that variously empha-sise clinical, legal, clinico-legal, and ethical aspects, and with cross-referencing into the corresponding pages of the handbook. This model of problem-based learning and working through real-life examples is recognised as highly effective in undergraduate and post-graduate medical education, as well as in legal education and law examinations, where the 'facts' are statutes and past cases, to which abstract reasoning and legal principles are applied. And we hope that readers of the casebook will find it of help in the context of forensic psychiatric practice, including clinico-legal practice.

Space within the second edition of the handbook does not all allow for more than the very occasional brief illustrative case vignette. The casebook fills that gap in resources for applied learning, with cross-referencing into the handbook given via the topics listed in the 'header' of each case, thereby allowing readers to test their knowledge, understand-ing, and ability to use the factual information given in the handbook on each case in the casebook.

The casebook sets out, in Part A, a general introduction to theories of decision-making and related guidelines, then applied to clinical, legal, clinico-legal, and ethical domains. This part includes a summary of the literature on rational and nonrational decision-making, including consideration of heuristics and bias, as well as of values-based practice, the latter going beyond what there is space to include in Part III of the handbook. And it is hoped that the reader will be able to use such discussion of how we all tend to think and behave in order to critique *internally*, in a 'fine-grain' fashion, the decisions to which they may come in the cases that are presented in Part B. That is, although it is not practicable comprehensively to relate detailed aspects of Part A to individual cases in Part B, it is suggested that the reader, or 'decision taker', view their decisions through the prism of the theory presented in Part A.

Part B contains a wide range of illustrative cases derived from the real-life experiences of the authors and others. In relation to which the reader is invited to consider certain decisions for themselves, and is guided to where further relevant information can be found in the handbook; before then reading a discussion of different approaches to the case that might be adopted. The aim is not to suggest that there is necessarily one right approach, but to offer potentially more than one justifiable approach, with consideration of the steps in decision-making leading to each, as well as description of the information, legal prin-ciples, and ethical rights or duties that are implicitly prioritised or privileged by each alternative justifiable decision.

This exercise is aimed ultimately at assisting practitioners to review the quality of the real decisions they take, or are about to take, or of the real decisions of others (the latter being of particular relevance to those involved in subsequent legal process, investigations, reviews, or inquiries, within the paradigms described in Part C). And within this, again the prism of Part A can be applied by the reader as a check on a decision either in the real world or made in a Part B case towards gaining assurance that whatever the eventual outcome may be, the process by which the decision was reached is of high quality and therefore robustly defensible.

Part C describes the various paradigms, both legal and nonlegal, within which real-life decisions that have been made are potentially critiqued *externally*, with particular reference to the extent to which each paradigm is capable of taking account of the fine-grain *internal* decision methods, and biases, that the decision theory presented in Part A describes. It concludes that the gold standard of decision critiquing is self-reflection.

In the many cases, which include clear and important legal aspects, the analysis of possible decisions will be of value not only to clinicians, including those offering expert evidence into litigation, but also to lawyers and judges who should thereby be better able to understand and/or expose the approaches used by clinician expert witnesses in their decision-making in real cases. This will include, for example, the solicitor representing a patient at a Mental Health Tribunal; the barrister evaluating an expert report or cross-examining a psychiatric expert witness, in any criminal or civil trial; and the judge assessing conflicting opinions provided by multiple experts in a civil case.

Hence the casebook seeks to offer clinicians the opportunity to improve the quality and consistency of their clinical, clinico-legal, and related ethical decision-making, and to offer legal practitioners a better understanding of the foundations of the clinical forensic opinions with which they are faced.

Finally, we hope that the format of the casebook, with its logical order of topics and case headnotes facilitating easy cross-referencing into the handbook, will enable readers to dip into a particular topic for speedy assistance, as well as facilitating its use in teaching and training programmes for all clinical and legal professionals.

The casebook expresses the mantra 'knowing information is only part of deciding'. And so we hope that it offers an essential practitioners' guide to decision-making in both clinical forensic and clinico-legal psychiatry.

ACKNOWLEDGEMENTS

Bee Brockman FRCPsych
Stephen Brooks FRCS *ob hospitio porcinam*
Anthony Haycroft BCL(Oxon) Barrister
Sanya Krljes MSc PhD
Catherine Penny MRCPsych LLM
Keith Rix MPhil MD LLM Hon FFFLM
Lucy Scott-Moncrieff BA, Solicitor
Mark Simpson
Lisa Whyte MSc
Hannah Kate Williams MB ChB BSc(Hons) MSc MRCPsych

We would also like to thank all the higher medical trainees in forensic psychiatry within the South London Higher Forensic Psychiatric Training Scheme who took part in psycho-legal workshops within which the some of the cases from this book were discussed and revised. Also those higher trainees who participated in psycho-legal workshops over the past two decades at both St George's, University of London, and the Institute of Psychiatry, Psychology and Neuroscience. The experience gained from this method of teaching gave rise to the concept of the book. Lastly, the casebook would never have been possible without the prompting, hospitality, and forbearance of Pete Stevenson, and colleagues of Oxford University Press.

CONTENTS

OUTLINE OF THE CASEBOOK

Part A of the casebook describes theories concerning what decision-makers do 'internally' in coming to their decisions in clinical and legal contexts, in terms of 'fine-grain' analysis that includes the role played in decision-making by values, as well as consideration of values-based decision-making.

Part B then presents a range of real-life clinical and clinico-legal forensic psychiatric case studies, and invites the reader to make decisions upon each, including through the prism of the theory presented in Part A.

As well as facilitating a continual process of evolution and improvement in one's own decision-making processes, such an exercise can also serve to inform anyone called upon to review the decisions of others, such as in supervision, grand rounds, case conferences, incident reviews, inquiries, or legal process.

However, it is **Part C** that explicitly considers *ex post* the various paradigms used that are 'external' to the decider, and the extent to which the method of each paradigm, including various legal paradigms, is intrinsically capable, or not, of adopting the 'fine-grain' critiquing as described in Part A.

Ultimately fine-grain critiquing of decisions is best undertaken by the individual deciders themselves; if they are able to allow themselves sufficient insight into their own thought processes, including insight into the role that their personal and professional values are likely to play. And this emphasises the importance of gaining a full understanding of the theory offered in Part A, both when dealing with the cases in the casebook and in real-life practice.

PART A
Decision-making

Good, effective, ethical decisions in the assessment, treatment, and management of patients in clinical contexts and defendants or litigants in legal contexts depend upon the strengths and weaknesses of the decision-making process used. Explicit reflection helps good decision-making in any area of medicine (and far beyond medicine), but is particularly necessary in forensic psychiatry and psychology because of the inherent scope for conflict between the clinical and legal perspectives on patients, defendants, and litigants when practising at the interface between those 'terrains', and because of the multiple overlapping, but distinct sets of values and ethical models that different actors (patients, families, clinical and legal professionals, courts, and others) bring to decision-making. Also, unlike most of medical practice, outcome should properly be conceived in terms not just of clinical outcome, for example in terms of QALYs ('quality adjusted life years') and DALYs ('disability adjusted life years'), but also LALYs, that is, 'liberty adjusted life years'.[1] Which is not only in the hands of legal process but is potentially heavily influenced by clinical decision-making, so that *clinical* decision-making will often have major *legal* implications: including sometimes 'antiliberty' implications (e.g. via medical recommendations for civil detention under mental health legislation, or its continuance, or via medical recommendations to criminal courts for sentencing, either for mental health care or for penal detention that may be increased in its length by way, at least partly, of medically founded risk assessment).

Clashes of values, whether between individuals or systems, are at the heart of most ethical and legal dilemmas; but these are not always made explicit, or may be categorised as 'facts' or 'practical' or 'obvious', when they are none of these things. And, although this is explored in the handbook, the casebook allows this to be addressed in more depth, and in more 'practical' terms, than is possible in Part III of the handbook: that is, both within Part A and within the cases of Part B.

Part A of the casebook briefly summarises some of the critical insights from a variety of theories and models of decision-making in situations where there is complexity and uncertainty, as well as ambiguity about the values at play. It describes the rational processes that we may fool ourselves into thinking dominate our decision-making, and the nonrational processes that actually underpin the vast bulk of day-to-day decision-making, including the ways in which our values influence and guide both. Still with such theory in mind, also related guidance, it then addresses practical decision-making strategies in both clinical and clinico-legal domains, the latter relating to criminal, civil, family, and mental health and capacity law. Where, in any legal domain, decisions are first clinical in nature, followed by decision-making in regard to the application of the clinical conclusions reached to legal questions posed, or evident, and always with heavy attendant ethical implications. Whilst in what may appear to be a solely clinical context, law will always require consideration (law lurks even in every ward round or case conference), including sometimes by way of modification of a proposed clinical decision.

---

[1] See Eastman N L G and Peay J (1999) Law without enforcement: Theory and practice, in Eastman N L G and Peay J (eds) *Law Without Enforcement: Integrating Mental Health and Justice*, Hart Publications, Chapter 1, pp. 1–38.

A.1

Decision-making theories

Rational decision-making

Before the Enlightenment of the eighteenth century, decision-making rested largely upon the time-worn pillars of faith, hope, and experience. As the Age of Reason progressed, however, scientists, philosophers, and mathematicians, who prided themselves on their rationalism, turned their attention to decision-making, and developed theories that reflected their assumption that it was no more than a purely cognitive reasoning process. Hence, rational decision-making theories focus on how decisions can be improved by more careful analysis and better thinking, with improvement being defined in terms of enhancing the expected utility of the outcome.[1]

There are three main strands amongst rational decision-making theories:

- Normative theories explain how to choose the 'best' available option.
- Descriptive theories explore (within a model) how decisions are actually made.
- Prescriptive theories set out techniques that can help optimise the chances of making good decisions.

According to *normative theories*, under ideal conditions, people should maximise their expected utility (roughly, the mathematical product of the probability of a hoped-for consequence and the worth[2] the individual attaches to it). 'Ideal' conditions require both that all the necessary information is available and that the person is able to weigh up that information rationally, so that decision-makers can use decision analysis to calculate the expected utility of all the options available, and then make the rational choice of the one with the greatest expected utility.

For example, a doctor seeking to help a patient decide between treatment options for hyperthyroidism would clarify the terms of the decision (e.g. Which of the available treatments offers the best combination of symptom-free life, risk avoidance, and side-effects?), and then draw up a 'decision tree' displaying all the possible options—perhaps

---

[1] This 'Benthamite' concept has been used in a wide variety of disciplines, perhaps most notably economics.

[2] The term *value* (in the sense of 'how great a good') is generally used in the decision theory literature instead of *worth*, but it has not been used in this section in order to avoid confusion with the related but more general meaning of *value* (in the sense of 'one of many types of good') used throughout the casebook.

no treatment, carbimazole, radioiodine implants, or partial thyroidectomy—in terms of the possible outcomes of each, their probabilities, and the utility the patient would attach to each outcome (e.g. 'a 50% probability of ten symptom-free years is worth more to me than a 1% chance of death from general anaesthetic and operative complications').[3] However this is a complex and lengthy procedure, which relies upon much intellectualisation of issues and familiarity with probability estimations, none of which comes easily to most people.

Descriptive theories recognise that human beings, even if still perceived to be utility-maximising 'econs' (members of the idealised species *Homo economicus*[4]), operate under a variety of constraints: limited time to make a decision, imperfect knowledge of the options available, fatiguability, competing priorities for resources, and so on—meaning that the most that can be achieved is 'bounded rationality'. Hence the individual is seen as actively solving problems, through purposefully directing their cognitive abilities towards an optimal solution *within those constraints*. And, as a result, descriptive theories emphasise the importance of fast and frugal heuristics: that is, rules of thumb that allow an approximate or good-enough answer to be obtained at far lower cost in terms of time, attention, and knowledge than the perfect utility-maximising answer.

Returning to the example above of the patient facing a choice of treatments for hyperthyroidism, imagine that the patient has already decided that their favoured treatment is a partial thyroidectomy. Their next choice might then be Which surgeon should I ask to perform my operation? A normative approach to this question would require the patient to exhaustively evaluate all possible surgeons, including, for example, in terms of the average morbidity and mortality rates of each (and perhaps other data too, e.g. the fee they would charge if the patient were paying privately for treatment). By contrast, a rational heuristic approach would make the task more manageable by way of 'satisficing': that is, stopping the search once a good-enough answer has been obtained. In this case, that might mean stopping as soon as one had found an available surgeon whose mortality and morbidity rates for partial thyroidectomies were below a preset cut-off, and whose fee was within the private patient's budget.

Another rational heuristic approach tackles the difficulty of combining conceptually different worths (e.g. survival, doctor's fee, symptom relief, and the hassle of taking a tablet every day for many years) into a single utility figure. For example, calculating how bad symptoms would have to be to justify a 1% lower chance of survival is difficult (since it involves comparing 'apples with oranges'). So, instead, each type of worth for each option is evaluated separately, and options discarded if any one worth is too low to be thought worthy of inclusion. And then once enough options have been eliminated in this manner, it becomes simpler to choose between the remainder.

Lastly, *prescriptive theories* set out criteria for good thinking, and methods that facilitate good decision-making. These include, for example:

- consciously recognising that a decision needs to be made and therefore information needs to be gathered;
- agreeing definitions of the decision to be made, and the criteria to be applied;
- avoiding distractions;

---

[3] Here 'utility' is closely related to the public health construct of 'quality adjusted life years' (QALYs).
[4] In fact, most descriptive theories acknowledge that people are not 'econs'; but, rather, employ numerous nonrational decision-making techniques, as explained in the next section.

- maximising the cognitive resources available (e.g. ensuring one is well-fed and well-rested, or, if the decision-makers have mild dementia or are very anxious, ensuring they are deciding whilst in a familiar environment with trusted people); and
- stating all options, worths, and evaluations explicitly.

Clearly such rational heuristics, and the techniques from prescriptive theories, can potentially produce some benefits in terms of better-quality rational decisions. However, they fail to capture both the psychological reality of decision-making and distortions from the pure rationality of *Homo economicus*, and therefore the gains, or avoidance of losses, in both welfare and liberty that can be made from understanding and harnessing nonrational decision-making processes. These are considered next.

Nonrational decision-making

It may seem hard to imagine a better place to find purely rational decision-making than in the rarefied atmosphere of a criminal court or tribunal, with its lofty ideals and rhetoric of justice, its adherence to strict rules of procedure, and with the verdict and sentence precisely calibrated to the evidence and the crime respectively. However, even in this acme of rationality, decision-makers have feet of clay.

For example, in 2011, Danziger and colleagues reported their examination of over 1,112 judicial parole rulings made by experienced judges during fifty sampling days in a period of ten months. They found that, at the start of each of the three sessions of work during the day, the probability of the offender receiving a favourable ruling was around 65%, and that this probability then tailed off consistently to nearly zero by the end of the work session. After a break and a meal, the probability of receiving a favourable outcome when the judge resumed work returned to 65%, and so on.[5] This relationship between case timing and outcome was highly statistically significant. And, in contrast, no such relationship was found between outcome and the severity of the offence, the duration of the original sentence, or the sex or ethnicity of the offender.

Lest any forensic clinicians reading this feel too smug, they fare no better when investigated by critical researchers.

In 1998 Ben-Shakhar and others[6] published research analysing psycho-diagnostic test results of clinician subjects, having given expert clinicians batteries of test results to analyse. Half offered the conclusion that the patient concerned suffered from 'borderline personality disorder'; the other half concluded that they suffered from 'paranoid personality disorder'. Within each round a particular diagnosis was suggested: in one round this was secreted within the background story that preceded presentation of the test results; whilst in another it was made directly within the instructions to participants. The suggestions had been allocated randomly. However, the researchers found that the experts rated borderline, or paranoid, personality disorder significantly more highly when that diagnosis had been suggested to them than when it had not been.

---

[5] Thus proving the wisdom of the quotation attributed to the legal realist Judge Jerome Frank: 'Justice is what the judge ate for breakfast.'

[6] Ben-Shakar G, Bar-Hillel M, Yoram B, and Shefler G (1998) Seek and ye shall find: Test results are what you hypothesize they are, *Journal of Behavioral Decision Making* 11(4):235–249 DOI:10.1002/(SICI)1099-0771(1998120)11:43.0.CO;2-X.

More generally, the assumption of rational decision-making theories that people can and do act as rational utility-maximisers, or 'econs', has been clearly and persistently criticised, originating in the alternative body of theory about decision-making known as 'prospect theory'.[7] One particularly trenchant criticism came from Amartya Sen (a Nobel Prize winning economist) who memorably skewered the notion by satirically describing two econs meeting on the street: ' "Where is the railway station?" he asks me. "There", I say, pointing at the post office, "and would you please post this letter for me on the way?" "Yes", he says, determined to open the envelope and check whether it contains something valuable.'

It is perhaps intuitively obvious that the rational processes described in the previous section do not capture the reality of real-world decision-making, and the studies cited above offer illustrative confirmation of this. However, it has taken many decades for research to tease out just what other mental processes people employ, in part because we deceive ourselves that we think rationally. These processes, described and explained in the following sections of the casebook include:

- unconsciously substituting an easier question for a difficult one;
- applying a causal model to a situation requiring statistical inference (leading to hindsight bias);
- unconsciously predicting answers rather than calculating them;
- selecting answers associated with narrative familiarity and cognitive ease;
- assuming that 'what you see is all there is';
- interpreting information in the light of first impressions ('the halo effect');
- representing categories by way of prototypes or exemplars;
- matching intensity across diverse, unrelated dimensions;
- ignoring sample sizes, base rates, and regression to the mean;
- applying a range of heuristics, including 'anchoring', 'availability', and 'affect';
- basing confidence on narrative coherence rather than statistical probability;
- ignoring 'outside-view' judgments in favour of unrealistically optimistic 'inside-view' judgments (exacerbated by the 'sunflower effect' and 'planning fallacy');
- socially preferring over-optimism to truth-telling;
- paying a premium to avoid uncertainty;
- preferring relative success to absolute success;
- 'loss aversion', and prioritising threats over opportunities;
- seeing more worth in something simply because you already have it ('the endowment effect');
- overweighting unlikely events ('the possibility effect') and underweighting likely ones ('the certainty effect'), and being insensitive to anything in between;
- framing choices too narrowly (leading to 'the disposition effect' and 'the sunk-cost fallacy'); and
- ignoring the insights of the experiencing self (leading to 'the peak-end rule' and to 'duration neglect').

Indeed, the many heuristics and biases that arise from these nonrational processes have been crucial to our evolutionary success as a species: without them, our ancestors would

---

[7] See Kahneman D (2011) *Thinking, Fast and Slow*, Penguin Books, p. 21 (see bibliography), which demonstrates the empirical errors in purely rational economic theory, and which laid the foundation for behavioural economics, the theories and empirical findings of which are directly relevant to clinical and clinico-legal decision making.

all have died on the African savannah, being eaten whilst still attempting to calculate precisely the velocity of the approaching leopard. However, in the world we now inhabit, their shortcomings (e.g. cognitive errors) can often outweigh their benefits (e.g. speed and ease of processing). To overcome this, we need to understand when and how these processes operate. And hence the next sections describe and explain them in detail, with examples given of how they can apply in forensic psychiatric practice, both clinical and clinico-legal. First, however, it is time to meet the main 'actors' of our cognitive processes which operate these heuristics: system 1 and system 2.

Dual processes: system 1 and system 2

How do you conduct your risk assessments?

Take a look at the list of facts about Kevin[8] in Box A.1.1. When you reach the end, summarise to yourself your personal assessment of how likely Kevin is to attack you in the next five minutes.

Box A.1.1 Facts about Kevin

He is aged twenty years.
He is homeless.
He uses alcohol and novel psychoactive substances.
He has been charged with rape and ABH.
His alleged victim was a young woman.
He allegedly raped her over a prolonged period.
He believes the devil is watching him.
He hears the voice of the devil telling him to kill.
He thinks he might have to kill you.
He is holding an axe.

Next, take a look at the artist's impression of Kevin over the page (Figure A.1.1). Again, summarise to yourself your personal assessment of how likely Kevin is to attack you in the next five minutes, based this time upon the picture.

Which risk assessment took longer? And how are the two processes different?

The process of absorbing and integrating the information in Box A.1.1 requires cognitive effort and, although fairly quick, takes an appreciable length of time. By contrast, your judgment on the imminent risk posed by Kevin when you glanced at Figure A.1.1 would have been immediate. The group of mental processes that you used when assimilating the facts is known as 'system 2'; the mental processes that you used when forming a judgment based upon the picture are known as 'system 1'.

One of the functions of system 2 is the generation of the sense of a conscious self[9]: the location of the 'I'. With our tendency towards self-aggrandisement, we assume that system

---

[8] Kevin is the protagonist in clinical cases 8 and 13. The facts in the box are taken from the point in case 8 at which he has not yet been admitted to hospital for treatment. You will be relieved to know that in case 13, he does not go on to kill the assessing psychiatrist.

[9] There is much psychological and philosophical debate about whether consciousness is truly a function of the mind, or simply an epiphenomenon.

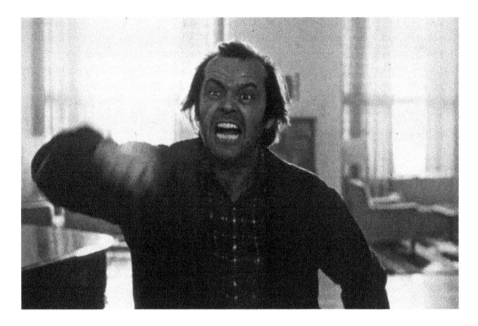

Figure A.1.1. Artist's impression of Kevin. **Used with permission from Warner Bros © 1980**
In fact, Jack Nicholson playing Jack Torrance in *The Shining*; used with permission (and with apologies to Kevin, who like all the characters in the casebook, is similarly fictional).

2 is in charge, and does most of the work. However, this is false: as Daniel Kahneman puts it in his classic work on this topic[10], 'the automatic System 1 is the hero'. Here are some of the characteristics of system 1:

- It operates *automatically* and *speedily*, without effort or conscious direction.
- It *orients* us and enables us to respond quickly to threats and to promising situations.
- When cognitive resources are overcommitted, it offers *shortcuts*; such as yielding to temptation, logical errors,[11] making selfish choices, and making superficial social judgements, all of which take effort to overcome.
- It generates *associatively coherent* responses: that is, combinations of thought, feeling, and physical state that reinforce each other,[12] and this supports associative memory, where ideas are stored in a network within which causes link to effects, objects to their properties, and items to their categories.

[10] Kahneman D (2011) *Thinking, Fast and Slow*, Penguin Books, p. 21 (see bibliography).
[11] For instance, believing a 'fact' (e.g. 'Professor Snape, whose judgement I admire, is opposed to Proposition X') simply because it supports a conclusion you believe true (e.g. 'Proposition X is a bad idea'), without doing anything to check the 'fact' (e.g. recalling from memory that you overheard Professor Snape speak warmly of a prominent propoposition X politician).
[12] Such as, perhaps, when prompted to remember your first youthful experience of intoxication, to feel a mixture of embarrassment, amusement, and disgust, and to experience a mild increase in heart rate and dilation of the pupils, on reading the phrase 'alcopop-induced projectile vomiting'. Associative coherence also explains why people who have been raped or sexually assaulted may feel compelled to cleanse their body, as an analogue for washing away the memory and sense of powerlessness, despite a conscious awareness that this may destroy potential forensic evidence and reduce the chances of a successful prosecution.

- It perceives events *without conscious awareness*, and *primes you to expect* whatever it associates with that event.[13]
- *Acquiring a skill* largely means 'programming system 1 to undertake this task without supervision from system 2'.

Here are some of the characteristics of system 2:

- It *allocates limited mental resources* to activities that require effort to process cognitively and/or emotionally.
- When system 2 is active, the conscious mind 'concentrates' and *experiences agency and choice*.
- Unlike system 1, it can *follow rules*, compare mental objects on more than one attribute simultaneously, and *make reasoned choices*.
- It can *multitask*, provided you have sufficient energy and other mental resources to meet the demands of the tasks combined.[14]
- Conversely, it can in favourable circumstances direct all mental resources to *a specific task*, so that you lose all sense of time, self-reflection, and awareness of surroundings.[15]
- It is *disrupted if attention shifts* (usually because of an alert from system 1).
- It can *influence the functioning of system 1*, by 'reprogramming' aspects of attention and memory (e.g. through establishing new habits).
- It turns selected impressions, intentions, emotions, and intuitions from system 1 into *new beliefs* and actions.
- It can *override system 1* with conscious effort.

System 2 is ponderous and inefficient by comparison with system 1, and it cannot substitute for it. The best that can be done is to recognise when circumstances make system 1 more likely to make a significant error (significant either because the stakes are high or the likely error great or both), and to override or reprogram system 1 in those circumstances. How to do this? One way is through the conscious adoption of values, to which we turn next.

---

[13] For instance, as you enter the interview room in the high-security hospital to assess a new patient for transfer to your service, system 1 notices (without your conscious awareness) a steam pipe adjacent to the door jamb, to which is affixed a notice that says 'Danger—high pressure'. You are now subconsciously primed to expect the patient to be volatile and at high risk of acting violently. You will tense up as you enter the room. The patient may notice this subconsciously and become more tense, and more likely to be aggressive than he would otherwise have been, creating the possibility of your expectation becoming self-fulfilling.

[14] Imagine you are walking an unfamiliar route in another town from the railway station to a prison, to assess a patient. A nurse from your ward calls you and asks urgently whether they have given your patient an overdose ('he's had the full daily regime of 1.5mg clonazepam four times over the past 24 hours, and we've just given 1mg PRN for a second time today, it's all on the prescription chart, but isn't that over the BNF maximum?'). You will almost certainly stop walking in order to calculate that the patient's total dose is 8mg in the last twenty-four hours, and to retrieve from memory the fact that the BNF maximum is (also) 8mg/day. Had the journey been familiar, or the sum immediately obvious (e.g. 1mg once daily plus 1mg PRN), you would probably have kept walking.

[15] Described by Csíkszentmihályi as an intrinsically rewarding 'flow state', and in popular culture as 'being in the zone'. Favourable circumstances include knowing what to do and how to do it; receiving immediate feedback on how well you are doing, so generating a sense of mastery; experiencing the task as challenging but your skills as equal to it; and being free of distractions. Flow states are what make hobbies that facilitate them so beneficial to mental health.

Values at the heart of decision-making

All of this detailed exposition of 'the associative system 1' and 'the cognitive system 2', and their differing foci within the mechanics of decision-making, would make it easy to think of values as distinct and separable from such processes. Certainly, the language used to describe values, and the literature within which they are discussed, is very different from that of the psychologists and others who have developed the concepts and methods of rational and nonrational decision theories. To switch to a culinary metaphor, this might lead one to think of values as the raspberry in a raspberry ripple ice cream: that is, albeit the raspberry is 'rippled' intimately throughout the ice cream, it is still possible to conceive of a vanilla ice cream that *lacked* such a ripple.

The casebook takes an entirely different position: values are the cream in ice cream, without which you simply cannot make genuine ice cream. In other words, the only way to avoid the influence of values is not to make a decision at all. Failing to acknowledge the role and influence of values in decision-making must mean that they operate unseen, leading to unresolved conflict, and potentially to poor-quality decisions.

To explain why this is so, it will help to clarify what is meant by 'values': stable motivational constructs or beliefs about desirable end states that transcend specific situations and guide the evaluation and selection of behaviours and events.[16]

People often refer to their values explicitly, or nearly so, when explaining or justifying their actions, decisions, and preferences to themselves or others (e.g. in reply to the question Why did you discharge Mr Smith from section when he's still symptomatic?, the relevant values are made clear in the response 'Because he had regained mental capacity and I think it's important to respect his autonomy, his right to choose whether or not he continues treatment'). And such explicit expression of values emphasises that they provide individuals with meaning that can be used to understand the world, and form the core of one's identity.[17] Indeed, particular values are sufficiently fundamental that many of them are recognised and understood universally across cultures.[18] Values are strong predictors of behaviours, including compliance with social norms, choice of one consumer product over another, and voting patterns.

What is ethically problematic, indeed dangerous, is to pretend that one's values do not influence one's decision-making; as if one could be 'value-free' in making what one thinks is a solely rational or 'cognitive' decision. That is, to make a decision without use of any 'cream', and to pretend that you have made 'ice cream'.

System 1 functions to preserve associational coherence and minimise cognitive dissonance, and in doing so, it forms, refines, and utilises the individual's values, the high-level associations between beliefs. It continually combines associated ideas, memories,

---

[16] Rohan M J (2000) A rose by any name? The values construct, *Personality and Social Psychology Review* 4(3): 255–277.

[17] Of course, not just professional identity but personal identity, since the latter does not disappear when you put on a white coat.

[18] The ten such universal values identified in Schwartz's original 1992 study across twenty countries were self-direction, stimulation, hedonism, achievement, power, security, conformity, tradition, benevolence, and universalism (a form of equality). The values conflict with one another and cannot be equally valued simultaneously, but they can be recognised and understood simultaneously. They can be plotted in two dimensions, one of individualism (e.g. self-direction) versus community (e.g. conformity), and one of openness to change (e.g. stimulation) versus stability (e.g. tradition). See Schwartz S H (2012) An overview of the Schwartz Theory of Basic Values, *Online Readings in Psychology and Culture* 2(1). https://doi.org/10.9707/2307-0919.1116.()

feelings, and physical states so as to create a coherent sense impression and intention that system 2 can then turn into belief and action (or choose to ignore and suppress). If a particular idea, memory, feeling, or state is not coherent with other things it has become associated with, it will be progressively de-emphasised and suppressed. The perceived worth ('decision utility') of possible behaviours that are not associated with the individual's values is lower than it would otherwise be, while the perceived worth of possible behaviours that are consistent with values is inflated. For example, in one study,[19] experimental subjects who endorsed the values of benevolence and universalism perceived a later opportunity to join an organisation that promoted community efforts to protect the environment as of greater worth than did those who endorsed the values of power and achievement.

Deliberate understanding and application of one's own values represents a prime means of overriding and reprogramming system 1, so as to maximise the benefit of, and minimise the harm caused by, undesirable use of the nonrational mental processes described in the following sections.

Ease, bias, and heuristics

System 1 loves to make work easier. By reducing the cognitive resources needed for a particular task, more can be achieved more quickly. System 1 uses associative coherence, and the heuristics and biases described below, to make things feel familiar, effortless, and implicitly right. Anything that promotes associative coherence will increase this cognitive ease, such as a repeated experience, an idea presented simply and clearly, a concept that you are already primed to expect, and being in a good mood. By contrast, stimuli that lack associative coherence cause cognitive strain, activating system 2 and making you more vigilant, suspicious, uncomfortable, and rigorous—a state in which you work harder and make fewer errors, but are less creative or intuitive.

Techniques to promote cognitive ease and facilitate acceptance of a message are widely known, particularly in disciplines such as marketing and politics. For instance, repeatedly presenting a message in a glossy form with high production values, using bright colours and vivid sounds, formed of simple words and memorable phrases, and associating it with familiar and trusted individuals will make most recipients significantly more likely to believe that message, even if it happens to be factually incorrect or misleading. If that message is particularly salient to the individual and accords with his values, the processes of associative coherence may then lead to other truthful but uncomfortable messages being rejected because they conflict with it. Overcoming such techniques requires activating system 2 so as to reassess and override the acceptance of the message by system 1.

Table A.1.1 lists many of system 1's processes, biases, and heuristics; how they can play out unhelpfully in individual forensic psychiatric contexts or scenarios; and what you can do about it. It does not cover the many ways in which these processes, biases, and heuristics are tremendously useful and should be allowed to operate unhindered (which would be a much longer table!).

In addition, there are some suggested general approaches you can take to minimise the opportunity for unhelpful operation of system 1:

[19] Feather (1995), and see also Brosch and Sander (2013)—see bibliography.

Table A.1.1 System 1's processes, biases and heuristics

Process, Bias, or Heuristic	Scenario	Response
Norms and causality System 1 creates *coherent causal stories* that link the information available. These are based in part on 'norms': what system 1 expects in a vast range of situations, arising from prior experience. If system 1 observes that X has occurred, and expects Y to occur next, then if Y does indeed occur, then system 1 will form the story that X *caused* Y, whether or not this is true (i.e. without any statistical or causal reasoning).	You lead a team responsible, amongst other things, for deciding whether and when to discharge patients from a secure ward to the community. Many of your patients have committed violent offences, and you are familiar with the assessment and management of serious violence. However, the rate of serious or fatal violence during the period in which your hospital follows-up patients is very low. When a particular patient with schizophrenia commits a homicide after discharge, you and the hospital management are shocked. You review the patient's history, and note the number of past instances of potentially fatal violence in circumstances very similar to the current homicide. You experience **hindsight bias**: it now *seems obvious* that, with that history, the patient would kill someone after discharge, and you wonder why on earth you agreed to discharge them.	Recognise the 'red flag' of 'obviousness'—and treat it as a trigger to engage system 2, and reanalyse the situation using statistical and causal reasoning. Search for relevant evidence to give you a **statistical baseline**, such as the rate of homicide by patients with schizophrenia.[a] Then use the BSCM (Baseline, Subjective, Correlate, Move) procedure (described later) to derive from this an estimate of how likely your patient truly was to do this. Next, consider what proportion of your patients have the same risk factors (e.g. the same past history of potentially fatal violent incidents) as this patient. Challenge system 1's assumption that those risk factors 'caused' the homicide. What was different about this patient from the others who did not commit homicide? If there is no readily identifiable difference, how can those risk factors have been causal?
Jumping to conclusions System 1 leaps intuitively to what seems the likeliest answer to a problem (sometimes referred to as **shooting from the hip**), and whenever this saves time and effort, the information available determines for you that the likely seeming answer is highly probable, and an occasional mistake is acceptable; this is an efficient process. However, if the available information is incomplete and/or mistakes are not acceptable, this process is counterproductive.	You visit your local remand prison to assess a man for treatment in a secure hospital. As you walk into the wing, an inmate comes up to you, unctuously offers to take your coat, compliments you on your suit, and relates your presumed attitude to your appearance to his own; pointing out the pride he takes in grooming himself, despite having to wear prison-issue clothing. You jump to the conclusion that he probably suffers from narcissistic personality traits, make your excuses, and walk quickly into the wing office to speak to the officer in charge about the assessment.	Recognise at the start of the assessment that you have already made a highly salient assumption about his clinical condition—do not dismiss this (it is useful information, both as an intuition that may be correct, and as counter-transference)—but try to put it to one side as information to be considered dispassionately later, rather than as a framework for analysing the new information you gather during the assessment.

A few minutes later, the officer guides you into the interview room, and you are surprised to see that the man you have come to assess is the inmate you met earlier. Your assessment from this point is coloured by your first impression of narcissistic personality, leading you to focus on his unstable, manipulative relationships and history of violence, and largely to dismiss as irrelevant his compliant behaviour in prison and the current symptoms of hypomania (this is the **halo effect** in action). You make no diagnosis of mental illness and do not recommend any treatment. Three weeks later, when he is floridly manic, a colleague reassesses him and arranges transfer to hospital.

Ignorance of regression to the mean

System 1's inability to adopt statistical or causal reasoning is particularly problematic in situations involving repeated observations, assessments, or interventions in which there is a degree of random variation, in which regression to the mean is likely to occur but cannot be accounted for by system 1.

You are responsible for the training of junior doctors in your area. After some criticism of training techniques from a new lecturer, you decide to study what works, beginning with trainees administering ECT for the first time. The study shows that those who are praised for achieving good contact and seizure duration have poorer outcomes on their second administration of ECT to the same patient, whereas those who do poorly on their first try and are criticised for it, typically do much better on the second administration. Without thinking too deeply about it (and without consulting the copious literature to the contrary!), you conclude that praise for good performance is ineffective as an educational technique, but criticism for poor performance improves results.[b]

Also, take into account other sources of information that may be less affected by this kind of bias. This might include the prison officers' opinions about his current condition and how it might have changed, as well as the opinion of any healthcare staff who may have seen him.

If possible, become familiar with the phenomenon of **regression to the mean** so that you automatically recognise situations in which it is likely; alternatively, recognise research, and other situations in which statistical reasoning is likely to be required, and ensure you consult a relevant expert before deciding how to interpret what you have observed.

(continued)

Table A.1.1 Continued

Process, Bias, or Heuristic	Scenario	Response
Answering an easier question If you are unable to answer a question, system 1 will typically **substitute** for it an easier question to which it already knows the answer (sometimes called the '**heuristic question**'). It will then translate this into an answer to the original question using **intensity matching across domains**, which is statistically invalid.	A patient on your ward has progressed well in treatment, and you are considering allowing her to step down to an open mixed-sex rehabilitation ward. You need to consider how likely she is to act in a sexually disinhibited fashion on that ward, and be at risk of engaging in inappropriate sexual activity with other, particularly male, patients. You do not know the answer to this question, and as you are not thinking about it too deeply, your system 1 substitutes it with the question, 'How sexually disinhibited does she seem to me?' Your answer to this is 'not very much', which is a low-intensity response that system 1 matches to 'low risk of sexual disinhibition on the rehab ward'. This is an unreliable conclusion, as the baseline rate of sexual disinhibition by patients in mixed environments is much higher than on your ward, and because it ignores her personal risk factors.	Spend a moment contemplating the question you need to answer, so that system 2 is activated and you are less likely to substitute a heuristic question. If you do end up answering a heuristic question (which is potentially valid and helpful e.g. if gathering information to answer the true question would take excessively long), analyse the result carefully and use statistical reasoning rather than intensity matching to estimate the answer to the true question. The BSCM procedure[c] can help you do this.
Affect heuristics A relatively extreme example of answering an easier question is when the heuristic question is based entirely on emotion—allowing how you feel about a person or topic to determine what you think about a particular question relating to him.	You receive a request to write a reference for a colleague who has applied for a new job. You also coveted the job, but decided not to apply when you learned they were going for it. You resent his general career success. Without specifically intending to, you write a reference that highlights his weaknesses, and ignores his strengths.	As with substitution generally, contemplate the question to be answered carefully, and seek specific evidence for the points you consider making, so that you are less likely to substitute the answer to the question 'How much do I like them right now?'

Anchoring

This process occurs when a possible value for an unknown quantity comes to mind before you estimate that quantity; system 1 will tend to accept the anchor value, and to **prime** you to evoke evidence in favour of it, and to dismiss evidence against it, and it requires effort to ignore it. Hence, if you perceive that you owe a debt or a favour to someone, then when dealing with them again you will be more likely to choose an option that allows you to repay the debt or reciprocate the favour (a form of anchoring known as **reciprocation bias**).

You are chairing a multidisciplinary ward review involving a patient, which is considering how much of his money the patient should be allowed to withdraw in cash and take on his overnight leave tomorrow. The patient opens the discussion by saying, 'I'll need at least £250, doc!' You know that this is a ridiculously large amount for one night, and suspect it would be spent on illicit drugs, but it still serves as an **anchor value**: you and others explain what factors mean that the total should be *reduced from £250*, rather than starting with a more reasonable baseline.

Recognise that the patient, intentionally, intuitively, or accidentally, has given you an anchor value and point this out to others (e.g. 'that's a useful suggestion, but before we consider that, we should think about ....').

Put it to one side in your mind, and seek objective evidence for an alternative starting point (e.g. what other patients have been allowed in similar circumstances, or what your organisation's policies recommend).

Availability heuristic

System 1 uses this pervasive heuristic to avoid the hard work of estimating the size of a category of frequency of an event, by considering instead the ease with which relevant instances come to mind (rather than the number of instances that can be recalled, which would be less unreliable). Memories that are personally salient, and involved drama, emotion, or hard work are particularly easily recalled, whereas the observed experiences of others are not—this is why everyone in the same shared house is likely to think they do most of the cooking or housework on behalf of the group, for example.

You are conducting a risk assessment of interpersonal violence towards future intimate partners. You ask the patient, 'How many times do you remember hitting your previous partners?' The patient intends to be helpful and truthful. He replies, 'Only two or three times—in fact, they hit me more than I hit them, I had to go to hospital several times because of the bruises they gave me.' The instances in which the patient was the victim of violence are far more painful and memorable to them, and (unlike memories of perpetrating violence) accord with the patient's self-image as a good and peaceable partner.

Recognise that invitations to estimate frequencies of emotionally and morally charged behaviours such as violence to an intimate partner are particularly likely to be influenced by the availability heuristic.

Specifically ask the patient to enumerate the instances in which he behaved violently towards previous partners—and keep prompting for more until you are sure he can recall no more.

Explain why he may find it hard to remember many instances: providing a reason for the difficulty of recall has been shown to increase effort and reduce the impact of the lack of ease.

(continued)

Table A.1.1 Continued

Process, Bias, or Heuristic	Scenario	Response
Representativeness heuristic The representativeness of an instance is the degree to which it conforms to the stereotype of the class to which it belongs (i.e. a Leica is highly representative of the class of cameras, but an iPad, even though it is just as effective a camera, does not conform to the current stereotype). System 1 cannot think statistically, so it judges how likely an instance is to belong to a class not by reference to the base rate (the proportion of the population that belongs to that class) but by its representativeness of that class's stereotype.	You work on a low secure unit. You are called to assess a patient for transfer from the hospital's psychiatric intensive care unit, who verbally abused and assaulted a nurse by slapping her face earlier that afternoon. He has no past history of violence, has never misused drugs, has no personality pathology, and his psychosis had begun to respond to antipsychotic medication. Nevertheless, he is tall, black, muscular, aggressive, and hostile, and so is strongly representative of your personal stereotype of the class of 'violent patients requiring treatment in secure conditions', and you recommend transfer.	Using the representativeness heuristic is associated with great cognitive ease: recognise the red flag of the 'obvious' conclusion that this man is a 'violent patient requiring secure care', and treat it as a prompt to state explicitly the evidence for and against his membership of that class of patients. Also, before reaching a conclusion, explicitly consider the relevant base rate: the proportion of patients with no prior history of violence, personality pathology, or substance misuse, who persist in violence beyond the acute phase of psychosis (which is low).
Conjunction fallacy This cognitive error occurs when, because of associative coherence, you estimate the combination of two events to be more likely than either event occurring alone, which is mathematically impossible to be the case. Such combinations are often distinctive[d] and more easily recalled, and therefore vulnerable to the **availability heuristic.** The most famous example of the conjunction fallacy is Kahneman and Tversky's fictional *Linda*: '31, single, outspoken, very bright, majored in philosophy, deeply concerned with discrimination and social justice, participated in anti-nuclear demonstrations'.	You write a report to the Ministry of Justice on a restricted patient's recent progress, in which you request permission to grant unescorted leave from the hospital, initially to be used within the hospital grounds. The patient, who has schizoaffective disorder, was convicted of manslaughter when in a psychotic state precipitated by drug use three years ago; he has responded very well to antipsychotic treatment, and has made no attempt to obtain alcohol or illicit drugs on the unit or during escorted leave.	Be alert to the possibility of combining possible events in such a way as to create a scenario that is particularly plausible (because of associative coherence) and therefore likely to be seen as more probable than it truly is—or conversely, a scenario that is so lacking in associative coherence that it is seen as much less probable than it really is. In this case, if you had separated out presentation of the risk of absconding from the grounds and the risk of using illicit drugs, and referred to specific evidence in making your assessment that the risk of each was low, you would have been less likely to have created a plausible scenario that worried the MoJ official out of proportion to its true probability.

The majority of respondents in a large survey thought it more likely that Linda was a bank teller who was active in the feminist movement than that she was just a bank teller, because the former is more **coherent with the associations** they each had to her story. In the abstract, it is easier to see that it cannot be more likely that both A and B are true about a person, than that only A is true.

Failing to make inferences

System 1 fails to update your beliefs on the basis of new, statistically valid information that conflicts with your existing beliefs and values (because to do so would reduce **associative coherence**): this is why so many users of socially tolerated drugs such as alcohol, tobacco, and cannabis may be aware of evidence of the damage to health they cause, but continue to believe that they personally will not suffer ill-health from them.

However, if the new information is presented in a way that appears **causally linked** to you, system 1 will infer a change to your beliefs and enable you to change your behaviour. So, for example, if you are told that an exam you are about to sit has a pass rate of 50%, you will be likely to think of reasons why you will be in the 50% of candidates who pass ('I usually score more than 50% so I should be fine' e.g.'); but if you are told that the exam has a pass rate of just 25%, you are more likely to **infer** that 'this is a particularly hard exam', and that therefore you might not pass, and change your behaviour by working harder at revision.

Without thinking too deeply about it, under the heading 'Risks during the proposed leave', you state that absconding from the grounds and using illicit drugs is a possibility, but the risk is acceptably low. You are surprised and disappointed when, several weeks later, you receive a letter from the MoJ refusing permission for unescorted leave 'because of the risk of absconding and using drugs'.

You co-facilitate a psycho-educational group for patients with a history of substance misuse. In one of the sessions, you present many facts about the harm done by drugs the patients commonly use (lung cancer caused by smoking tobacco, psychosis caused by smoking cannabis e.g.), and the participants undertake exercises that show they understand, accept, and can use the information to answer questions. However, you are disappointed to find, some time after the course, that none of them has changed their behaviour.

Recognise that in order to change behaviour, the participants need to infer from the sessions that they personally should change their behaviour, so that any statistical information you employ should be presented in a way that appears causal to them. You might do this, for example, by using stories of real or imagined people who conform to participants' stereotypes of 'people like me', who have suffered the ill-effects that you have described.

(continued)

Table A.1.1 Continued

Process, Bias, or Heuristic	Scenario	Response
WYSIATI System 1 automatically assumes that What You See Is All There Is, and is incapable of taking into account the possibility of information that it does not have, even if you are aware that such information might exist and be highly relevant. This leads to **narrative fallacy**: flawed stories of what happened in the past, based on inadequate and incomplete information, that generate false expectations for the future.	You are a senior consultant, shortlisting candidates for interview for a new consultant post in your service. You have done this many times before, and your impression is that on every occasion you and your colleagues have selected the best available candidate, who has gone on to become an excellent new colleague. You do not think deeply about the fact that you have no experience of working with the candidates you did not appoint. You read a poorly constructed CV, written in an awkward style with imperfect grammar. The first page mentions a basic medical degree in the 'qualifications' section and some relevant experience at a junior level, but shows no evidence there that the candidate possesses the essential higher professional qualification for the post. You discard the CV partially unread and recommend rejection, with the note 'does not meet essential criterion of possessing MRCPsych or equivalent'.	Develop systems of work that automatically prompt you to seek relevant evidence that is not immediately apparent. In the current context, this might mean using an application form and person specification that make obvious the essential criteria and require candidates to state explicitly whether or not they meet each criterion. Recognise the 'red flag' of 'summary dismissal', as indicating that you may not have sought all the relevant information before jumping to a conclusion. In this case, neither a well-constructed CV nor (arguably) perfect English grammar is essential to being an excellent consultant, and reading the CV all the way to the end with an open mind would have meant you realised that the candidate had in fact passed the MRCPsych exam, and had performed exceedingly well in a number of challenging senior posts.
Overconfidence Once system 1 has constructed an associatively coherent story, you feel cognitive ease and a sense that the story is *obviously* true. This leads to false confidence in the predictions generated by that story, and distaste for the reality that the world is in many respects chaotic and unpredictable. (The desire for order that arises from this distaste also leads to **chance bias**: seeing spurious and supposedly meaningful correlations in pure co-incidences.)	You are a highly experienced expert witness, called upon frequently to give evidence in often high-profile criminal trials on the mental states of defendants at the time of their alleged offences. You are usually, though not always, instructed by the prosecution, and the vast majority of the defendants you determine as not meeting the criteria for a mental condition defence (e.g. diminished responsibility, insanity, or automatism) go on to be convicted by the court of the offence charged.	Accept that, simply by virtue of being experienced in your field, you are at high risk of overconfidence.[8] Recognise the 'red flags' of the defendant seeming 'very familiar' in nature, and the conclusions seeming 'obvious'. Ensure you engage your system 2, and explicitly think through the evidence for possible alternative conclusions in detail, both clinically and clinico-legally; the latter by considering every limb of each of the legal tests involved, not just the limb(s) that spring to your mind as being obviously the most relevant.

Such coherence is more likely when your views are reinforced by others of like mind around you (the phenomenon of **groupthink**), or when you are influenced by an authoritative, charismatic and/or likeable individual who has spoken before you, to follow their views (**the sunflower effect**).

Conversely, **inferences** are not drawn from facts that challenge the coherent story, and those facts are effectively ignored.

In any professional sphere, you are typically in touch with the sense of uncertainty and unpredictability as a new trainee, but steadily become overconfident as you gain knowledge and expertise.

Also make use of the system 2s of others by asking for their view on expert opinions you have offered in past cases, in a structured fashion that requires them to consider the evidence for and against your opinion. Minimise the sunflower effect by requiring participants to summarise their views on paper to themselves before anyone speaks. This might mean gaining peer review within an expert witness chambers, for example, or within a peer group case discussion. The fact that clinico-legal opinions given in cases are necessarily 'individual', and cannot properly be the product of 'group thinking', determines that expert witnesses tend to work independently, which can result in failure of self-critique.

For more junior expert witnesses, being supervised, or mentored, will be important, although the fact of this must be made plain in your reports. Indeed, even as an experienced expert witness, you should sometimes consider discussion with a senior colleague in regard to any difficult case, or one where you think you may be at particular risk of bias, albeit you should make plain in your report that you have done so.

You assess a middle-aged man who is charged with murdering his housemate when apparently psychotic. He looks very much like many such defendants you have assessed previously, and you overlook the apparent lack of any recorded psychiatric history, assuming that you are simply the first psychiatrist to assess him properly. You make a diagnosis of schizophrenia and confirm that his psychotic symptoms are likely to have been present at the time of the alleged offence; however, you then argue that they were not sufficiently severe to found the defence of insanity, or the partial defence of diminished responsibility, because in your interview he was able to demonstrate that he knew that he was killing his housemate and that this was wrong, and because his abnormality of mental functioning did not, in your view, substantially impair his ability to form a rational judgment.

You are aghast when evidence is then introduced of a report from a defence expert demonstrating that the defendant undoubtedly suffers from an orbitofrontal astrocytoma, which often causes disinhibition and impulsivity. The jury accepts the contention of the other expert witness that the tumour would have substantially impaired his ability to exercise self-control, a limb of the test for diminished responsibility that you had entirely ignored. After conviction, the judge criticises you from the bench for what she describes as your 'arrogant and slapdash' approach, and the defence barrister complains to the GMC about your inadequate professional practice in the case.

(continued)

Table A.1.1 Continued

Process, Bias, or Heuristic	Scenario	Response
Intuitions versus algorithms Experts like complexity within their field (because they understand it, or at least think they do, and it can seem to lend credence to their opinions), and they typically apply clever, complex analyses and solutions, including 'thinking outside the box.' However, a clear majority[h] of studies have found that simple statistical models, in which a small number of factors are given equal weight, are superior to expert judgment in predicting outcomes in a variety of fields. Moreover, presented with the same information on more than one occasion, experts often give different answers because of unnoticed stimuli influencing system 1; whilst simple statistical models give consistent predictions.	Assessment of the risk of future violence is a well-known example of this phenomenon: it is widely accepted that simple actuarial models such as the VRAG[i] and OGRS[j] are more accurate and reliable than unstructured clinical judgment, provided that they are used appropriately (e.g. that the subject fits the reference group used to develop the model). However, the more general point of the relative unreliability of unstructured expert opinion has not been widely accepted, even within forensic psychiatry.	Whenever possible, make use of structured instruments and procedures that enable you to found your clinical judgment upon reliable, including statistical, information, such as the HCR20v3 in the case of violence risk assessment. If no such instrument is available, employ a framework or structure that prompts you to state explicitly the evidence you have taken into account in reaching your judgment, and the weight you have given to it, such as Shared Decision-Making (with the patient), the Clinical Decision Support Tool, or the Situated Clinical Decision-Making Framework. If no relevant framework is available, consider sketching your own simple framework (perhaps just a list of headings) that prompt you to consider and weight all relevant evidence.
The outside view Familiarity leads insiders to search for evidence relating to a question within their own experience—moreover, memories of their own experience which tend to take credit for past successes and overlook or explain away past failures (**ignoring your own track record**). Outsiders, by contrast, lack this familiarity and experience, and evaluate the question by reference to a much broader **reference class**.	You are a junior doctor who has worked at Hospital X for three years. On considering the question 'What should I offer this acutely suicidal patient?', you decide, without thinking about it too deeply, 'I'll refer to the A Team because that's what we usually do here.' By contrast, when you move to a job at Hospital Z three months later, where you have no experience of how such patients are usually treated, you are likely to fall back on a much wider class of evidence, such as the NICE recommendations on suicide prevention and treatment, and the recommended treatment for any mental disorder you may have diagnosed.	Recognise when you have developed such a degree of familiarity with a person, situation, or institution that you are at risk of using your own past experience as the sole guide to decision-making. Adopt a structured approach to decision-making (perhaps linked to a structured approach to making clinical notes at the same time) that prompts you to consider relevant evidence from first principles in coming to your decision.

As a result, the inside perspective will often be over-optimistic, whereas the outside perspective is more realistic. This is exacerbated by the fact that such optimism is often **socially valued**. For example, a hospital's internal estates department may estimate that it can complete a much-desired new building project within a pleasingly small budget and short timescale—this is known as the **planning fallacy**. External consultants, alive to the fact that a high proportion of such projects encounter unexpected delays and obstacles, forecast a much longer timescale and recommend a larger contingency element in the budget.

And adopt the perspective of an outsider as part of this—or, if appropriate, explicitly include outsiders in making the decision. For instance, this could mean involving patients, [k] carers, and lay representatives in designing and implementing service improvements (sometimes called co-design and co-production). Before deciding on large and risky projects, consider holding a '**pre-mortem**': a group discussion that hypothesises that a year has passed after you implemented the current intended plan, and the outcome was a disaster, and that seeks to explain what could have gone wrong.

Risk and loss aversion

A purely logical decision-maker would always choose the option with the highest **expected utility** (see 'rational decision-making' above), and would calculate utility based on the absolute worth to them of each option.

Most people, however, have a degree of aversion to risk and will pay a premium, or accept a lower return, in order to avoid uncertainty; and they also evaluate the worth of an outcome not in absolute terms but **by reference to the previous outcome**. So that, for example, a given state of wealth will be seen as pleasant if it follows a gain, but as unpleasant if it follows a loss, with the degree of displeasure associated with a given loss being

You are a clinical leader responsible for introducing a new policy on the pharmacological treatment of a particular condition. Compared to regular treatment, drug X costs half as much, is twice as effective, and has a better overall side-effect profile (it commonly causes transient nausea, which dissipates by day five, and it has only one serious side-effect, which can be detected in advance and therefore prevented by sufficiently frequent blood tests). You are very excited about drug X coming onto the market, and you have told many colleagues about its benefits, raising their expectations.

Recognise when the nature of the uncertainty in a situation is likely to inspire risk aversion and/or loss aversion.

'Under-promise and over-deliver': talk up the possible costs and talk down the expected benefits (while still communicating that the latter outweigh the former), so that you set expectations such that most patients and doctors will be pleasantly surprised by the outcome (i.e. set their reference point such that their experience counts as a gain).

(continued)

Table A.1.1 Continued

Process, Bias, or Heuristic	Scenario	Response
perceived as greater than the degree of pleasure that would be obtained by an equal gain: this is loss aversion.l,m The reference point may also be 'what you expect the outcome to be', or 'what you feel the outcome ought to be' (e.g. what you feel entitled to)—so even a smaller gain than you believe you deserved is experienced as a loss. Taking the status quo as your reference point leads to **status quo bias**: perceiving the costs of change as outweighing the expected benefits. Put another way, this is the **endowment effect**: you value what you already have more highly than you would if you did not have it, and put more effort into keeping it than you would do into obtaining it.	Six months after recommending making drug X available on the hospital formulary, you are dismayed to find that it has seldom been prescribed for patients who would be suitable for it, and that even when prescribed patients have frequently discontinued it after a few days. Your colleagues come to see the drug as useless in practice, despite the research evidence for its benefits. The expected utility of treatment with drug X for suitable patients seemed obvious to you, but to those patients and those treating them, the change in treatment to a new and unfamiliar drug involved uncertainty and inspired risk aversion. Also, prescribing it is more complicated than of its predecessors, requiring doctors to organise and check the results of many blood tests, which for them is a loss in time and effort. Moreover, you had not prepared your colleagues to warn patients about the likelihood of an (albeit minor) side-effect: and the unexpected nausea is experienced by patients as a loss from their previous nausea-free state, which outweighed the (objectively much greater, but uncertain) benefit of future symptom reduction.	Minimise the endowment effect by reducing the perceived costs of change as much as possible. For example, this could mean agreeing with your Pharmacy Department (which will benefit from the reduced expenditure in its drug budget if drug X is widely prescribed) that for the first six months, pharmacists will manage the additional blood tests, including monitoring and communicating results, so that doctors (who make the prescribing decisions) do not have to do so.

The rare and exotic

When system 1's perception of an event or case is particularly vivid and emotionally arousing, this promotes the availability and cognitive ease, and can lead to an excessive response to a rare event, such as a **moral panic**.¹¹ Instances are more likely to seem vivid if they follow an instance that is very different in some way (this is **contrast bias**).

If a particular outcome stands out in this way, your attention is drawn to it, and you over-weight its likelihood and do not evaluate the full range of alternative outcomes that make up the denominator in your estimate of frequency (the **denominator effect**).

You work in a rehabilitation service in a high-security hospital, where you are responsible for the care and treatment of an elderly man who exhibits paedophilia, and who gruesomely raped and murdered his three step-daughters, all aged under thirteen years, thirty years ago. His case led to changes in the law and practice relating to relevant police procedure and to local authority safeguarding, and his offences are still vividly remembered by people at large, and referred to intermittently in the media.

He has responded well to treatment and rehabilitation. He is now frail, suffering from congestive heart failure and emphysema, and having had several small ischaemic strokes. You and the rest of the multidisciplinary team have conducted a very thorough risk assessment over a considerable period of time, using structured clinical judgment, with evidence from multiple sources, and you have gained a second opinion from an external clinician. You have had all of this information reviewed, and your risk assessment explicitly approved, by a committee of peers at the hospital. Your firm conclusion is that he poses a low risk of sexual, violent, or any other form of offending, and that he should be permitted to step down to a lower level of security, with a view to possible eventual release into the community under supervision.

You write to the Ministry of Justice recommending approval for transfer but (as on every previous occasion you have done this) permission is refused.

Recognise that the decision-makers in the Ministry of Justice are likely to be influenced by the denominator effect in this instance, because of the exceptionally vivid and emotional associations of your patient's past offending. They are also likely to respond to their perception of the public and media reaction to news of your patient's transfer, and, while it may be inappropriate for this to affect your clinical decision-making, it is legitimately a matter for *them* to consider, given their duty to protect the public from serious harm.

In order to minimise the degree to which they are affected by the denominator effect, you should present your request in a way that promotes careful evaluation of the scenarios that do *not* involve him raping or murdering any more children. That is, instead of simply stating the reasons for your collective assessment that the scenario of reoffending is very unlikely, set out scenarios (e.g. compliance with the less restrictive regime in a lower security setting, leading to granting of and successful use of escorted and then unescorted leave) which you assess as being likely, and your reasons for believing this. Present evidence showing what *proportion* of comparable patients, and perhaps also an estimate of *how many* individual patients,° went on to succeed after decisions were taken to allow them to step down.

(continued)

Table A.1.1 Continued

Process, Bias, or Heuristic	Scenario	Response
Narrow versus broad framing Most people are more comfortable considering a series of decisions as single decisions taken in isolation (**narrow framing**) rather than a set of decisions considered jointly (**broad framing**) since this reduces the apparent complexity, and the required cognitive load, and facilitates leaving more of the decision-making to system 1.[p] However, the risk aversion, loss aversion, and endowment effects described above have much greater adverse effects upon outcome when they operate on every single decision, rather than when spread across a set of decisions. For example, someone buying and selling goods in a market is far more likely to lose money overall if they aim to make money on every individual trade (and therefore consistently avoid lucrative but risky trades, and gamble on avoiding losses[q] rather than accepting small certain losses), whereas if they were to focus on their average performance over (say) each month's worth of trades, they would be able to tolerate losses on several trades, seeing them more than cancelled out by gains on other trades.	You are the clinical leader of a multidisciplinary team responsible for making decisions on leave and discharge for (unrestricted) patients. You are acutely aware of the limitations of risk-assessment technology, and the fact that you cannot accurately predict whether a patient will abscond, use drugs, relapse, reoffend, or otherwise harm themselves or others while on leave or after discharge. You frame each decision on leave or discharge narrowly, and over time as occasional patients have bad outcomes that you regard as unacceptable, you become paralysed in your decision-making, and highly reluctant to agree to leave or discharge because you cannot be sure there will be no bad outcome. Eventually you find your patients complaining to the tribunal about your risk aversion and apparent unwillingness to allow them to make progress, and your hospital management pressurises you about the long lengths of stay and low throughput of patients on your ward.	Take a step back from each individual decision. Recognise that you are causing more harm to patients than you are preventing by stopping the occasional incident of absconding, drug use, or reoffending, for example—just as does the neurosurgeon who never resects any patient's brain tumour and therefore denies him the chance of recovery because of the possibility that the patient will die during surgery. You can end your decision-making paralysis by framing your decisions more broadly, and focusing on the frequency of bad outcomes across all decisions on leave and discharge, rather than on the outcome of each individual decision—and by including in your analysis the bad outcomes of unnecessarily restricted liberty, and failure to provide a treatment that can only be provided in the community or in a less secure setting. Consider adopting (individually, or at a team, service or at an institutional level) a **risk policy** that reduces the heartache of the occasional bad outcome by demonstrating that it improves overall outcomes in the long run, within an 'audit' model.

The sunk-cost fallacy

This is another instance of loss aversion related to narrow framing: the tendency to continue to invest additional resources in a failing project when objective analysis suggests that better investment opportunities are available.

It is motivated in part by the desire to avoid **anticipated regret** (a form of psychological loss) caused by the fact that it is more coherent and easier to contemplate an unusual, vivid event that would make the project a success after all, and its cancellation something to be regretted, than it is to contemplate the progressive, gradual failure of the project that would make its cancellation something to be relieved by.

It is exacerbated by the **bias towards action**: in that people have stronger emotional reactions towards outcomes caused by action rather than those caused by omission or inaction (e.g. to the patient dying during the operation, as opposed to the patient dying because you did not operate).

You are a highly specialist psychotherapist who has seen a particular patient for individual sessions for two years. You have felt on the verge of a psychological breakthrough with him for the past year. You care greatly about all your patients, and you are committed to giving them the best chance of recovery.

As evidence mounts of lack of change in their attitudes and behaviour, you double down on your investment in the patient, offering him twice-weekly instead of weekly sessions, and seeking to persuade him not to 'give up on himself'.

Your supervisor expresses concern on behalf of the multidisciplinary team about your inability to take on new patients, and your seeming obsession with this one particular patient. Eventually they send you on sick leave, saying that you have become 'burnt out' and that your clinical judgment is no longer objective, and they appoint a new psychotherapist to work with patients on your ward.

Listen to the judgments of others on the success or otherwise of your endeavours, especially when they conflict with your own.

If you find yourself coming up with facts or opinions that 'explain away' their dissenting judgment, try stating explicitly both the evidence in favour of their position and the evidence in favour of yours, and evaluate each objectively.

Routinely take part in group and individual supervision or case discussion arrangements, and train yourself to act on the judgments of others, especially when it feels most uncomfortable (lacking in associative coherence) to do so.

(continued)

Table A.1.1 Continued

Process, Bias, or Heuristic	Scenario	Response
Experiencing versus remembering When we use our experiences as evidence for future decisions, we do not use experiences directly, but only our memories of them. Because system 1 represents sets (in this case memories summarising many sense impressions) by their averages, norms, and stereotypes, those memories are dominated by the most intense part of the experience and by the final part of it (the **peak-end rule**). The length of the experience is irrelevant to how the memory of it is evaluated (**duration neglect**). This means, for example, that most people will choose to re-experience a longer unpleasant experience, instead of a shorter one, if they remember the longer one as less awful.[r] As a result, we learn to maximise the quality of our memories, rather than the quality of our future experiences per se.	You are a doctor at the end of three-years' core training in psychiatry, facing a decision about what role to apply for next. You look back on the rotational posts you have worked in, and one stands out for you: a job in forensic psychiatry with several moments of high excitement (observing evidence being given at the Old Bailey; jointly assessing a man alleged to have committed a high-profile homicide; and successfully leading a safe seclusion review of a patient who believed you were the devil and wanted to eat your heart), which ended with a particularly memorable farewell party. You consider applying for higher training in forensic psychiatry.	Bear in mind that your memory of forensic psychiatry will be dominated by those moments of peak intensity and by the end of your experience, you will tend to ignore periods of tedium or minor displeasure, no matter how long they lasted. Before committing yourself, make an effort to recall aspects of the experience throughout the post: What did you think of your day-to-day duties? How did you feel about the slow pace of change for each patient; the low turnover of patients; the long delays and bureaucracy for restricted patients? If the moments of excitement are what motivate you, were there enough of them in any given stretch of time to be fulfilling in the longer term?

[a] In E&W, between 2003 and 2013, 346 people with schizophrenia committed homicides, according to the National Confidential Inquiry into Suicide & Homicide; say 35 per year. NICE estimated in 2014 that 220,000 people in E&W had schizophrenia. Therefore, each year, around 35/220000 = 0.016% of people with schizophrenia commit homicide.

[b] This may seem like a ridiculous scenario—but it really happened, in the context of flight training for Israeli military pilots (cited in Kahneman D and Tversky A 1973. On the psychology of prediction, *Psychological Review* 80: 237–251.)

[c] 'Baseline, Subjective, Correlate, Multiply,' see clinical case 16.

[d] We tend to over-weight distinctive (interesting, surprising) information, and under-weight common (familiar, humdrum) information. This is **information bias.** Likewise, we under-weight highly likely events (the **certainty effect**), and over-weight unlikely events (the **possibility effect**); this is observable in new medical students, who are quick to consider the presence of 'small-print' diagnoses and have to be taught that 'common things are common'. We also have too few decision weights, so that probabilities intermediate between unlikely and likely are commonly lumped together.

[e] A related consequence of this process is 'consistency bias': once you have behaved in a particular way in a specific situation, behaving differently would reduce associative coherence, so you are likely to behave in the same way again, even if you correctly recognised the first time around that your chosen behaviour did not lead to the optimal outcome.

[f] This is a classic example of a failure to reason statistically and to substitute an easier question for a hard one. Your average score in similar tests might be well over 50%—say it's 65%—but this is not conclusive of the question 'Will I pass?'. What your system 1 has done is answer the easier heuristic question, 'Will I score more than 50%?' and matched the high intensity of your response to

that ('Yes, I almost always score over 50%.') to give a similarly confident answer to the true question. The passing *rate* of 50% means that the highest-scoring 50% will pass, and if 50% or more of the candidates score more than your score on the day (e.g. 65%), you will fail.

g In other words, draw from the evidence that experts in general become overconfident in their professional ability, the inference that you personally are at risk of such overconfidence: do not allow the lack of associative coherence of this fact (i.e. its conflict with your self-image as a wise and high-performing psychiatrist) to lead you to ignore it.

h Around 60%, according to Kahneman and Tversky. (*Thinking Fast and Slow*, Chapter 21).

i Violence Risk Appraisal Guide.

j Offender Group Reconviction Score.

k Patients are 'outsiders' in this context because they do not share the specific experience, assumptions, and beliefs that staff members of the institution have acquired.

l Research in the field of gambling suggests that most people only take a bet when probability-weighted gains amount to at least 1.5 times the possible (probability-weighted) losses. Separate research suggests that the administration of D^2 dopamine receptor agonists reduces loss aversion and leads to riskier decision-making. Loss aversion can outweigh risk aversion: facing a choice between a certain loss and a larger but merely possible loss, many people will take the risk of the larger loss, even when this has a lower expected utility than the small certain loss. This can turn a manageable failure into a disaster.

m A specific category of loss aversion is the prioritisation of threats over opportunities. This is hard-wired into system 1, and one of the factors behind your instant response to Kevin's picture in 'nonrational decision-making' above, and the fact that you probably recoiled fractionally when you first saw it.

n For example, a country drastically restricting immigration because of a small number of widely reported sexual assaults on vulnerable citizens by recent immigrants, particularly those conforming to a stereotype of an 'alien' or 'dangerous' immigrant.

o Focusing on the absolute numbers of individuals will promote a greater weighting of the associated outcome than will focusing on the proportion or frequency. For the same reason, you could present evidence on the rate of bad outcomes such as reoffending in terms of proportions and frequencies rather than absolute numbers, to reduce over-weighting of that outcome.

p **Values blindness** is a particularly relevant instance of narrow framing: overemphasising a single value objective (e.g. the risk of future violence by a patient), rather than being able to balance multiple potentially competing value objectives (e.g. symptom reduction and improvement of quality of life, alongside risk reduction).

q This aspect of loss aversion caused by narrow framing leads to the **disposition effect**: the counterproductive tendency to sell winners (on which you will make a profit, albeit a smaller one than if you had held the asset for longer) rather than losers (on which you will make a loss, but a smaller one than if you hold it for longer).

r In one experiment, for example, subjects chose to repeat a trial involving 90 seconds of discomfort (holding their hands in 14°C water for 60s then 15°C for 30s) instead of one involving merely 60 seconds (14°C for 60s only).

1. Anxiety and stress increase the chance of relying excessively on system 1's shortcuts. Approach important tasks in as relaxed a state as possible, and minimise the likelihood of interruption.
2. Ensure the time available is adequate to the task.
3. Recognise elevated or depressed mood states in yourself that will tend to reduce cognitive capacity or affect perception of values or weighing of evidence, and consider postponing the task if possible.
4. Accept that uncertainty is inevitable in most decision-making in forensic psychiatry, and do not seek to drive it out (which will lead to false certainty and overconfidence).
5. Always mentalise about your thought process. Ask yourself, what cognitive steps have you taken? Why do you think what you now think?

Taming intuitive predictions: the BSCM procedure

As described above, system 1 is unable to reason statistically or causally, and so, when asked to make a prediction, it has to substitute an *evaluation* of the evidence (e.g. the evaluation of the heuristic question as 'not very sexually disinhibited' in the 'answering an easier question' section of the table above). The BSCM procedure is a reliable and straightforward way of making good use of valid statistical reasoning in such situations, with minimum effort.

Step 1.   Identify a relevant reference class, for which the distribution of outcomes is known, or can be found, with reasonable confidence. For example, in relation to the question posed in the table above, 'How likely was/is my patient with schizophrenia to kill someone after discharge?', a suitable reference class is 'people with schizophrenia'.[20] Assess the distribution of outcomes for the reference class. As described in footnote 1 on page [30] above, 0.016% of people with schizophrenia commit homicide each year. This is your statistical **baseline**.

Step 2.   Put this to one side, and then make your own **subjective**, intuitive estimate of the answer to the question, based upon whatever singular information you have that you consider relevant to the issue. In this example, particularly given that you approach it with hindsight, your subjective impression might be 'high-risk patient', which might at most amount to '10% risk of homicide in a year'.

Step 3.   Estimate the degree to which the factors you have incorporated into your subjective estimate capture *all* the factors that will influence the outcome concerned and therefore **correlate** with the true answer (put another way, estimate your ability to predict that true answer, based upon the information available to you). In this example, you might perhaps think that you have incorporated around 30% of the possible factors, or that your subjective estimate has about 30% positive predictive value.

Step 4.   Incorporate your subjective estimate by starting with the baseline figure and **moving** towards your subjective estimate by the correlation factor you estimated in the previous step. In this example, the baseline figure was 0.016%, and you should move it 30% of the way towards your subjective estimate, meaning that your final estimate is $0.016\% + 0.3 \times (10\% - 0.016\%) = 3.01\%$.

---

[20] 'Patients with schizophrenia who have just been discharged from hospital' would be an even more suitable reference class, but research findings on the outcome of killing versus not killing other people in this more specific group are not readily available at the time of writing.

This is a far better estimate of how likely your patient was to kill someone than your subjective estimate, let alone your initial intuitive thought that the killing was, in retrospect, 'obvious'.

Having incorporated appropriate statistical and causal reasoning into your decision-making using the BSCM procedure, or otherwise, and having mentalised about your thinking process so as to minimise the impact of any unhelpful biases or heuristics, how do you then come to a final decision? This is where the explicit consideration of your values is most helpful, and it is to this that we now turn.

Values-based decision-making

Values-based decision-making (VBDM) is an approach to decision-making in health care that involves identifying and understanding the issues that are most important, and mean most to all those involved in the decision-making process. It is not a theory in itself of how people make decisions, akin to those explored earlier in this Part of the casebook (there must be some 'process' used to get from 'problem' to 'decision'), but an approach to making decisions that complements the evidence-based approach[21] that most clinicians instinctively use. That is, VBDM is an invitation to be *explicit* about the values that are in play and how they influence the decisions you take, which may, for example, clash with the values emphasised by other stakeholders. It thereby also allows reflection upon how to weigh the various values that are accepted as underpinning principled bioethical decisions-making.

Awareness of personal values matters so much because those values underpin one's personal choices and sense of authentic identity. Social, cultural, ethnic, and professional values may also, in turn, strongly influence your choices, either directly or through influencing your personal values.

The commonest ethical dilemmas arise in health care when the *patient's* values clash with the doctor's values (see e.g. clinical cases 13 and 17),[22] usually about treatment. And notably, in a recent legal case in England and Wales, it was deemed that the value to a patient of knowing all the treatment choices available, even the risky ones, outweighed the doctor's value investment in what he considered the best treatment (the so called *Montgomery* test[23]). In that case, the UK Supreme Court said that health care professionals needed to have a dialogue with patients so as to explore their different values perspectives.

In addition, ethical dilemmas often arise when, for example, professional values (as articulated by professional codes and regulations) clash with the *personal* values of clinicians (see ethical cases 10 and 17) or their contractual obligations, where the *employer's values* may clash with *professional* values (see ethical cases 8 and 13), giving rise to cognitive dissonance and anxiety, or even anger. These kinds of dilemma are particularly common in organisations that encourage their employees to have a kind of 'value neutral' state of mind at work, as if that were even possible. Or where there are *different values expressed within a clinical team* (clinical case 16; ethical cases 12 and 14).

---

[21] The originating author of VBDM, Bill Fulford, would say that although facts and values are both evidence, the facts are more obvious.

[22] The case examples from the cases in Part B referred to are example cases and do not represent a comprehensive list of Part B cases set against the issues discussed in this Part A.

[23] *Montgomery v Lanarkshire Health Board* [2015] SC 11 [2015] 1 AC 1430.

In summary, therefore, VBDM encourages you to develop explicit awareness of the values you hold, and/or are applying to the problem at hand, so as to avoid personal values remaining, to yourself or others, 'subterranean'. Beyond this, it encourages you to think about the values of others involved in the decision: especially the patients under your care, but also the colleagues with whom you work.

VBDM was originally developed from the perspective of an ethical dilemma between two persons (e.g. in regard to whether or not to detain a person who doesn't want to be detained), but it has been developed for use in teams where clashes of value arise between different professional decision-makers (e.g. whether or not to give a patient leave, as in clinical case 17 and ethical case 12). Exploration of the values of the different stakeholders can help to identify and explain the meaning of both 'agreement' and 'dissent', and so can reduce feelings of anger and distress. And, at the level of organisational dynamics, VBDM can help to ensure that perspectives are not overlooked.[24]

Five stages of values-based decision-making

VBDM invites you to identify the ethical dilemma you are facing and ensure that all relevant parties (stakeholders) are involved in your decision-making process; to have a dialogue that clarifies different values perspectives; to identify clashes of values that underpin people's views and choices, together with the intended and potentially unintended consequences of their position; to help the group come to some kind of consensus about what is a good-quality decision and commit to it; and to communicate that decision in a way that acknowledges dissent but makes clear why one option has been deemed best. Box A.1.2 summarises these five stages: clarifying, comprehending, committing, choosing, and communicating.

Box A.1.2 Five stages of values-based decision-making

Clarifying your perspective
Comprehending your values
Committing to what is most important
Choosing the best-fitting option (taking the decision)
Communicating it effectively

Clarifying your perspective

In order to clarify your 'values perspective' on a decision to be made you need to take a step back and reflect upon the values that are consciously important to you in relation to that decision, especially the feelings and beliefs that seem obvious or unarguable to you. You need then to try to do the same thing from the point of view of other people's perspectives. Of course, it goes without saying that the patient's views and values must be part of the clarification process.

Although careful reflection can highlight to you other people's feelings and beliefs, in practice, the best results come from making space and time for honest discussion between the different parties, it being made clear that openness and transparency are welcome and

---

[24] As occurred in Mid Staffordshire Hospitals (see Report of the Mid Staffordshire NHS Foundation Trust Public Inquiry: Ref: ISBN 9780102981476, HC 947 2012-13, the Francis Report).

deemed helpful, and that all stakeholders need to be involved, no matter how junior or inexperienced.[25] When consulting others about their perspectives, it is important to try to avoid comment, debate, or disagreement since, at this stage of the process, you are trying to facilitate awareness and understanding of different perspectives, not judging or evaluating them.

By clarifying the different values-based perspectives you will make it more likely that dialogue in the process of making decisions will be meaningful because there will be mutual understanding, and you will also be able to identify assumptions, biases, and prejudice in your own thinking. And this stage should also help you to 'frame' the decision, including identifying the scope of what needs to be decided, bearing in mind the complex interrelationships between aspects of a decision. It should also help you to own your particular role in the decision, and give you the confidence to maintain your position (if appropriate) if you face resistance later on, as you will understand how you came to form your own views and the implied decision.

Depending upon the gravity of the decision to be taken, and the time available, you may at this stage go on to gather further information.

Comprehending your values

This stage involves expressing to others what values underpin your view about the decision to be made, and hearing them reflect back to you what they understand of your values, and their own values perspective. Depending on the time available, you should engage in dialogue with others in order to work out what values are most important in the given situation, and how they apply in that situation. Even in emergency situations, when time seems very short, you should attempt to have some sort of dialogue about the values involved in the situation at hand.

In such a dialogue, avoid assuming that when someone expresses a high-level value (such as 'fairness' or 'freedom') you share an understanding of what that means in the context of the decision to be taken. One way to do this, whenever someone uses such a term without explaining it in context, is for someone else in the group to share their understanding of what that person meant by the term.

You may need to think explicitly about who is not represented or available for discussion, and what values they might have identified. And this is especially true in relation to patients.

Committing to what matters most

Within this stage you and the other stakeholders need to work out which two or three of your identified values are the most important in the context of the decision, and which may indicate a course of action. If you are on your own, you need to try to imagine yourself in the shoes of other relevant people, and what they might say was most important from their perspective. It may be especially important to try to imagine a values perspective that you cannot support or that you profoundly disagree with, but with which you know others may identify.

Wherever possible, identify where there is consensus on important values, and, where there is disagreement, the meaning behind it.

---

[25] Although clinical experience gives a professional the advantage of both knowledge of technical detail and also of 'having experienced something similar before', ultimately proper application of VBDM is not based ultimately upon experience but upon clarity of the exposition of differing values and their clashes.

Choosing the option that fits best and taking a decision

In VBDM, the best decision from your perspective will be the one that has most integrity with the values you have identified as most important. Within this stage, you will test each possible decision or option against the most important values, thinking in particular about the intended consequences of each option and considering the possible negative or unwanted consequences of each decision.

During this process you may identify other options that you had not considered previously, and so evaluate these against your most important values too. Again, wherever possible, identify areas of consensus and disagreement, and demonstrate how they have been considered and either accepted or rejected.

Communicating your decision

Having worked through these stages (even if they have all been done in a short period of time within your own mind, for a less significant decision or when there is no time for a longer process), you should be able to explain your decision credibly to others. Your explanation needs to show awareness of the personal values involved in your decision,

Table A.1.2 Process, reflection, and outcomes of values-based decision-making

Step	Process	Reflection	Outcomes
Clarification	Stepping back Thinking of other people's perspectives	What's important to me? What seems obvious or unarguable? What do I/others feel strongly about?	Increasing awareness of values perspectives and how they differ
Comprehension	Opening dialogue about values perspectives	What values are in play here? Why do the perspectives differ?	Understanding why there is agreement and disagreement about values
Committing	Identifying the values that are going to drive the decision-making process	What will be the consequences of this decision? What might not be obvious to me?	Developing consensus Involving patient (if clinical) in the process
Choosing	Ensuring that all voices are heard if a group process Documentation of discussion	Asking, how might this choice be seen by others?	Opportunity for review of values
Communication	Sharing the process and the outcome	What values have not been honoured in this decision? What negative outcomes will happen that others have to bear?	Honesty and transparency about values and consequences; communicate integrity and enable others to commit to action

awareness of the values perspectives of others, and how these have influenced your professional view of what is the right decision to take. This kind of honesty about values communicates your commitment to personal, as well as professional, integrity, and is an important quality in leadership roles. It also enables others to implement your decision.

In communicating your decision, you will also need honestly to address any negative consequences of your decision, and acknowledge that there may be those who cannot support your decision from their values perspective. You may need to make time and space for the expression of distress and anger that arises from a decision that does not honour other peoples' values; in mental health settings, it is patients whose values are most often not recognised or taken full account of, but professionals may also feel distress if their values are not honoured by the decision.

Table A.1.2 shows the process, reflection, and outcomes of these five principles.

Decision sequencing

The foregoing discussion has been couched largely in terms of single scenarios requiring single decisions. In clinical reality, however, any decision taken gives rise to a new scenario, which often requires a further decision. This can extend to 'rolling' decisions and scenarios, with new scenarios occurring in response to decisions taken (or from changed clinical circumstance that supersede a previous scenario in the absence of any decision having been taken).

As described in more detail in Part C, when externally critiquing decisions (usually with outcomes that are deemed 'bad'), methods such as Root Cause Analysis are used to review the sequence of events and decisions that led up to the outcome, to identify which specific circumstances and decisions were crucial in causing the bad outcome.

A.2

Decision-making in practice

Clinical decision-making in both clinical and clinico-legal practice

Accepting all of the theory already described concerning how decisions are, should, and should not be taken, what advice can be offered on practical clinical decision-making, whether it is directed at clinical intervention or at assisting lawyers and courts to address defined legal questions?

Basic principles

It might be thought that all that needs to be written here is, 'follow the rules of ordinary good clinical psychiatric practice'. However, as we have already suggested, all medical practice is subject to both heuristics and bias, as well as to the role of values, and all—but particularly the latter—is *especially* so in a forensic context. Hence, for example, some diagnoses under consideration in clinical assessment inherently 'contain' less facts than do others, and so leave more room for value judgment (and values conflict); so there is much 'cream' in the ice cream, and other ingredients are sometimes 'thin'. For example, the 'fact to value' ratios of psychiatric diagnoses vary greatly, which bears directly upon the potential for the role of values to determine their 'use'.[1] And consideration of the difference between diagnosing dementia and personality disorder immediately serves to make the point.

Hence, even before getting to the point of 'mapping' a defendant's likely mental state, arising from a particular diagnosis, onto a given legal definition or test (see later), which perhaps contains an *obvious* potential for value judgment, the mere making of the diagnosis itself is potentially open heavily to value judgment, and especially so in relation to some diagnoses. So there can be widely varying degrees of 'inter-rater agreement' in the making of different types of diagnosis clinically (e.g. schizophrenia versus personality disorder). Indeed, some psychiatrists may even take a 'values position' per se on particular diagnostic categories in a forensic context, by, for example, refusing even

---

[1] See generally Fulford KWM et al (2006) *Oxford Textbook of Philosophy and Psychiatry*, Oxford University Press; also Fulford KWM et al (2013) *Oxford Handbook of Philosophy and Psychiatry*, Oxford University Press.

to acknowledge 'personality disorder' in the context of court process (or some even in clinical practice).

Even more is the foregoing true where it is not solely 'diagnosis' or 'mental state description' that is offered to the court but 'formulation', since clearly formulation, which offers an 'understanding' of the defendant, or litigant, is 'looser' and *even more* open to inter-rater unreliability, including via the role of values.

It might be said, of course, that psychiatrists should therefore stick to 'diagnosis and mental state description', and eschew 'formulation'. However, a crucial aspect of both clinical forensic practice and offering expert psychiatric evidence is commonly that of addressing 'causation'. Hence, for example, a particular diagnosis and mental state description might be suggested as likely to have been 'present' at the time of a killing, but the court will then understandably ask 'so what?'; that is, 'what is the relevance of the mental condition to (e.g.) the killing?' Now clearly there is almost never a 'scientific' basis for offering an opinion on causation, even where, for example, the defendant suffers from substantial brain damage (since there may have been other additional nonmedical determinants of the offence than solely alteration of decision-making or behaviour directly attributable to a specific location of brain damage). Rather, all that can be offered is evidence as to 'narrative'; that is, an answer the question 'how does the condition contribute to the overall narrative of the killing?' (where there may e.g. be both 'normal' and 'mentally abnormal' contributors to the narrative, and where there may be disputed narratives between the defence and prosecution). This requires the offering of 'formulation', or an understanding, of both the mental condition and the offence; albeit the nature of formulation, being distinct from either diagnosis or mental state description, must be made plain to the legal recipient.

And clearly in solely clinical forensic practice the need for 'narrative' and 'understanding' of both the patient and his offending behaviour are equally necessary, particularly in regard to risk assessment and management.

Categories of clinical decision-making

This is not the place to rehearse comprehensively the literature on clinical diagnostic decision-making and guidelines. However, it is important first, at least, to distinguish between decisions concerning (1) *data collection* (what to collect e.g.) and (2) *the method and extent of direct clinical assessment*; leaving aside, for the moment, *diagnostic decision-making*.

Data collection may seem straightforward at least in regard to assessment directed at solely clinical purposes; put simply, be as comprehensive in data collection as circumstances and resources, including time, allow. However, in clinico-legal practice, the legal context may determine that investigations should be pursued beyond what would be justified in ordinary clinical practice. For example, whereas in ordinary clinical assessment for a potential diagnosis of a degenerative brain condition it might be adequate, or even good practice, not to immediately request imaging or neuropsychometry, rather to 'watch and wait', where the diagnosis, or its absence, is legally relevant the case will not wait for time to give the answer. And certainly in serious criminal cases, and especially in capital cases, the maxim *'leave no stone unturned (now)'* applies. Whilst, in the opposite vein, data *availability* is often particularly an issue in the clinico-legal context, in that it can be restricted, at least in part, by legal process (see e.g. ethical case 9). This can have implications for how robust is the clinical conclusion that is, or can be arrived at.

In clinico-legal practice, what is crucial is that there is as little contamination of clinical method as possible, in terms of contamination of investigative method by the legal context.

We say, 'as possible' because, as already described, some data collection may not legally be allowed. For example, in regard to either, or both, diagnosis and/or reconstruction of the defendant's likely mental state at a relevant time, an important source of clinical data might be a witness in the case to whom you are told you do not have access, and may not be granted access (e.g. if you are instructed by the defence and the witness is a prosecution witness). In some circumstances it may be possible to *gain* access to such a witness: for example by giving an assurance that you will not ask questions beyond such as are directly clinically relevant. However, on occasions data may be *both* medically and directly legally relevant, so that the data remains unavailable to you, beyond simply the witness statement (which may not be in a form, or sufficiently so, or comprehensive enough, to serve effectively as clinical data, so as to be clinically fully useful). Or there may be evidence that is legally privileged and that is not therefore available to you in any form or circumstance, even though you may be aware of its existence, or even content.

The foregoing said, the maxim must be 'function clinically as normally as possible given, or despite the legal context'; where the clinical decisions to be taken range across deciding what data to collect; how to assess the defendant clinically; what 'tests' to apply or request; and how to approach making a diagnosis or determining a relevant mental state description, or formulation.

Clinical assessment

Turning to the process of clinical assessment per se, it may assist to rehearse what an official source advises clinicians. This will serve to ground assessment for both clinical and clinico-legal purposes in 'ordinary' clinical decision-making, and to expose where alterations or restrictions are imposed by way of legal context within specifically clinico-legal practice.[2]

For example, NHS Scotland has produced a brief guide to clinical decision-making written for nurses, midwives, and allied healthcare professionals,[3] which addresses the principles of clinical decision making; the core skills of decision making; the decision making process; and the power of shared decision making;, it opines, reflecting much of the theory already described above, 'decision making can range from fast, intuitive, or heuristic decisions through to well reasoned, analytical, evidence-based decisions … there is a spectrum of decision making; at one end of the spectrum we use our intuition and experience to make decisions, where there is typically a high volume of simple decisions to be made. At the other end of the spectrum, there may be complex decisions to be made, where the level of uncertainty is high and an analytical and an evidence-based approach is needed to support the rules-based heuristics or experience we have gained over time in "similar" situations.'

The guidance adds, 'Good, effective clinical decision making requires a combination of experience and skills, including … critical thinking; that is, *removing* emotion from our reasoning,[4] being "skeptical", with the ability to clarify goals, examine assumptions, be open-minded, recognise personal attitudes and bias, and the ability to evaluate

---

[2] Of course sometimes assessment that is directed at solely clinical purposes can then be applied, even unexpectedly, to a clinico-legal purpose, and this can give rise to ethical difficulties (e.g. the patient may have told their doctor something that, as a defendant, they would not have told a medical expert).

[3] See www.effectivepractitioner.nes.scot.nhs.uk.

[4] This surely is a counsel of unachievable perfection.

evidence … plus evidence-based approaches: using available evidence and best practice guidelines as part of the decision making process … and sharing your learning, and getting feedback from colleagues on your decision making' (emphasis added).

The latter aspect of the advice emphasises one obvious difference between decision-making in ordinary clinical and in clinico-legal contexts, in that assessment in the latter context is characteristically clinically individual (albeit there can, and should be *ex post* 'peer review' across cases of a clinician's practice). Indeed, it is perhaps necessarily so in that the clinician gives their own expert opinion, not that of a team (although where assessment is conducted by a clinical team, for example as an inpatient, and the designated expert then gives an 'individual' opinion, they will probably have taken account of the expertise and opinions of clinical colleagues). And herein lie ethical risks arising from being, or becoming over time, 'a lone expert wolf'.

The same NHS advice continues, '(use) feedback from others, and the outcomes of the decisions to reflect on the decisions that were taken in order to enhance practice delivery in the future. It is also important to reflect on (all) your … decision making strategies to ensure that you hone your decision making skills and learn from experience.' And here, although this may properly be applicable to clinico-legal practice, reflection cannot operate in quite the same way that it can in ordinary clinical practice, including forensic clinical practice.

The advice continues further, 'There are many factors involved in clinical decision making and each of the core skills has the potential to impact effective decision making. In an ideal world, decisions would be made objectively, with a full set of evidence, an endless bank of resources, no time pressures, minimal interruptions, decision support tools to hand and plenty of energy to handle any decision making situation at any time of the day. However, this is not always the reality.' Yet in a forensic context, especially in regard to serious criminal offences, the counsel must indeed be 'leave no stone unturned'.

Perhaps of crucial importance in a forensic setting is the guidance advice 'Reflect back on a recent decision you made—did you make the judgement and decision objectively, did you use all the data and evidence to hand? Did your personal attitudes or biases have a part to play in the decision? … And examine your own decision making patterns.'

Clinical assessment towards diagnosis and mental state description for legal purposes

There are distinct aspects of assessment, involving both direct clinical assessment and reviewing of other clinically relevant information; with decisions required in regard to the detail of each aspect.

First, as already indicated, it is necessary to decide what *sources of information* can potentially be relevant to determination of diagnosis and mental state(s) (related to whatever time is relevant to the clinical or legal questions(s) at hand). As detailed in Chapter 4 of the handbook, on forensic psychiatric assessment, there will be a range of sources of information potentially capable of such relevance, and the first decision is to determine what sources should be considered. This may include, for example, past medical records, plus witness statements and police interviews, as well as the custody record. However, what is crucial is to make the decision based upon 'bias' towards over-inclusion. Sources that prove irrelevant can be discarded, but sources not considered will remain unknown in terms of their relevance (risking the 'WYSIATA' heuristic); whilst the mere fact of 'selection' lays the foundation for an enhanced risk of bias in the assessment. Finally, great care should be taken to avoid selectivity in seeking out, or using, the various potential sources of information, because of the risk of bias via selection.

Second, when it comes to *direct clinical assessment*, the manner and detail of questioning is crucial. And here the first rule is to make the assessment, as far as possible, with 'wilful blindness' as to the legal relevance of any particular clinical findings to which you may come, since an obvious source of potential bias in your clinical assessment may arise from awareness of the impact particular clinical findings may have upon the legal outcome. Hence, the expert should be 'wilfully unconcerned about the legal outcome'.

Third, as regards making decisions about *further investigations* (see again Chapter 4 of the handbook), the approach should err once more towards over-inclusion, which will likely enhance the reliability of the final clinical conclusions reached, whilst also offering a safeguard against frank, or inferred bias, expressed within the manner of selection between various possible further investigations. And, notably, such further investigations may well require the expertise of other clinicians (e.g. a clinical psychologist or neuro-radiologist) or indeed full clinical assessment by another psychiatrist with specialist expertise (e.g. a neuropsychiatrist).

All of the foregoing will then lead to a decision as to what *diagnoses and mental states*, often also *formulation*, are potentially 'in play': that is, worthy of consideration in terms of 'differential diagnosis' (to use classical medical terminology). Since only uncommonly is there just one certain diagnosis or mental state. And, where the evidence does indeed not point to just one clinical conclusion, it will be necessary to lay out for yourself the points for and against the competing conclusions, as well as deciding upon how best to present to the court such competing conclusions (see below concerning decision-making in regard to report writing). And finally, experts will need to address explicitly the likely validity of their favoured clinical conclusion (or of competing conclusions).

If the clinician or expert cannot themselves decide upon one favoured conclusion then it is not at all unreasonable, indeed it is right, to present the competing contenders, with the arguments in favour and against each, and then to leave the court to determine which should be alighted upon. That is, in a legal context, although the issue is a solely clinical one, if the expert cannot be fully confident in coming to a conclusion, the issue should be left to legal determination, even though this may feel alien to you as a doctor.

The latter infers another topic in that, especially but not solely, where there is a question concerning whether the defendant might be malingering or exaggerating mental symptoms (see criminal law case 12), it will be important to address this directly within your clinical assessment (and then include a section of the clinical diagnosis aspect of any report, for example to a court of Mental Health Tribunal, on *validation*, i.e. setting out in detail what factors support, or tend to contradict, the clinical opinion to which you have come, see below).

Related to the latter point is the question *When is a small or restricted quantity of data too little to be a basis for offering a clinical opinion?* This is not an uncommon question with which to be faced in the jurisdictions of less developed countries, with less developed mental health and other medical services, and often greater difficulty gaining access to both past medical and other records and informants. There is no simple answer to the question. However, in essence the proper response is in terms of coupling your opinion with an estimate of its likely reliability, with explicit recognition that the reliability of the clinical opinion expressed is dependent upon the data upon which it is based, and the nature of any gaps there may be. And, unless there is a gross lack of information, it should usually be possible to offer an opinion, clinical or/and clinico-legal, but always with a caveat concerning its likely reliability. Indeed, the clinician, also lawyer, should always be aware of the maxim 'absence of evidence is not evidence of absence'. This said, there may be a 'floor' of limited data below which no reasonable clinical conclusion can be reached.

A variant of the latter issue concerns *retrospective assessment* (see criminal law case 15): that is, consideration of the bases upon which a mental state that occurred in a defendant, or patient, at some earlier point than when they are clinically examined in retrospect. In this context, it is not unheard for a forensically inexperienced psychiatrist to say, 'I can't say what was the defendant's mental state when they killed because I wasn't there.' This is a naive, and unhelpful, response. Since it is *entirely possible* for an expert to use all available data so as to reconstruct retrospectively, as best they can, what was an individual's likely mental state coincidental with given behaviour, albeit with proper warnings about validity and reliability, and it is *necessary* both clinically, for example for risk assessment and management, and for the courts, that they do so.

Almost finally, it is good practice to express any diagnosis in terms of one of the two accepted international classifications of mental disorders, DSM-5 and ICD-11. This will exert personal diagnostic rigour certainly upon the expert, including in terms of consistency across cases, lay a clear foundation for diagnostic discussion with other experts, and aid the court in both understanding the basis upon which any diagnosis has been made and in determining proper routes to challenging that diagnosis. Albeit, as the handbook cautions, there are dangers of misapplication of the two accepted classificatory systems to legal process (especially DSM-5), or of deliberate adversarial 'misunderstanding' of them. The same rigour should be pursued in solely clinical practice, and not just because many patients will have tribunals.

Finally, but now we veer very clearly towards clinico-legal *reporting* of findings (see below), there will have to be decisions made about *how best to explain* to a lay audience, which may ultimately include a jury, the clinical conclusions to which you have come. Here the first rule is to avoid jargon as much as possible or, at least, if you need to use it in order to facilitate communication with other experts in the case, go on then to offer a simple lay description of what the term used means. And, in laying out in your report the relevant clinical opinions to which you have come, keep in mind that you will, almost certainly, need to explain very much in lay terms in oral evidence, especially if there is a jury in the case, what these various terms mean. Given that much psychiatry is abstract, a useful approach is to use concrete analogy to get over abstract clinical notions. And, even though you may not choose to use any such concrete analogies within the report, at least describe your clinical conclusions in a fashion that lays the ground for some means of offering an easily understood within oral evidence.

Clinico-legal decision-making

The immediately foregoing section dealt with clinical decision-making in both a clinical assessment and treatment settings and in regard to clinical assessment as the basis for provision of expert evidence to a court or tribunal. We turn now to decision-making in the further stages of clinico-legal practice within a case. And in doing so we adopt explicitly the further headings used for each case in Part B of the casebook: 'Legal', 'Clinico-legal', and then also 'Ethical' (the immediately foregoing section of this Part A having been relevant to the 'Clinical' heading of any given case in Part B).

Law

It is clearly not the role of experts to determine for themselves what are the legal questions, definitions, or tests to which their clinical findings should be applied. However, it *is* the responsibility of experts to ensure that they have clear and comprehensive legal instructions, so far as they are, or can be, capable of determining this, and this duty emphasises the need to have a real understanding of relevant law, both so as to be able to 'understand' what they are told and to be aware when instructions may sometimes not be adequate. So that, where experts do not understand the instructions, or suspects that they are not comprehensive, they must ensure that there is a dialogue with the instructing lawyer sufficient to rectify this.

In the cases presented in the Part B we lay out the law relevant to each case, usually as it is in all four domestic jurisdictions, and/or the reader is referred to such law in the handbook. However, in practice of course, what the expert is told of the law within a case will be dependent upon the instructing lawyers.

One difficult, often ethically difficult, question arises where the particularly experienced expert becomes aware, when dealing for example with a clinico-legally inexperienced lawyer, that the lawyer is missing a question of importance. And here it may be sensible, and acceptable, to ask legally intelligent questions of the lawyer about their instructions to you, as a means of focusing them on questions that you are aware are likely to be important. So that within the cases in Part B we sometimes 'set the case' by way of giving poor legal instructions, where part of the learning aspect of the case is to *recognise* that the instructions are inadequate, so that you need to decide to go back to the lawyers to ask for better or clearer instructions.

Finally, in serious criminal cases there should be appointed very experienced counsel, and so you should ensure that you receive, directly from them, and at an early stage, detailed advice that includes the relevant legal questions, with explicit reference to any related statutes or case reports. However, even in capital cases, counsel are not always at this level.

> ### Clinico-legal
>
> Having determined the likely diagnosis and mental state at some relevant time(s), and being informed of both the relevant law and what are the legal questions within the case, you the expert must apply your mind to 'mapping' your clinical conclusions onto the legal questions that you have been asked to address (see 'psycho-legal mapping' in Chapter 2 of the handbook). That is, directly addressing the relevant legal questions by reference to the mental state findings to which you have come, in relation to whatever time point is legally relevant. Where you can choose to map onto the law of your own domestic jurisdiction or to test your clinico-legal skill by also mapping onto another domestic jurisdiction or even onto some other common law jurisdiction you may research (see *Preface*).[5]
>
> Here it might be thought perhaps that the process is automatic and requiring of no 'decision-making'. However, in practice, first, there must be a decision taken concerning which of the clinical conclusions to which you have come (diagnosis, mental state description, or formulation) are *relevant* to the legal questions at hand, and then what should be the *manner of presentation* of those clinical conclusions in relation to the relevant definitions or tests (i.e. the manner of the psycho-legal mapping).
>
> Deciding about how to address the clinico-legal issue(s) may go beyond deciding merely about presentation, however. Although the law of expert evidence requires, almost ubiquitously, that an expert should not offer opinion on 'the ultimate issue' (e.g. guilt or innocence), sometimes this requirement may not be entirely unambiguous in its observation or the court may itself bend the rule or the legal test may be so simple that the boundary between clinical and legal seems almost to vanish (i.e. no 'mapping' at all appears to be required).[6]

[5] Two criminal cases, 16 and 17, are written in the law of a Commonwealth jurisdiction.

[6] An example of this situation from comparative jurisprudence is contained within Section 44 of the Norwegian Criminal Code, wherein legal insanity is equated with medical psychosis. Hence, there is no required intermediate step involving a decision about the 'responsibility implications' of a given abnormal mental state.

In order to illustrate these alternative situations, consider first *insanity*, in relation to which almost always the expert is allowed or required to give an opinion on whether the defendant did not, for example, know that what they were doing was 'wrong' (see criminal law cases 17 and 18). Yet what does 'know' mean? What about the defendant who was so psychotically driven at the time of the alleged acts that they were unable effectively to pay attention to knowledge that they would otherwise have that what they were doing was wrong? Does such lack of appreciation amount to 'not knowing'? Now surely that is a legal question, yet it is not uncommon, almost apparently required, for experts to give an opinion on insanity in a way that can leave them to adopt their own understanding of the law, sometimes not even noticing that they are doing so.

Similarly, in many jurisdictions it has become almost accepted practice that, in consideration of the partial defence of *diminished responsibility* (see criminal law cases 5, 7, 8, 9, 10, and 11), the expert may, almost should, offer an opinion not only on whether there was an 'abnormality of mind' but on whether that abnormality of mind was such as 'substantially impaired the defendant's mental responsibility', rather than solely describing the defendant's likely mental state concurrent with the killing and leaving the court solely to translate that into addressing the moral question. Indeed, before reform of the defence in English law, the Court of Appeal explicitly approved the practice. Yet in so doing the expert both seems to take on the role of the jury and also opens themselves up to cross-examination on all of the evidence in the case that the jury will have to decide upon. So, in addressing that defence, experts must often draw their own boundaries: that is, decide how, clinico-legally, to express their opinion in regard to the second limb of the defence.

The latter example raises a more general question: if the legal definition at hand is loose, how do you deal with such latitude in the expression of your opinion?; recognising that such latitude allows in the expert's own values (see criminal law case 16). Where, by contrast, a tight legal definition offers greater certainty in clinico-legal mapping; albeit that the lack of room for the exercise by the court of discretion may, if the definition is highly incongruous with clinical constructs, infer the potential for infringing natural justice.

Or in addressing whether a defendant had been *capable of understanding the police caution* (see criminal law case 25), the expert will have to decide whether solely to describe the defendant's likely mental state concurrent with the administering of the caution, or whether to answer the ultimate question. Here the court will be very likely to require them to do the latter. Yet without expressing knowledge of what degree of understanding is, in law, required, or whether the law requires 'continuing' understanding, and the ability to keep the caution in mind throughout the interviews, how can they properly do so?

In almost entirely similar terms, you will, as an appointed expert, often be asked to express an opinion upon whether a defendant is *fit to plead* (see criminal law case 3), when to do so may require a detailed understanding upon your part of, and more crucially judgment upon, the complexity of the evidence in the trial, to which the defendant will have to respond.

Or whether, having assessed a defendant to be abnormally *suggestible* and/or *compliant* (criminal law case 2), you are prepared, when asked, to opine upon whether his confessions to the police are 'reliable'. The first two constructs are quasi-clinical, whereas the latter is solely legal, and open to jury determination beyond taking a view about any expert evidence offered to them.

Where another expert, for example a clinical psychologist, is instructed by the same side as you and is reporting direct to the court, you will need to decide how much of their report, if any part, to repeat in your own report. Here, usually, summarising their findings will be sufficient and necessary, so as to be able to relate them to your own clinical findings and psycho-legal mapping.

In summary, the legal definition at hand may be 'tight' or 'loose', and may be more or less (in)congruent with relevant medical constructs. So that the required psycho-legal mapping may be highly/poorly focused (depending upon the tightness of the legal definition) and varyingly (in)congruous with relevant medical constructs.

Ethical

The latter types of issues naturally infer ethical decision-making (under 'ethical' we subsume 'professional practice' issues). Indeed, such decision-making will be necessary potentially across all three of the stages already discussed, even the stage dealing with law, since as will already be apparent, there may be ethical decisions to be taken in regard to your actions in respect of your communication with the instructing lawyers concerning what legal questions, tests or definitions are in play (see above).

In this respect we refer the reader to Chapter 15 of the handbook concerning the identification of the myriad potential ethical pitfalls that exist within assessing and presenting clinical information for use in legal process, often reflecting the profoundly different methods and constructs of medicine and law. In the cases in Part B, we sometimes offer information intended to be suggestive of particular ethical issues that require identification and then decision-making. Or we explicitly raise particular ethical questions. However, rather than repeating here examples of ethical issues that it may be important to address, and ways of deciding upon them, again we refer the reader towards detailed reading of Chapter 15 of the handbook.

Finally, in criminal law there is a duty not merely on defence lawyers to be aware of and to pursue possible consideration of the relevance of a defendant's apparent mental condition in relation to a wide variety of legal issues but also, in natural justice, on the prosecution to be so concerned. Yet this can be overlooked because, in most situations, the law, either per se or in practice, focuses upon the defence raising such issues. This disparity can spill over into the attitude of expert psychiatrists appointed by the prosecution—in that, for example in relation to the partial defence of diminished responsibility, because it is for the defence to raise the issue, and for the prosecution potentially to rebut it, this can be mirrored not only in the sequential instruction of defence and then prosecution experts but also in the attitude of each, certainly the latter.

Because it is indeed for the defence to raise a range of legal issues that require expert psychiatric evidence, most of the cases in the casebook are written in terms of instruction by the defence. However, where the expert is instructed by the prosecution it is incumbent upon them to apply exactly the same approach to clinical assessment and clinico-legal opinion formation as they would apply were they to have been instructed by the defence. Hence, the cases should be seen as equally constructed and relevant had the expert been instructed by either side. Indeed, the pursuit of nonbias demands it.

Cases

How to use the cases

As already described, whereas the handbook offers information, the casebook offers assistance in using information in practice. This is expressed through variation of the method commonly used in postgraduate medical education of setting problem cases, plus questions to address; with suggestions overleaf of how the case might be approached. Hence, in each of the cases described in Part B, we offer a case description, comprising clinical, and often also legal information, also sometimes with explicit ethical aspects, and pose questions to address. This is then followed by suggested approaches to deciding upon answers to the questions posed.

The cases take the form of 'short cases', in that neither the description of the case, nor the discussion of suggested ways of responding to it, are at all exhaustive or even comprehensive. That is, they are not 'long cases' as used to be adopted in the old-style medical 'final' or membership examinations or, indeed, in an important other casebook in the field of general psychiatric ethics.[1] Rather, they are designed to prompt the reader to recognise major issues, and ways in which they may be responded to; albeit we hope this will go beyond *mere* raising awareness of the issues, since the meat of the work is in the decision process.

Also we do not offer 'dynamic' case descriptions, in terms of asking the reader to answer initial questions, and then posing further details of the case beyond what was first posed. That is, we do not pose any 'decision sequencing' (as we described it above). However, the reader may wish to pose for themselves 'what if?' questions, beyond the case as set; that is, having worked through decisions on the case as set, they may wish to pose further questions, such as supposing the outcome of my decisions is X, or alternatively Y, how would I *then* decide further at *that* stage?

It follows that it is not suggested ever that any specific questions are the only possible questions arising from the case as it is described. However, they are the ones that we have alighted upon to offer for your consideration, and so you may wish to add in other questions of your own to address. Similarly, we do not suggest the approaches to responding to the questions we outline are the only ones that are justifiable. Indeed, the reader may profit from, and enjoy, pointing out to themselves approaches that we might seem, to you, to have missed.

So it is important to emphasise that we do not offer a 'correct answer' to each case, clinically, clinico-legally, and/or ethically; indeed, we often offer alternative answers, which must be decided between. Rather, we try to demonstrate the *justification* for each possible answer (if more than one is proposed) that might be arrived at, clinically, clinico-legally, or ethically. Put simply, this is in terms of 'show your workings', given that the quality of an opinion lies not in the opinion expressed but in the process by which it was reached, and in its underpinnings and justification.

The cases are also chosen to be practical, in that they are intended to represent situations that we hope will be recognised by clinicians to be real within ordinary daily forensic practice, and they are responded to, in the answers we offer, in a similar practical fashion. So it follows that, in being so practical, no attempt is, or in the space available can, be made in the answers offered to invoke detailed theory of decision-making as it is expressed in Part A. Rather, in regard to any particular case that you may address, you

---

[1] Dickenson D and Fulford K W B (2000) *In Two Minds: A Casebook of Psychiatric Ethics*, Oxford University Press.

may wish to view your responses through the prism of theory described in Part A. Perhaps thereby exposing for yourself the heuristics and biases, as well as the role of values, that you might have brought to the case. That is, in your interpretation of the case description, in your clinical and clinico-legal responses to it, and in your identification of and responses to the ethical issues inherent to the case. Put simply, the reader may wish to pose the question, after having made decisions about the case, How did I get to that decision? or even, how did I get to *that* decision!

So we would urge you the reader to 'fine grain' critique the decision process that you underwent in coming to your responses to the case, in terms of Part A methods of decision-making, including the role of values.[2] Aimed towards addressing what is a valid critique of the decision process; that is, a *clinically* valid critique (by contrast with an external critique that might originate in e.g. legal process, see Part C).

The cases are offered within sections of Part B, distinguished according to the predominance of *clinical*, *legal*, *clinico-legal*, and *ethical* issues within them, and as regards legal, they are distinguished into criminal, civil, and mental health and capacity law categories. However, it is important to emphasise that *every* case contains all of the categories of aspects (including often more than one category of legal aspect). For example, even a ward round decision that appears to be solely clinical will have, lurking behind or within it, not only ethical but also legal aspects, even if these are not evident (and they might become so at a later stage when e.g. the decision is challenged retrospectively). So the sections of Part B serve merely to aid the reader in using the book practically.

There are within specifically clinico-legal practice recognisable '*psycho-legal case types*' that represent a particular combination of diagnosis, or mental state abnormality, *and* a particular legal question. That is, each is a particular exemplar of a type of psycho-legal 'mapping' (mapping of a given mental state description onto a given legal definition). And we have tried, in choosing clinico-legal cases, to capture particularly common, or problematic, psycho-legal case types: that is, case types that give rise to common, or particularly problematic issues at the interface of psychiatry and law, and/or ethical conundrums.

Similarly, we have tried, within the clinical cases, to choose often either/both common sets of issues or/and particularly complex and problematic ones.

Given that *all* cases do contain clinical, legal, clinico-legal, and ethical aspects, we therefore address each in terms of all of these categories. And, in addition to each case having a title, which describes the core issues of the case, there is a summary of the specific topics, or issues, arising in each of the four categories within the header to each case, with cross-references to the handbook. We hope that this will serve to allow you the reader to look through the 'menu' of cases in order to select fields and topics in relation to which you believe you would benefit from experiential education and training. Alternatively, you may wish to look at some case that appears to have aspects in common with a real case with which you are, or have been faced with in your practice: that is, a case that looks to be of a similar clinical or psycho-legal case type.

Each case therefore comprises first, a *Case Description*, which includes set questions, followed by suggested answers, in terms of responses that are *clinical* and/or *legal* (knowing the relevant law), and then the *clinico-legal* stage (concerned with mapping the clinical findings onto the legal questions, definitions, or test), and we then add text on *ethical*

---

[2] Of course, many methods of *external* critiquing of decisions made will not indulge in such fine grain critiquing; albeit their capacity and tendency to do so will vary with the method adopted (see Part C). And this emphasizes the importance of clinically based fine-grain *self*-critiquing.

issues. In just a few cases, the nature of the case, and the issues it presents, is such that it is more convenient to merge two or more of the three stages just described.

As already described, many of the criminal clinico-legal cases are written in terms of instructions from defence lawyers. This is not, of course, to suggest that forensic psychiatrists should be 'defence-minded'. Rather, it is because, in very many circumstances, the burden of raising some form of defence, or other issue, based upon mental disorder, falls upon that side. However, of course, any psychiatrist instructed by the prosecution should properly address the clinical and clinico-legal issues uninfluenced by the side instructing them, including often putting themselves in the position of asking, how would I respond if instructed by the defence or prosecution?

As described in the preface, although the law described in each case is that of one, or usually all, of the UK & Irish jurisdictions dealt with in the handbook, most case are set out so as to allow the reader to test themselves clinico-legally in relation to jurisdictions that are not their own, or indeed in relation to any Commonwealth common law jurisdiction.

There are cases in which it appears clear, or at least likely, that data and opinion from other experts (e.g. clinical psychologists or neuro-radiologists) is required. And where this is so, we address what are reasonable ways of incorporating into your decision-making, both clinically and clinico-legally, such data and opinion as are beyond the expertise of the instructed psychiatrist, but which are relevant to the opinion they express within their own discipline.

Finally, as we write in the postface, we should welcome responses from readers to the cases presented, and to the approaches we suggest towards addressing them, including of course constructive criticism.

B.1

Clinical cases

When is a case a 'forensic' case?

Themes: *mental symptoms relating to risk of harm to others and sexual offending (p.62), formulation of offending risk (p.146), 'forensic caseness' (p.20), and specialist forensic versus general psychiatric management (p.8) [C]; violent thoughts absent criminal offending (pp.322, 466) [L] and detention for depression (p.474) [CL]; and injustice through lack of resources (p.276) [E]*

Case description

You are a forensic psychiatrist working in a community forensic team, and are asked by one of your colleagues to assess a young man called Martin, who has been treated by your colleague for depression.

You review the records and see that the presenting problem began two years ago, when Martin was twenty-three years of age. He talked then to his GP about having violent thoughts, including imagining killing people he saw in the street, which, in the context also of depressive symptoms, precipitated his referral to general psychiatric services. And since then he has also described to his psychiatrist thoughts of raping women he has known who have rejected him.

Your colleague has established, so far as possible, that Martin has not taken any action in relation to these thoughts, nor does he have any criminal record. He also says that Martin's mental state has seemed improved with antidepressants. However, the referral has been prompted by Martin's disclosure that recently he has been accessing (he says legal) pornography sites on the internet that have sadistic content.

Questions

1. Should you recommend that your forensic service provide treatment to Martin?
2. If so, what treatment?
3. If not, what advice will you give about Martin's management within general mental health services?
4. What other clinical, legal, clinico-legal, and ethical issues does his case pose?

Clinical

The theme of this case is 'forensic caseness'; that is, what aspects of a case make it appropriate for a specialist forensic psychiatric service to take over management, rather than leaving monitoring and management solely with general clinicians, albeit offering advice?

First, and most obviously, is the question of what danger Martin poses to others, and the role of a forensic psychiatrist in the assessment of his risk of harm to others. Although all psychiatrists train to assess such risk, and understand the basic components of risk assessment, the forensic psychiatrist has additional expertise, particularly in regards to sexual offending. This being by dint of specialist training and use of clinical techniques and schedules, plus 'daily acquaintance' with violence and sexual offending, since their clinical practice focuses on linkage between mental states and violence risk, in general, and in an individual. Indeed, forensic psychiatrists rarely see patients who do *not* pose a risk of serious harm to others. They are also usually better resourced to assess and manage the risk of serious violence or sexual offending than are general services.

In their training and practice, forensic psychiatrists focus on understanding violence as a complex human behaviour, expressed in terms of a wide range of routes by which people come to harm others, and the contribution of different kinds of psychopathology, also ordinary criminogenic factors, to violence, including sexual offending and violence. They treat risk as dynamic, recognising that it can rise and fall, depending on what factors, both intrinsic and extrinsic to the patient, are present at any given time, including the mental state of the individual, drug and alcohol usage, plus the person's situational context, cultural values, social pressures, and the legal constraints upon them. Ultimately they formulate the individual's offending and its risk.

Second, forensic psychiatrists have particular experience of how clinical signs, symptoms, and diagnosis relates to law and legal process, as well as having greater acquaintance with working in relation to justice agencies, including the police. Hence forensic psychiatrists have a role and are experienced in translating clinical formulation into legal processes.

Thirdly, forensic psychiatrists usually have access to specialist, secure inpatient services, as well as to specialist community services, acting as gatekeepers to such expensive resources. And they use their experience of managing a range of patients at risk of expressing violence, or other offending, including *potentially* in regard to a patient like Martin.

Finally, in a case that does not warrant on-going management by specialist forensic psychiatry services, those services still have an important role in assisting other professionals and organisations better to assess and manage the risk of offending, and to manage staff anxiety.

Mental Health Trusts are subject to high levels of scrutiny, and mental health professionals (whose patients inevitably includes a small group of people at high risk of suicide or violence) naturally feel anxiety about being criticised, or even disciplined, for failing to prevent or anticipate serious untoward events. Gaining an opinion from a forensic psychiatrist may show that the potential for serious harm to others has been taken seriously, which is anxiety-relieving. Indeed, this may result in 'over-referral' to, and misuse of specialist forensic services. General adult colleagues may also hope that the forensic service will take the patient into its care, which will fully relieve them of anxiety. So, at an organisational level, medium and high secure hospitals act as anxiety-relievers for the wider community as a whole.

There are therapeutic centres that offer treatment to people who use pornography, usually based upon an addictions model: for example, in the UK, the Portman Clinic and the Lucy Faithfull Foundation. But the numbers of those potentially in need vastly exceed what is available. And there is no evidence that the standard sex offender treatment programme is likely to be of value to Martin.

In this case, there is nothing obvious that the forensic services can add to the management of the patient by direct clinical involvement. However, they can assist their general adult colleague with a more structured risk-assessment if that has not been done, such as the HCR20v3, including 'risk formulation', or application of a specialist sex offending schedule, and completing this may help the general adult team feel more empowered and confident in managing the case, based upon better monitoring of the risk that Martin may present as time unfolds.

It is also clinically relevant to remind colleagues that 'violent thoughts' per se have not been identified empirically as reliable or valid predictors of violent behaviour in populations of patients. The fact that Martin is discussing his thoughts at all is *prima facie* evidence that he sees his thoughts as a problem that he wants help with from professionals, which is itself protective against actual violence. This does *not* mean that Martin's thoughts can be dismissed, and that he can be discharged, just that actuarially; Martin is more likely to hurt himself than others, especially if he does transgress the criminal law.

It *could* be argued that Martin's risk is escalating, in that the use of internet pornography represents a move towards enacting his thoughts in the external world. However, there is little empirical evidence to support this, beyond retrospective case studies of individuals who have gone on to offend (so it is not known how many individuals have violent thoughts but never act upon them). Moreover, the empirical calculus is skewed because we know the numerator (the number of people caught using illegal pornography) but not the denominator (the number who look at concerning but legal pornography). There is also a view (not yet refuted) that use of legal pornography may help contain concerning thoughts and feelings, and further, that rape fantasies are culturally acceptable in mainstream movies and videos.

What would *really* help would be for Martin to undergo psychotherapy in which he can explore these feelings and thoughts, assisting him not to act on his thoughts but also giving clinicians a better understanding of the risk they represent.

The formulation of Martin's violent thoughts is probably that they are related to his low mood, and may reflect externalisation of the anger and hostility often found in depression. A few sessions with an experienced therapist would allow for an extended formulation to be developed, helping both Martin and his team to understand his depression, and the function of his violent thoughts. This is a case where a good-quality intervention now might reduce service usage long-term, and reduce everyone's anxiety.

What will be crucial for good and safe management will be having sufficient resources to achieve the intervention; if there are not, the forensic community team should not/cannot try to fill the gap.

Legal

Martin has not yet committed a crime, provided he is not accessing illegal pornography sites or downloading unlawful material. Even if Martin were to obtain a weapon, this would not be a crime (unless it were an unlawful firearm, or he carried it in a public place). He has made no threats to others, having only described thoughts of harming others. So there is currently no basis for disclosure of any clinical information to the police.

Clinico-legal

Although Martin has a mental disorder, there is nothing to suggest that it requires assessment or treatment in hospital. If in the future the risk of harm to others escalated, his mental disorder and need for hospital treatment would determine whether he could be legally detained.

Ethical

The most pressing ethical issue in this case, at least in the UK, is likely to be resource allocation. Some Trusts are unable to spend money on experienced therapists who can work competently with unusual and risky patients—or may have no community forensic service at all. This results in services not being provided, so that people like Martin are left alone to cope with their distress and the potential for their risk to escalate.

The most likely outcome here is that Martin will fall between all the service 'stools'; too anxiety-provoking for inexperienced therapists in IAPT and general psychology, but not risky enough for forensic services.

If Martin does not access the right help, there is a risk (of unknown degree or time scale) that his enacting of fantasies will escalate, and he may start to look at illegal pornography. At this point, he may well then 'get detected', arrested, and probably convicted, and so acquire a criminal record, which will have potentially massive effects upon his social and professional life in the future. If you were Martin, or Martin's family, you might well ask if this is fair, just, or humane.

2 Use of behaviour without conviction within risk assessment

Themes: *valid data for risk assessment and their quality and weight (p.166) [C]; 'nature of mental disorder' and risk assessment (p.470), legal admission with unproven facts (p.382) [L]; clash of medical and legal paradigms within risk assessment (p.354), and choice of method (p.174) [CL]; injustice by careless determination or use of 'facts' (p.304) and avoiding 'defensive risk assessment', inflicting 'harm' and 'wrong' on patients (p.322) [E]*

Case description

You are asked by a solicitor to provide an independent report for a mental health tribunal hearing of a man detained on a restricted hospital order. Henry, aged forty-seven, was detained in hospital after he was found guilty of assault occasioning grievous bodily harm on a female stranger: he broke her jaw and several ribs by kicking her, after pushing her to the ground. She also claimed that he had pushed up her skirt and had tried to sexually assault her, but he was not charged with this. Henry was considered to be mentally ill on arrest, and an urgent Mental Health Act assessment at the police station found him to be psychotic and in need of admission for assessment. This was confirmed when he was remanded to prison and he was transferred to his local medium secure unit, where he remained. Henry later accepted that he had been mentally ill at the time of the alleged offence, and he followed legal advice to plead guilty to GBH. He was happy to take medication and attend a variety of psychological therapy courses.

This is Henry's first tribunal hearing. He wants to be conditionally discharged to a local mixed-sex hostel where other patients from the unit have been successfully placed. However, recently nursing staff have raised concerns about Henry's sexually inappropriate behaviour with women: he is sometimes over-familiar (offering them endearments, and complimenting them on their appearance), and at times critical and dismissive of some female staff when they ask him to do something. Henry dismisses these concerns, saying that the female staff are prejudiced against him because he is an 'old-fashioned man'.

At a MAPPA meeting the police raise the alleged sexual assault, and disclose that Henry was one of a number of local men investigated for a series of brutal assaults and rapes. However, there was insufficient evidence to prosecute him.

When you interview Henry, he presents as mentally well. He accepts the need for medication and supervision, and expresses regret about the harm he caused his victim. He is adamant there was no sexual element to the index assault and is outraged that you have now raised this and the alleged series of rapes when neither were an issue at trial. He becomes hostile and accuses you of bias.

Questions

1. How should you address Henry's perceived risk of sexual offending?
2. What other clinical, legal, clinico-legal, and ethical issues does his case pose?

Clinical

If Henry is mentally well, then it may not be appropriate to continue to detain him in secure conditions to receive treatment; the 'least-restrictive' principle should mean that if it is clinically appropriate, and does not increase the risk he presents, then you should support conditional discharge.

However, assessing his risk of sexual offending after discharge is far from straightforward, involving deciding what data can and should be used. It will be important to determine the degree to which Henry's psychosis was thought to cause his offending behaviour, including whether any possible sexual element was included in the formulation of his risk, and the extent therefore to which successful treatment of his psychosis might reduce or eliminate his risk of violent and/or sexual reoffending.

Neither the sexual allegation by the victim nor the alleged rapes are proven facts. The case therefore raises the question of how to select and weigh information as the basis for clinical risk-assessment. Unlike in a court, which applies 'adversarial' method, you should apply 'investigative' method. So, clinically one can and should include all information received, but not necessarily giving it all equal weight. For example, whilst noting the nursing anxieties, disputes with staff are common in long-stay residential care; behaviour perceived as sexually inappropriate might in fact have been old-fashioned courtesies (grounded perhaps in thoughtless sexism, but without any intent to be sexually inappropriate); and some staff do have a rather brusque personal style.

Hence, when conducting a risk assessment, the assessing psychiatrist must choose what data to include and how to weigh it. So one might give the comments about sexually inappropriate behaviour a low weight for the reasons above, and the allegations of rape a similarly low weight because they are unproven. (You could request medical records covering the period of the alleged rapes, and if they show that Henry was likely to be psychotic at the time, this might influence your formulation of those allegations.)

At the tribunal hearing, Henry's solicitor might reasonably argue that these points are not legally proven and therefore should not be included at all. However, you might argue that clinical assessment operates on the basis of *patterns* of behaviour informing risk, and that a risk assessment is valid, or not, taken as a whole, not on the basis that each individual contributing piece of information used is proven.

An additional approach would be a psychological assessment of his sexual preferences and attitudes, on the ground that any sexual offending might be driven by attitudes and proclivities, even if those are only expressed when Henry is disinhibited during psychosis. If this is not available within the treating service, you might recommend that the solicitor consider obtaining this independently.

Finally, assessing functional links between mental illness and sexual offending is complex. Most violent sex offenders have no diagnosis at all, and those who do usually exhibit severe personality dysfunction. And the therapeutic interventions indicated for sexual offending risk are very different from those currently on offer to Henry, and are often not available within an ordinary MSU.

If the tribunal were to conclude that Henry poses a risk of sexual violence to women, then his treatment plan would have to address this, and he would arguably no longer be ready for any form of discharge. Indeed, he might have to be transferred to another secure service that can provide specialist treatment.

Legal

The legal issue for the tribunal will be whether Henry has a mental disorder of a nature or degree that makes it appropriate that he continue to be detained in hospital, and whether appropriate treatment[1] is available. More generally, Henry has the right to a fair hearing under Article 6 of the ECHR.

---

[1] What counts as suitable or appropriate treatment for the different legal tests in each jurisdiction is explored in clinical case 15.

Since 'nature' and 'degree' must be considered separately (disjunctively),[2] and 'nature' includes the course and consequences of Henry's illness, 'appropriateness' depends not solely upon how unwell Henry is now, but also upon the risk he would present if conditionally discharged. Henry's solicitor will seek to argue that Henry does not pose a risk 'as a result of his disorder'; or that, if he does, it can be managed in the community, and that the allegations are legally irrelevant to the tribunal's decision about discharge.[3]

Clinico-legal

Unlike legally, clinical risk-assessment is valid, or not, based upon data taken as a whole, not by summing its parts. And it is likely that the clash of paradigms will be resolved by tribunals and courts in favour of this approach in relation to expert evidence.

However, Henry can argue that his disorder is no longer of a nature or degree that warrants detention, perhaps even that he no longer has a mental disorder.

Your report will only be used by the solicitor if it is helpful to Henry's case for release, which may depend on your opinion on risk (and therefore upon what information you include and what weights you apply), even if your opinion is that he should be conditionally discharged. And so, if you choose to include the allegations and find significant risk of sexual offending, your report may be kept confidential from the clinical team and tribunal, unless you decide that the threshold for breaching confidentiality is met.[4]

Crucially important is that your own risk assessment and evidence is transparent in its methods, as well as its conclusions, including the extent to which your assessment relies upon unproven allegations or similar information and what weight it has given them.

Ethical

It is unjust for citizens to be denied their liberty without good evidence, and a legal process that fairly examines that evidence. In forensic mental health care it might seem unjust to treat a patient for one kind of offending risk, and then to introduce concerns about a new and different kind of risk of offending, just at the point at which the patient applies for leave or discharge; injustice that might seem compounded were it to be driven by professional anxiety about public criticism and consequent 'defensive risk-assessment'. (Anxiety can and should be relieved by transparent expert process, including the 'mapping' of clinical conclusions onto the relevant legal tests. As always, security lies in the maxim 'show your workings'[5].)

This may be especially problematic within long-stay residential settings, where offending behaviour is generally controlled, so that risk assessment is often based upon observations by professionals of subtle social interactions between staff and patient, where it tends to be only the professional's view that counts; the patient's view often being seen as subjective, unreliable, and biased towards, at best, gaining liberty and, at worse, subverting security.

Carrying out a good-quality risk assessment raises many ethical challenges, mainly because it can cause harm to the person being assessed. Such harm may be justifiable: for example, although patients often feel aggrieved at their loss of liberty when detained, this is usually justified by the benefit that will accrue *to them* through treatment, aside from the public benefit of risk reduction. It is unethical to use poor-quality evidence in making risk assessments, thereby treating patients unfairly, exploiting their vulnerability, and it is part of the forensic psychiatrist's ethical duty to ensure that the information they use is of the best possible quality.

---

[2] *R v Mental Health Review Tribunal for South Thames, ex parte Smith* [1998] *The Times* 9 December.

[3] This used to be straightforwardly the medicolegal position on factual evidence (as distinct from expert opinion): it had to be proven. However, the recent Parole Board case of John Worboys, a taxi driver who allegedly drugged and raped scores of women in addition to the small number he was convicted of raping, caused a public outcry because it did not take into account those allegations in its assessment of his likely risk of harm on release. This has led to a review which may change the legal position, at least in Parole Board hearings. See *R v Parole Board & SS Justice, ex parte DSD, NBV, Mayor of London and News Group Newspapers Ltd* [2018] EWHC 694, in which the Parole Board's original decision to release Mr Warboys was quashed.

[4] *W v Egdell* [1990] 1 AllER 835.

[5] This raises an ethical concern about any move, following *Worboys*, to give allegations some factual weight in legal proceedings: if 'facts' cannot be properly challenged in court through being proved, this increases the chance that the legal process will not be fair to the detained person or defendant.

3 Risk assessment–clarifying the risks of harm to be assessed

Themes: *violence versus anger and aggression and types of violence (p.26) [C]; legal context of risk assessment (p.664) [L]; consent to assessment, report ownership and use (p.660) [CL]; and 'false positives' and risk aversion in risk assessment (p.322) and inadequate training and experience, psychologist or psychiatrist? (p.308) [E]*

Case description

You are a clinical forensic psychologist instructed by the Parole Board to carry out a risk assessment on Vincent, who is twenty years old and is detained in a Young Offender Institution. He was convicted of wounding with intent three years ago, after a drunken argument with a stranger outside a bar. Both became physically aggressive, and Vincent hit the victim in the neck with a broken beer bottle.

Vincent has several previous convictions for violence, including one for robbery (of a stranger), one for violent disorder, and one for common assault (of an ex-girlfriend). He enjoys going to football matches with friends and fighting opposing fans. He has committed various street robberies to fund his cocaine habit.

Vincent wants help to control his temper: he dislikes becoming angry with loved ones, such as his mother and girlfriend. He has demonstrated remorse for his index offence, saying he loses control when arguments escalate; he often feels ashamed by his behaviour, particularly hitting his girlfriend.

In interview with you he presents as agitated, and prison staff report that he can appear aggressive and intimidating. However, in his three years in custody he has not been violent. He has successfully completed Controlling Anger and Learning to Manage it (CALM) programmes, as well as treatment for his alcohol and drug use.

Questions

1. If you are a forensic psychiatrist, should you take instructions in the case?
2. If you do, how should you assess Vincent's risk?
3. What other clinical, legal, clinico-legal, and ethical issues does Vincent's case pose?

Clinical

Vincent has been convicted of four different types of violent offences, and has reported carrying out other violent acts that went unpunished. He describes different motivations for violence during his life, involving different types of victim and relationships with them. His case therefore offers a reminder that violence is not a homogeneous construct, but a complex human behaviour with many causes that can take many forms and have a range of meanings.

A risk assessment aims to (a) identify the possible types of harm; (b) determine the likelihood of each, within a given timescale; (c) identify scenarios of heightened risk; and (d) lead to a risk-management plan.

Severe violence is rare: many individuals with historical or current risk factors for violence will never be severely violent; by contrast, minor aggression is very frequent.[6] There is therefore a high rate of 'false positive' predictions for serious violence. This complicates assessment of the risk of severe violence, even where the individual has a history of such violence, making individual case formulation crucial. This must separate out unlikely scenarios of further severe violence, and highly likely scenarios of minor aggression.

The risk assessment should distinguish actual violence, threats of violence, thoughts of violence, and fantasies of violence. Violence is not synonymous with anger, aggression, or hostility, all of which are distinct emotions or behaviours with different meanings. Not all angry people are aggressive, and aggression may be appropriate in certain regulated settings (e.g. some sporting events), whilst hostility may be an appropriate response to a threat, based on past experience.

Another useful distinction is between 'instrumental' and 'reactive' violence. Instrumental or 'proactive' violence is unemotional, and calculated to achieve some end: for example, in armed robbery, using the weapon may be calculated to increase the chances of successful escape with the loot; gang members may habitually use violence as a deliberate tool to manage their illegal activities. Reactive violence is often an emotional response by an individual with antisocial personality traits to a situation that is threatening, frustrating, or otherwise intolerable to them.

An overlapping distinction is whether violence is premeditated, or impulsive and unplanned, although they are not mutually exclusive (a premeditated idea of killing one's partner may be acted on impulsively following an argument as impulsive violence is more likely when a person is disinhibited by mental disorder or substance use.

Vincent can present as hostile and intimidating towards prison staff, but has not actually been violent to staff or to fellow prisoners. This may indicate a degree of self-control (a protective factor), but the persistence of his hostility suggests that his attitudes are rigid (a risk factor).

A significant concern in Vincent's case is the diversity of his violence and offending. He has used violence instrumentally to commit robberies and in football-related fights, but he has also employed violence in relationships, accompanied by high levels of emotion. He has attacked strangers and partners, and he has convictions for nonviolent crime, which suggest more general antisocial attitudes. He falls into the category of youths whose violence persists into adulthood, rather than the much larger group who violence is limited to adolescence, and it is possible that he has some degree of callous and unemotional personality traits.

Protective factors in Vincent include his expressed concern about his violence, his reported sense of shame, and his engagement with CALM and substance misuse programmes. Future risk management should focus on these strengths, as well as minimising risk factors such as contact with antisocial peers.

Another risk factor to explore is exposure to adverse childhood experiences, such as parental mental illness, physical abuse, and neglect, because exposure to high levels of childhood adversity predicts future persistent severe violence. Vincent's propensity for violence may be related to unresolved distress from childhood trauma, and/or symptoms of untreated PTSD from past severe violence he has experienced, perhaps resulting in hypervigilance to threat, or even paranoia. If you find this to be the case, you could recommend interventions to improve his emotional regulation and distress tolerance.

[6] Severe violence and minor aggression are thought of by some authors as 'over-controlled' and 'under-controlled' violence respectively. Much research focuses on selected samples of severely violent individuals who have often been convicted of violent offences; it is much more difficult to carry out research on those who only commit 'under-controlled' minor aggression.

Legal

As regards to what data can be properly included in a risk assessment, and what weight attached to what data, see clinical case 2.

Legal ownership of your report is determined by who requests it of you, which, in turn, affects to whom it may be, or will be, disclosed. As you are conducting the assessment for the Parole Board, it will be automatically made available to all parties. Were you to be instructed by Vincent's lawyers, then it should not be disclosed to anyone else without Vincent's consent (other than where there are grounds for breaching his confidentiality[7]).

Once used, by whatever route, your report may be of assistance to Vincent's offender manager and the mental health in-reach team, aside from its relevance to any parole hearing, now or later.

Clinico-legal

The Parole Board must address the risk of future offending by Vincent, and your report should be directed towards this, including by way of recommending what release conditions would minimise his risk of further offending.

Ethical

There are several ethical concerns about risk assessment which relate to the principle of justice. First, there is a risk of 'false positives', inferring that prisoners like Vincent may be subject to unnecessary detention or enhanced security, and be impeded in their progress towards release. Second, in anxious organisations like prisons, professionals readily become risk-averse, and can be reluctant to give due weight to positive factors (and to over-emphasise risk factors), which again tends to make the process unjust. Third, it is clearly unjust for prisoners to be subject to risk assessments by anyone whose work is biased or of poor quality. Lastly, Vincent's consent to the assessment should be based upon a clear explanation of its potential conclusions and how it might be used.

Finally, if you are a psychiatrist rather than a psychologist, you should consider whether you have skills that are appropriate for the case, particularly if there is no mental disorder. One view is that doctors should only assess cases where there is a potential diagnosis; another is that skills relating to violence assessment and management are generic to all forensic specialties. As will be apparent from the detail of clinical method and required knowledge above, the skills required go beyond medicine or psychiatry: so any doctors accepting instruction must be confident that they possess those skills to a sufficient level.

---

[7] *W v Egdell* [1990] 1 AllER 835.

4 | Risk assessment–information needed and obtaining it

Themes: *risk assessment and report for Parole Board (pp.170, 696) and information sources and use of information (pp.142, 356) [C]; criteria for release, ownership and disclosure of report (p.660) [L]; risk versus protective factors, recommending release conditions (p.589) [CL]; and limits of confidentiality (p.320) and responsibility to the Parole Board, psychologist or psychiatrist? (p.298) [E]*

Case description

You are instructed by Adam's solicitors to provide a report for a parole hearing. Adam is fifty-two years old and currently in a category B prison. Twenty-six years ago, he pleaded guilty to the murder of a good friend, whom he had known since childhood. The offence took place whilst he was out drinking with the victim, and the victim's partner, who had previously been Adam's partner and is the mother of his two children. There was an argument, and Adam stabbed his friend nineteen times. He received the mandatory life sentence, with a minimum tariff of nine years.

Adam reports being in care from age ten, which suggests possible familial neglect or abuse; he also reports sexual abuse by staff at the children's home.

Adam has now been detained for seventeen years beyond his tariff. He had previously been transferred to a category C prison, from which he absconded. He had also been released on one occasion, five years ago, but was recalled due to breaking the conditions of his licence, after he used a prostitute and failed to return to his hostel by his curfew time. He has participated in various prison 'lifer' programmes, with mixed reports about his engagement and involvement.

You are also informed that Adam has made two superficial suicide attempts in the past, after he had been transferred between different institutions, and that he seems to be struggling with his identity as a life-sentenced prisoner and the challenges of being released into the community.

Questions

1. What clinical, legal, clinico-legal, and ethical issues does this case raise?
2. If you are a forensic psychiatrist rather than a psychologist, should you take instructions in the case?

Clinical

The primary role of the report is to provide risk assessment based upon formulation of Adam's past violence, using (i) a clinical interview; (ii) collateral information, both historical and contemporary; and (iii) appropriate instruments.

In order to provide a high-quality report, you will need good information from a variety of sources, so as to provide narratives of Adam's psychological development, adult life events, and offending behaviour, as well as his adult personality.

The interview will provide information about Adam's mental and physical health and his childhood, including childhood neglect and adversity, and any conduct disorder or violence before the age of ten (all of which are associated with violence).

The interview should also cover history of violence and other offending, including his developmental trajectory. Adam reports starting to offend violently while in his teens, suggesting he is in the group whose violence tends to escalate, rather than wane, in adulthood. It is also important to determine the range and diversity of his criminal history, and the influence of substance misuse and peer relationships.

The third focus should be upon the homicide itself, and Adam's view of it. Homicide victims may have a relationship with the perpetrator, or be strangers; so the relationship between Adam and his victim requires close investigation. Adam had two important attachments at one point in his life: a good friend, and a partner with whom he fathered two children. Both these attachments underwent a major change, which is likely to be relevant to the homicide. So you will need to understand the timing of the changes in his relationships with his friend and his ex-partner, how relational loss affected him, and his attitudes towards his ex-partner and their adult children now. You will need to ask about any arguments with, or violence towards, his partner and his friend. You will also want to know whether there had been any other attachment disturbances, such as bereavements, before the offence.

The next source of information should be evidence from the trial, including the judge's sentencing remarks, and the depositions and relevant reports if possible. You will need to know whether mental disorder, or a psychiatric defence, were considered pretrial, even if they did not give lead to him putting forward a mental condition defence (instead, he pleaded guilty).

You will need information about his progress in prison, including his behaviour and relationships. There may well be a very large 'parole bundle' for you to read (it would be a hostage to fortune not to know the bundle in detail); pay particular attention to past evidence of problematic behaviours, such as prison adjudications and past parole hearings. It appears that Adam has made good relationships with prison psychologists over the course of his sentence, but has not participated well or consistently in standard offending behaviour programmes. Address the meaning of his superficial suicide attempts.

You should conduct your own risk assessment using clinical material and structured risk-assessment tools like the HCR20v3. There are also more specific tools that can be used with different types of offender (e.g. sex offenders or perpetrators of domestic violence) which do not seem likely to be useful here. The prison dossier will include psychology reports, risk assessments based on a system called OASyS, and probation reviews that will assist with this. You will also need to look at his adjudication record, which will tell you about his relationships with the prison and staff, and you should speak to professionals who know him, such as his offender manager (OM), his personal officer, the chaplain, or others he identifies. You know that Adam has been considered a low risk of harm to others because he has been released twice before, and this finding is unlikely to have changed (though you do not necessarily have to accept it). The more likely risk is that of rule-breaking and noncompliance with conditions, and this is an issue worth exploring with Adam and his OM.

Legal

The fact that you are reporting at the request of Adam's lawyers should not affect your opinion, but it may affect how and to whom the report is disclosed.

Seeing him for his solicitors, you will have to gain the agreement of Adam's solicitors to disclose the report to anyone else, unless you consider that not to disclose it would create a significant risk of serious harm to others.[8] You may not disclose the report without consent just because you consider it to be in Adam's interest to do so. (If you had been seeing him for the Parole Board, you would have needed to make this clear to Adam, explaining the limits of confidentiality.)

---

[8] *W v Egdell* [1990] 1 AllER 835.

Clinico-legal

The Parole Board must address the risk of future offending by Adam, and your report should assess this, and recommend what conditions would be needed to minimise his risk of further offending if released.

Much may depend upon whether the OM is recommending release, to where, and on what conditions. It will be important to consider Adam's engagement with professionals and his participation with interventions that have been offered to him. As you are being asked about future risk, you will need to know what plans have been made regarding accommodation if discharged and what professional and personal support will be in place.

It will also be important to refer to external protective factors (e.g. support from local psychiatric services, if appropriate), as well as any protective (or risk-enhancing) relationships with friends and family.

If you were to conclude that Adam has a personality disorder, you might consider referral to one of the community Pathfinder Offender Personality Disorder (OPD) services for high-risk offenders with PD, which reduce the risk of recall and reoffending. These services provide consultation and joint working with health, probation, and other professionals, and may also provide some limited clinical interventions. Adam should have been screened in to the OPD pathway in prison if a PD diagnosis was made (and there should be an existing basic formulation and evidence of previous discussions about his needs).

Finally, you will need to decide whether, in your report, you will address the 'ultimate question' of whether to release him, or will only summarise your risk assessment and recommendations for conditions on any release.

Ethical

The main ethical issue is respect for justice: your role in the process, and your commitment to truth, honesty, impartiality, and respect for the quasi-judicial parole process.

You should make plain to Adam that you are independent, not representing his interests, even though instructed by his solicitor—and that your report could reduce, rather than enhance, his chances of release.

As regards whether you should take the case if you are a psychiatrist and not clinical psychologist, if there is sufficient suspicion of personality disorder, or other mental disorder, then you may have relevant expertise, provided your skills and knowledge are not merely adequate, but comparable to the ideal expert.

Hospital back to prison transfer—impact of values on decision-making

Themes: *diagnosis (p.144), formulations impacting on management (p.146), and schizophrenia versus personality traits in offending (pp.73, 78) [C]; clinical and legal narratives (p.358) [L]; transfer between prison and hospital (p.506) [CL]; and ethical conflict within teams (p.312) and ethical decision-making 'within the formulation' (p.288), resource allocation [E]*

Case description

Jay is a twenty-eight-year-old man diagnosed with paranoid schizophrenia who has been transferred to his local MSU from prison. Whilst serving a sentence for robbery, Jay displayed aggressive behaviour, and seemed very paranoid. He complained of hearing voices telling him to harm himself and others, and his speech seemed incoherent. He has had two admissions to the MSU in the past, mainly because of being unmanageable in a PICU. The prison in-reach team said that his schizophrenia had responded well to antipsychotic medication in the past, including clozapine.

You are a new consultant taking over Jay's care. You meet him and his family, who tell you that child psychiatrists diagnosed him with ADHD, conduct disorder, and borderline learning disability (confirmed by his medical records). They also say Jay has used cannabis, cocaine, and amphetamines since his midteens, and has multiple children by different partners. The police confirm that Jay has offended since his early teens, with convictions for theft, driving offences, and minor assaults. His longest sentence was twenty-eight days, for assaulting a policeman.

You discuss your findings with the multidisciplinary team, and together review the notes of Jay's past admissions. Different MDT members formulate Jay's problems differently. Your view is that his offending is primarily (if not exclusively) related to his mental deterioration since his first psychotic episode. Others see his psychotic episodes as related to emotionally unstable personality traits, with poor affect regulation and impulse control, complicated by missed education and mild cognitive impairment. They think his capacity for reality testing breaks down when he is under stress and using drugs, such as happens in prison. They note that the robbery took place a month after his girlfriend had left him for another man, and concealed where she was living, so that he was unable to see his young son. Finally, they point to his history of childhood conduct disorder and drug use, before his first psychotic episode.

Some of the team wish to transfer him back to prison, now that he is mentally well, on medication; your view is that he should remain in hospital and be rehabilitated into the community from there.

Questions

1. How might a different diagnosis or formulation from your own affect management?
2. How should you address the disagreement within the team?
3. What other the clinical, legal, clinico-legal, and ethical issues arise in the case?

Clinical

Diagnoses in medicine are hypotheses about the meaning of signs and symptoms of disease. They also represent a shorthand by way by which professionals can easily communicate; so that, for example, the diagnosis of pneumonia is recognised and identified in the same way around the world. Diagnoses are also grounded in epidemiology, and categorise the patient within the population.

Diagnosis is arguably more complex and open to dispute in psychiatry than in the rest of medicine: partly because most psychiatric diagnoses rely primarily on subjective symptoms rather than objective test results, and partly because diagnoses can be made on signs of disorder that are disputed by the patient and others, such as delusions or 'antisocial' behaviour. In addition, although there is international agreement about many psychiatric diagnoses, some behaviours and 'symptoms' are viewed differently in different cultures. That is, diagnoses are grounded in values as well as facts (whether observed behaviour amounts to variation from an accepted norm e.g. is a value judgment). Some psychiatric diagnoses, most notably personality disorder, have very low 'fact-to-value ratios', and are therefore particularly vulnerable to the influence of the psychiatrist's personal, sociocultural, and professional values, as explored in detail in ethical case 14).[9]

A formulation is, by contrast, an account of how an illness, disorder, or behaviour arose in a particular individual: and psychiatric formulations tend to be a structured narrative understanding of the patient's condition, rather than an explanation or categorisation, and are therefore different from the less value-laden formulations of other medical specialties.

Formulations in forensic psychiatry contribute to risk assessment[10] (as when identifying the perpetuating factors for risk reoffending e.g.). In offering an account of how a person's mental disorder led them to act criminally, a particular formulation can grant access to mental health services (e.g. admission to hospital for psychosis), or deny it (e.g. because of a focus on a condition such as psychopathy). It can also lead to a reduction in adjudicated responsibility for a crime, or conversely to stigmatisation and blame.

Legal

Law adopts its own narratives of offending, expressed in juries' verdicts and judges' sentencing remarks and decisions, including not just the type of sentence (therapeutic or punitive) but also the degree of punishment.

The narratives adopted by judges and others, such as the Ministry of Justice (MoJ), may be informed by clinical formulations but may ultimately lead to different conclusions. For instance, as a matter of public policy, the legal construct of 'voluntary intoxication' usually holds people responsible for their actions when in that state, and overrides any medical view that intoxication is an abnormal brain state, or that dependence can impair a person's ability to choose not to use a drug.

Mental health law can effectively allow treatment to 'trump' punishment (through sentencing by hospital disorder, or transfer of a sentenced prisoner to hospital for treatment), but only if the justice ministry agrees that transfer is in the public interest—another legal construct that can over-ride medical opinion.[11]

---

[9] See the extensive writings on this offered by KMW Fulford, including in Fulford et al (editors) (2015) *The Oxford Handbook of Philosophy and Psychiatry (Oxford Handbooks)*, Oxford University Press.

[10] To the extent that some risk-assessment tools specifically include a stage at which information must be compiled into a formulation, such as the HCR20v3.

[11] In England and Wales the most famous example of this is the 'Yorkshire Ripper', who, though unanimously diagnosed as suffering from schizophrenia, and recommended for transfer to Broadmoor, was nevertheless held in prison for eighteen months after conviction by the then Home Secretary, 'in the public interest'.

Clinico-legal

When Jay is diagnosed with paranoid schizophrenia in prison, he is transferred to hospital and likely to be seen as a 'patient' not a 'prisoner' (and perhaps less to blame for his offence). Moreover, a diagnosis of schizophrenia usually implies continuing treatment and rehabilitation beyond the point of recovery from psychosis.

The law allows Jay to be remitted back to prison after sufficient treatment. But crucial to your decision whether to recommend remission is the formulation of his mental deterioration and perhaps, arguably, also his offending.

Your own formulation of Jay suggests that he had a lifelong relapsing mental illness (paranoid schizophrenia), and that lack of medication led to relapse in prison. His mental illness meant he did not work, and was therefore homeless, hungry, and liable to steal; further, it made him vulnerable, and perhaps also less culpable for his offending. Your formulation supports further treatment in hospital, followed by discharge and community supervision when his sentence expires, combined with regular medication: this should keep him well and out of trouble.

Other team members' alternative formulation is that Jay's difficulties are related to dysfunctional personality traits that impair his capacity to make and maintain close relationships and to regulate his impulses and affect. On this view, there were several reasons for his offending: a desire for money for drugs, alcohol, and/or food; impulsivity; and a lack of regard for possible consequences; as well as low IQ and lack of education. This formulation links his psychotic symptoms to an exacerbation of emotionally unstable personality traits, without ruling out schizophrenia as an underlying cause for the psychosis; noting that psychosis commonly coexists with personality traits or disorder in forensic populations. On this formulation, both economic and emotional stress will increase Jay's risk of offending, and the management plan therefore should include psychological treatment to address his relationships with his girlfriend and family, his new role as a father, his poor emotional regulation and anger management skills, and that he should receive help finding accommodation and avoiding drug use—all of which can be done from prison.

Ethical

Differing formulations arise from application of not only differing clinical data bus also differing values, or weighting of those values. The formulation adopted will affect how Jay's problems are perceived and managed.

Ultimately, the most significant ethical implications of using formulations in forensic psychiatry relate to their impact on professionals' ways of viewing an individual's behaviour, risk to others, and way of being in the world.

Beyond the formulation adopted, the ethical principle of justice is also relevant. Jay has already been convicted, and it is not the role of clinicians to take a view on criminal responsibility in any case. However, justice includes fairness in the allocation of healthcare resources, and you are aware of other psychotic prisoners awaiting transfer to your MSU, who could be admitted if you remit Jay (and others like to him) to prison, notwithstanding your formulation that he warrants continued treatment in hospital.

There is no single right answer to any of these ethical conundrums; rather, there are different justifications for different courses of action. And the quality of an ethical decision lies not in the decision taken but in the ethical reasoning behind it, and in its justification.

Different team members often bring different personal and professional values to their formulation of a case and the decisions to be made, and this may infer conflict. A values-based practice approach (as discussed in part A and other cases) may assist in elucidating the ethical foundations of any disagreements, and deciding upon a course of action.

6 Forensic low secure versus general intensive psychiatric care (PICU)

Themes: *defining a case as 'forensic' (p.20), essential differences between forensic and general PICU services (p.12), and objectives of forensic care (p.352), staff skills [C]; informal admission to secure ward (p.478) and legal bases and protection [L, CL]; care quality and ethical principles, respect for justice processes (p.300), and tension between care and coercion, shared dialogue, making tension creative and humane (p.324) [E]*

Case description

Chloe is a twenty-one-year-old woman who developed a relapsing and remitting psychotic illness two years ago. Recently she was found shouting and chanting in the street, and she assaulted the police officers who tried to detain her for assessment, though they were not injured, and she was not charged.

She was admitted to a PICU, and whilst there assaulted two older female staff, by punching them in the face. She has been referred to your forensic low secure service.

Questions

1. What is your view of the role of your forensic low secure service?
2. What distinguishes forensic from general mental health care, both low secure and community care?
3. How will answering the forgoing inform your assessment of a proper response to Chloe's care need?
4. What particular ethical problems attend secure forensic treatment and care?
5. What other clinical, legal, clinico-legal, and ethical issues does Chloe's case pose?

Clinical

Effectively, you are being asked to think about the essential role of a forensic low secure service, given the staff needed to carry this out to a good standard.

It might be argued that the primary clinical task is to stabilise Chloe's mental state with appropriate medication and nursing care, and, if this cannot be safely achieved in a PICU, to admit her and then later return her to general services. Albeit even if she is prosecuted for the assaults committed in hospital (which is unlikely[12]) a conviction does not automatically make Chloe's a 'forensic' case (see also clinical case 1).

---

[12] Police are sometimes reluctant to recommend prosecution of patients who assault others whilst detained in hospital, unless the assault is serious, despite the official position of the Royal College and the NHS that such patients should be prosecuted.

Arguably the essential task of any forensic service is to offer longer-term treatment to those whose mental states lead them to present a significant and/or persistent risk of serious harm to others, in order to restore health and to minimise the risk of harm to others. This will usually occur in a secure hospital or prison, but can be in the community, after discharge from hospital or release from prison, or as an alternative to admission.

Delivering such care requires a range of professionals with a variety of experience and competences, beyond that seen in a PICU, with attention paid to physical health, to the nature and the meaning of Chloe's violence, and to Chloe's pro-social skills and strengths.

Unlike in a PICU, ideally all staff in a forensic service will have specialist training in the origins and meaning of violence and other offending behaviour and in risk assessment and management, including encouraging more pro-social attitudes. Also, most forensic services will have higher staff-to-patient ratios than general inpatient services, usually also with access to more occupational therapists, psychologists, and psychotherapists, including art, dance, and music therapists.

Legal and clinico-legal

The danger of admission to a secure forensic service is that patients can lose their freedom for long periods (sometimes much longer even than if they had been imprisoned following conviction).

So that patients must be expertly legally represented, and have access to an independent advocate, forensic staff have a duty to explain that the service is concerned with risk reduction as much as with their welfare, and how, for example, this may limit confidentiality.

Forensic psychiatrists should be explicit in talking to patients about the ethical ambiguity of this position, and trainee forensic psychiatrists need to acquire the communication skills necessary to enable them to discuss a patient's potential for harm to others clearly, compassionately, and honestly.

In summary, the clinico-legal culture of any forensic service is usually quite different from that of general services, including PICUs and nonforensic low secure services.

(Notably, most secure services will not admit patients 'informally', because the service is designed for those who need detention and constraint, and it can undermine the security of the unit to have informal patients in such a setting.[13] It can also cause bad feeling between residents, as well as leading to inadvertent coercion of informal patients.)

It would be unwise to admit Chloe to your unit unless you are confident that she both cannot be safely managed in the PICU and crosses the threshold of need for it.

---

[13] The Barrett Inquiry found that allowing patients to be admitted informally to the medium secure unit concerned was a material factor in the absconding of the patient concerned and thus the subsequent homicide he committed. NHS London (2006) *Report of the Independent Inquiry into the Care and Treatment of John Barrett.*

Ethical

Important quality indicators of secure care are based on ethical principles. They include respect for justice processes, because patients are detained and vulnerable to coercion, and respect for autonomy and best interest as defined by the patient, as well as others. All within a shared dialogue between patient and team about treatment, achieving valid consent to treatment if possible.

The forensic psychiatrist who is Responsible Clinician (RC) is often the *de facto* leader of the multi-disciplinary team. He has a role in enabling others to do their work well. As well as leading discussions on complex issues relating to confidentiality, relational security, balancing welfare and justice, and ensuring that different value perspectives are heard and explored, especially ones that cause dissent within the team.

Forensic care involves a tension between care and coercion, and the skill is to make that tension both creative and humane. Although many patients admitted to secure care understandably feel anxious and angry on admission, the whole team have a role in helping Chloe, if admitted, to understand how managing her risk is part of achieving better mental health, and that her detention is an opportunity, not necessarily a punishment.

7 A worked example of structured risk-assessment using HCR20v3

Themes: *risk assessment using structured tools (pp.168, 170) [C]; robbery (p.426), sentencing (p.442), and dangerousness, mitigating and aggravating factors (pp.672, 638) [L]; applying risk assessment within sentencing, distinguishing dangerousness and risk (p.672) [CL]; and use of risk assessment for punishment (p.322) and avoiding mitigating (p.298) [E]*

Case description

Ahmed is a nineteen-year-old man from Pakistan who has been convicted of robbing an older female stranger, and referred to you for a presentence psychiatric report. You are asked to address his risk of future violence. He does not come from your forensic catchment area.

Ahmed came to the UK aged ten and was brought up by his maternal aunt. His parents live in Pakistan, and he has not seen them for nine years. He left school at age sixteen years and has never worked. Just prior to his offence, he found out that his mother had been diagnosed with cancer.

Ahmed has no previous convictions, and this is his first time in custody. In prison, he has undergone adjudications for fighting on several occasions. He has never used alcohol or drugs. At the time of his arrest he was in a longstanding relationship, but his girlfriend has now left him, and his family disowned him once he was convicted. He has never before seen a mental health professional.

Clinical assessment indicates that he has an average IQ, is moderately depressed, has low self-esteem, and is concerned about his future. There is no evidence of impulsivity or hyperactivity. He demonstrates very limited insight into why he committed his offence, or its impact upon his victim. He says that he wanted to fit in with his peers, who appear to be mostly negative, antisocial, influences upon him.

Questions

1. What process will you adopt in completing an assessment of his risk of further violence?
2. What is your assessment of the risk of violence in the medium term?
3. What should you otherwise recommend to the court?
4. What other clinical, legal, clinico-legal, and ethical issues does Ahmed's case pose?

Clinical

A structured risk-assessment using the HCR20v3 will help in this case. The case does not immediately suggest that you should have any clinical role with Ahmed but the process of addressing legal questions will, by necessity, involve a clinical encounter.

Your HCR20 assessment indicates few historical (H) risk factors: for example, no history of previous offending, offending when young, substance use, 'psychopathy', or major mental illness. However, there is a history of caregiver disruption (i.e. possible early maladjustment) and poor school achievement plus employment problems. On the clinical (C) scale, Ahmed has limited insight into his offence, but he does not demonstrate procriminal or antisocial attitudes, and he is willing to accept interventions offered to him. As regards risk-management (R) factors, Ahmed is currently in custody, which has probably increased the risk of mental health problems such as depression, and perhaps also therefore his risk of minor violence, whilst the stress of the feared sentence is likely to be exacerbated by concerns about his mother's health. A past protective factor, the support of his girlfriend and extended family, has now been lost. Were he to be released into the community, this lack of support, and his continued association with antisocial peers, would be additional risk factors.

You conclude that there is at present a moderate risk of a further act of violence in the short-term, should Ahmed be released into the community. Your primary 'scenario' is of a further impulsive assault or robbery in the presence, or under the influence, of his friends, with the aim of impressing them, acquiring money, or expressing anger and frustration. You note that his lack of a serious mental illness or personality disorder reduces the general validity of the HCR20 assessment (as the HCR20v3 was not developed for use on people with depression alone), but your clinical judgment, based upon your own experience, is that the findings are likely to be valid for Ahmed.

There is a deeper question here: why did this particular person commit this particular offence against this particular victim? Is the choice of an older female victim relevant, given what he had just learnt about his mother? These outstanding questions suggest the need for a narrative formulation of Ahmed's offence. This will take time, and possibly the involvement of a psychologist or psychotherapist, but doing so might allow a higher quality of risk assessment, as well as offering improved ways to support and treat Ahmed.

As you are not to treat Ahmed for his depression yourself, you should recommend referral to his catchment area general psychiatrist, and in the meantime ask the prison psychiatrist to initiate antidepressant treatment.

Legal

Sentencing Ahmed will include the judge considering his degree of culpability, and the severity of harm to the victim, which together indicate the 'starting point'. There will then be a process of examining the presence of aggravating and mitigating factors, plus a reduction of sentence for a prompt guilty plea. There will be specific consideration of 'dangerousness'.[14]

Clinico-legal

It should be made plain in your report that further psychological investigation might refine your risk assessment, but that you are presenting your current findings in the expectation that the court will not consider it so as just to remand him for longer for additional investigation.

The judge is required to give reasons for the sentence; he will use your risk assessment and risk-management recommendations in his consideration of legal 'dangerousness', and of aggravating and mitigating factors (your report may effectively present evidence of these, but should not appear to advocate either type of factor). It is often helpful to set out your recommendations conditionally (e.g. 'if Ahmed were imprisoned, I would recommend …; if he were to receive a community sentence, I would recommend …'). If any of your recommendations involve action by another psychiatric service, you should consult them before submitting your report (or even advise the solicitor to instruct the local psychiatrist to prepare their own report).

---

[14] This term is often used in the criminal justice system, as if there were a character trait of inherent dangerousness. Experts should encourage judges to see risk of violence as contributed to by factors both intrinsic and extrinsic to the offender, plus their interaction, and that risk management involves attempting to influence these factors.

Ethical

Assuming that it is ethically appropriate to conduct this risk assessment knowing that it will be used for sentencing (an issue addressed in ethical case 18), you may need to consider including the possible conflict of interest between your role as a doctor and your role as an expert for the court; potential bias arising from 'being a doctor'; and the intrusion of personal values, perhaps especially if you are from a different cultural or ethnic background from Ahmed. (These issues are explored in clinical case 27 and ethical cases 1 and 10.)

8

Secure hospital versus prison—psychosis, PD, and substance misuse

> **Themes:** *psychosis (p.72), personality disorder (p.78), substance misuse (p.76), and risk assessment for sexual offending (p.172), prison or hospital (p.184) [C]; transfer to hospital during remand (p.506) and aggravating and mitigating factors in sentencing (p.442) [L]; reports for risk-based sentencing (p.670) and evidence about determinants of rape, clinical bases for disposals (p.62) [CL]; and justice and resource allocation, link between disorder and offence (p.276), suicide prevention (p.322) [E]*

Case description

Kevin is a twenty-year-old man charged with rape and ABH. There is good evidence that he violently attacked a young woman, a stranger, behind a railway station; the assault was severe, prolonged, and involved rape with objects. He also broke her nose. The assault ended when passers-by intervened.

At arrest, Kevin gave a coherent interview to the police; but he smelt of alcohol. He claimed that the victim had consented to the various sexual activities, but also implied that he knew she had not. He told police he had been sleeping rough for three weeks, drinking heavily, smoking cannabis, and taking spice. Nothing about his demeanour or answers at interview, or at assessment by the Forensic Medical Examiner, suggested he was mentally unwell. He has no previous criminal record. Kevin was remanded in custody.

Kevin's family were contacted for information. They were hostile and reluctant to discuss their relationship with Kevin. They said that, over the last two years he had been increasingly withdrawn and occasionally aggressive, which they had put down to drug abuse. They added that when younger he had 'got in with a bad crowd' at school. He left school at age sixteen years and then went to college, where he completed a BTEC in mechanics. His drug use then increased, and his mother and her partner threw him out of the house a month before the alleged offence. They want nothing more to do with him.

You are the local MSU consultant. The prison mental health team ask you to assess Kevin with a view to admission. They have observed him apparently responding to auditory hallucinations and expressing persecutory beliefs about the Devil watching him. He has smashed a mirror and cut himself repeatedly, and they now believe he is at high risk of self-harm and suicide. They have prescribed antipsychotic medication, which he takes reliably, and which has calmed him.

Questions

1. What are the clinical, legal, clinico-legal and ethical issues in the case?
2. What alternative courses of action are there, and how might each be justified?

Clinical

The first clinical decision to take is whether Kevin should continue to be assessed and treated in the prison healthcare centre, or transferred to a hospital bed, and if the latter, at what level of security? This may depend not only on his current risk to himself, and the need to prevent escape during remand, but also on your view on his mental state at the time of the offence, which could have implications for his trial.

If you conclude that Kevin has suffered a brief psychotic episode associated with imprisonment, and is now well on medication, then he can continue to be treated in prison. Although you may decide that a brief transfer to hospital is needed to prevent relapse, so that he remains well for trial. This would also facilitate a comprehensive formulation that could be of use at trial and sentencing. Or you may conclude that he has an underlying functional psychotic illness and should be admitted for a longer period of time.

If you find evidence of personality disorder, this may have contributed to his motivation for the alleged offence (and may also mean you should refer him for the OPD programme in prison).

Inferring motivation from any diagnosed mental disorder is relevant to clinical risk-assessment. It is also relevant to the trial: the prosecution will argue that the offence was driven by 'bad' motives such as antisocial attitudes and misogyny, whereas the defence will argue for motives arising from mental illness, or 'released' by psychosis. So the records of any admission will be viewed as potential evidence at trial or sentencing, and you may be asked to testify at least as a professional witness.

Transfer to hospital during the remand period would best enable you to assess his risk of future violence, which will inform his security need, in hospital or prison, at sentence. However, the prison team may also want to be reassured about Kevin's risk of suicide and self-harm. So there may be considerable debate between your team and the prison team about whether Kevin's risk to himself can be safely managed in prison.

In summary, in deciding whether to admit during the remand period you will need to make decisions about the likely validity of the prison diagnosis, whether Kevin is still psychotic, whether the psychosis is likely to be more than 'brief', his current treatment needs, his risk of harm to others, and his suicide risk.

Legal

Relevant sections of mental health law allow for patients to be admitted to hospital during various stages of the criminal justice process. Whilst on remand, transfer from prison for treatment[15] (if the criteria are met and the justice ministry consents) is usually preferable from the clinician's perspective to a court remand for assessment because the latter orders allow only time-limited detention. It is not necessary to demonstrate any link between prisoners' disorder and their alleged offence. If and when Kevin's mental state improves whilst on remand, then he can be remitted back to prison.

If you did not recommend hospital admission and Kevin were to kill himself in prison, your decisions, and those of the prison, would be scrutinised closely, at an inquest, inquiry or even civil court hearing, should his family allege that you acted negligently (see civil law 1).

It is very unlikely that even determining that Kevin was psychotic when he offended would give him access to a mental condition defence, in that he is unlikely to be deemed to have been unable to form the relevant intent; although it may be deemed relevant to sentencing.

Clinico-legal

If, during an admission, you conclude that Kevin does have a functional psychotic illness that needs treatment, then if he is convicted you may decide to recommend a hospital order with restrictions if he is mentally ill at the time of sentencing. This is, in principle, unrelated to the question whether his mental disorder contributed to the offence. However, in practice, it will be difficult to assess and manage

---

[15] For urgent treatment on remand, s48/49 MHA in E&W, art54 MHNIO, s15 CLIA in RoI (no Scottish equivalent).

the risk he may pose if there is no clinical formulation linking his mental disorder to the offence, and in this case, you might indicate to the court the possibility of a 'hybrid order'[16] or plan for temporary transfer to hospital, if he is sentenced to imprisonment.

Your diagnosis and risk assessment will probably be used by the court in sentencing, whatever recommendation you make, particularly if it is considering a hybrid order, as the law in England requires it to do if there is evidence of mental disorder.[17]

There is little empirical evidence about the nature of sex offending, how to formulate it, and its relationship with mental disorder. And this can lead to a wide range of clinical views, each with different legal implications for defendants and victims. Rape is a complex crime of violence, with varied motivations. The connection with mental illness is obscure, and there is good evidence that most rapists do not suffer from any mental disorder.[18] So, although the clinical formulation within your risk assessment may have a profound impact upon the defence and/or prosecution narratives in sentencing, the evidence base for it will be weak.

Clinically, it is not safe to assume that someone who is psychotic on remand was psychotic previously, although the oddness of Kevin's alleged offence, and the lack of previous violence convictions, should cause you to look for any evidence that he might have been in a disturbed mental state at the time. However, most men convicted of rape do not have a mental illnesses of any sort; may not even be paraphilic or otherwise criminal; and the violence that is known to be associated with paranoid psychosis is not normally sexual in nature.

Many people are mildly antisocial and misuse substances, but hardly any commit acts of serious and prolonged violence. And, in Kevin's case, an abnormal mental state, if there is evidence for it, will be a strong explanatory variable (even if not the sole relevant variable). Although the court will likely see a drug-induced psychosis as an aggravating factor; even though, if any underlying disorder is managed well, this could enable better long-term risk management than a prison sentence.

Ethical

There are other ethical questions to consider in respect of admitting people in Kevin's situation to medium security.

One ethical issue is fairness, in terms of resource allocation, since there are many prisoners who are suicidal and/or psychotic,[19] but far too few secure beds for all of them to be admitted and that there might be a case for concentrating on those who are not yet convicted, given that defendants need to be in the best possible mental health at trial. However, it could also be argued that prisoners who are mentally ill and distressed should be in hospital not prison, especially those who have an enduring psychotic illness. And this argument is stronger now that more prisons have access to programmes for treating personality disorder.

Alternatively, prisoners should only gain access to secure treatment beds if there is a link between their mental disorder and their offence and therefore a greater chance of risk reduction through hospital treatment. However, it may not be easy to separate out the causal contributions of psychosis, drug intoxication, and personality dysfunction. Moreover, causation is ultimately an issue for the court, not the psychiatrist, to determine, and mental health law admission criteria make no reference to the cause of an offence.

The remaining ethical issue concerns the duty to save life by preventing suicide and self-harm: if the risk of harm is great enough, hospitals should perhaps support prison healthcare services if they are unable to manage that risk safely.

[16] s45A MHA in E&W (hospital and limitation direction); hospital direction under s59A CPSA in Scotland; no equivalent in NI or RoI. These orders combine a prison sentence and immediate transfer to hospital.

[17] *R v Vowles* [2015] EWCA Crim 45; *R v Edwards* [2018] EWCA Crim 595 (27 March 2018).

[18] See, for example, Scully D (2013) *Understanding Sexual Violence: A Study of Convicted Rapists*, Routledge.

[19] A landmark English study carried out in 1997 found rates of psychosis of 7%–14% amongst prisoners, and found that up to 27% of prisoners had attempted suicide in the past year (Singleton N et al (1998) *Psychiatric Morbidity Amongst Prisoners: Summary Report*, Office of National Statistics).

9

Risk assessment: founded on the PCL-R

Themes: *paranoid schizophrenia (p.73), antisocial personality disorder or psychopathy (pp.82, 90), risk assessment using PCL-R (p.137), and interaction of disorders in enhancing risk of violence (p.134) [C]; care in reporting test results (p.684) [CL] and ethical connotations of psychopathy (p.340) [E]*

Case description

Michael is a twenty-two-year-old man convicted of manslaughter on the grounds of diminished responsibility for killing a stranger on a bus. He has diagnoses of paranoid schizophrenia and antisocial personality disorder, plus a history of misusing cannabis and cocaine. He is currently in a high secure hospital.

The basis for the successful diminished responsibility defence was the combination of paranoid schizophrenia and antisocial personality disorder, and he is detained for treatment of both disorders.

Michael's parents separated when he was young, and he grew up with his father. He has no contact with his mother. He attended mainstream school but was repeatedly excluded for aggressive behaviour, including from primary school; he left at age fifteen years with no qualifications. Michael reports a number of important jobs, which he left as they bored him, and he would like to be a lawyer when discharged from hospital. However, his notes indicate he has not worked since leaving school. He has numerous convictions dating back to age fourteen, including for burglary, theft, possession of cannabis, and ABH.

On psychometric testing by a clinical psychologist, he has an average IQ, and personality tests show elevations on the clinical subscales of depression, paranoia, and substance misuse.

Michael's reports from clinical interviews are not always consistent with his records or reports from other professionals and family members: his story changes depending upon his audience. He is derogatory about the clinical team and says he can 'play the system'.

You have specific training in the PCL-R and have therefore been asked by a colleague to conduct a PCL-R-based risk assessment. You find Michael easy to talk to and engage; he makes frequent jokes. He presents as narcissistic and grandiose, and appears to place his rights above those of others. When talking about his index offence, he says that the victim deserved to die as he should have 'minded his own business', and 'he was smirking at me'. He blames his victim for his own loss of liberty and laughs when he talks about his offence.

Questions

1. What are the clinical, legal, clinico-legal, and ethical issues presented by the case?

Clinical

Homicide convictions are not always associated with high risk of future violence, and you will address a range of risk factors.

You need to exercise caution in interpreting what Michael says at clinical interview, as his self-reports are variable and inconsistent with other accounts. He may be deceptive, or be an unreliable narrator because of mental illness. Collect as much information as possible from different sources, including previous reports such as school records, GP notes, social care records, and previous psychiatric and psychological reports.

The most reliable and widely used measure of psychopathy[20] is the PCL-R. There are several PCL-R items particularly relevant to Michael, beginning with factor 1 (affective/interpersonal) items, including a grandiose sense of self-worth, pathological lying, cunning and manipulative behaviour, lack of remorse or guilt, emotional shallowness, callousness/lack of empathy, and failure to accept responsibility for his actions. His factor 2 (antisocial/lifestyle) items include need for stimulation, lack of realistic long-term goals, irresponsibility, poor behaviour controls, early behavioural problems, juvenile delinquency, and criminal versatility. This may be sufficient to exceed the cut-off score for psychopathy.

Within the PCL-R it will be useful to differentiate between symptoms related to his mental illness and those related to his personality. Since, for example, insofar as his grandiosity is part of psychosis, it may be reduced by successful treatment.

Legal and clinico-legal

You find that the overall score on the PCL-R suggests that Michael is at high risk of reoffending on discharge or release, and would be likely to become even more difficult to manage on the ward or the wing were his mental health to improve, with more frequent altercations.

A finding of psychopathy has no immediate legal significance, but it is a risk factor for reoffending that may influence future release decisions. No interventions have been proved to reduce psychopathy scores, and so interventions will be focused on risk management and treatment of any comorbid conditions.

Michael has comorbid schizophrenia and substance misuse. These are risk factors for future violence independent of psychopathy, especially if he has little or no insight into his need for treatment. The fact that he attacked a stranger also suggests that he may be at higher risk. Hence, the clinical complexity in Michael's case lies in the combination of, and interaction between, his multiple pathologies.

Ethical

The PCL-R should only be utilised by those who have been trained in it; and with the patient's consent.

The term *psychopath* has acquired a pejorative connotation, implying ethical concern that Michael will be stigmatised, and perhaps considered untreatable or unreformable, by some services if so described. Hence reports used for risk assessment and decisions on release should be cautious about how the term is used, and be explained. Some authors do not report test scores for this reason, instead citing where the person sits on a statistical distribution.

There is ethical diagnostic concern relating to personality and developmental age. Some argue that personality does not become stable until the late twenties. Michael is only twenty-two-years-old, and so his personality may change. In particular, some of his lifestyle/antisocial features, such as a need for stimulation, lack of realistic long-term goals, and poor behaviour controls, may decline naturally as he matures.

---

[20] Psychopathy is not a diagnosis within DSM 5 or ICD 11; it is in effect a subset of antisocial and narcissistic personality disorder that emphasises particular mental characteristics, notably callous and unemotional traits.

10 Risk management–brain injury and prison offender programmes

Themes: *traumatic brain injury (p.112) and prison offender programmes (p.220) [C]; imprisonment for public protection (p.448) and Parole Board (p.582) [L]; rights to, and advice on programmes accounting for disabilities (p.230) [CL]; and injustice in use of imprisonment for public protection (IPP) (p.296) [E]*

Case description

Roger is a fifty-five-year-old man currently serving a sentence of IPP.[21] He was convicted of wounding with intent for attacking his girlfriend. His tariff was three years; he has been in prison for eight. He shows signs of cognitive impairment, as well as low IQ.

The Parole Board has determined that he poses a high risk of reoffending against future partners, refused to release him, and recommended that he undertake certain prison offender treatment programmes[22] before his next hearing.

He is from a large family in St Lucia, and grew up on a plantation. He did poorly at school and has borderline literacy. He experienced several head injuries in his teens from fights and accidents, although never lost consciousness or required inpatient hospital treatment. He worked on the plantation and with his father in a local quarry.

He emigrated to the UK aged thirty-six years. He has since been unemployed and in receipt of benefits. His first conviction was for shoplifting food because of hunger; he has since been convicted of seven public order and domestic violence offences, including an assault for which he served a short prison sentence. He says he does not want to do the prison programmes because he does not like groups. He insists that his assault on his girlfriend was justified because she cheated on him.

You are a consultant forensic psychiatrist asked by his solicitor to assess his ability to utilise the programmes because he does not accept responsibility for his offence and refuses to participate in treatment.

Questions

1. What clinical, legal, clinico-legal, and ethical issues are raised by this case?

---

[21] These sentences in E&W were abolished with effect from 2013 but continue to apply to those sentenced before then. Equivalent 'ICS' sentences still exist in NI.

[22] Such as Enhanced Thinking Skills (ETS) or Building Better Relationships (BBR).

Clinical

Traumatic brain injury (TBI) can lead to persistent effects on behaviour, emotions, and/or cognition; it can also impair memory, attention, concentration, planning and organisation, self-awareness, self-control, and social judgement. Such deficits have been linked to an increased risk of criminal behaviour, and make it difficult for the individual to engage effectively with the criminal justice process.

Many offenders have literacy problems, and shame about this may stop some from engaging. Roger's history of TBI, and the fact that he went to a special school, raise clinical questions about his memory function, affect regulation, and cognitive flexibility, whilst significant impairment of executive function might explain both his lack of engagement with rehabilitation programmes and his entrenched attitude to his offence.

Your assessment must include neuropsychological tests of intelligence and cognitive function (by another expert if you do not have the right training) to provide evidence of the presence or absence of TBI and its type and degree. These should include tests of frontal lobe function (looking at cognitive rigidity and planning ability), memory, and literacy. They should be valid for people from Roger's cultural background.

Brain imaging is unlikely to assist, as TBI in men such as Roger is usually mild to moderate and unrelated to a particular single injury.

You should consider whether other risk factors are present that will amplify Roger's risk of violence to future partners, such as misogynistic attitudes towards women, and substance misuse. You could use a structured tool for partner violence such as the Spousal Assault Risk Assessment.

Evidence within the criminal justice system has also highlighted that offenders with TBI may be more vulnerable to those around them.

Roger's general mental health may also need attention: stigma and stereotyping can lead to a failure to look for mood disorders in Afro-Caribbean men, and mood disorders are a risk factor for intimate partner violence, especially in older men.

Legal

The Parole Board often makes recommendations on steps towards release, which are usually incorporated into sentence plans by the OM. Such recommendations must be reasonable and appropriate to the offender, also available. There has been concern that the Parole Board recommends courses that prisoners on IPPs, in particular, have no hope of accessing, because their prison cannot provide enough places on them, or in which they cannot participate because of their particular disabilities. In the case of *R (Weddle) v Secretary of State for Justice*,[23] the court stated that it was unrealistic to expect a prisoner to complete unsuitable programmes. The Parole Board should also consider the limited evidence that the programmes reduce risk.

The Bradley Report (2009)[24] commented that sentence plans must be 'realistic and attainable in order to be effective in providing offenders with an opportunity to address offending related factors and reduce risk'. It also commented that they should not contain a list of activities that 'may' be helpful.

[23]   *R (on the application of Weddle) v Secretary of State for Justice* [2013] EWHC 2323 (Admin).
[24]   *Bradley Report* (2009) 294278 1p 2.5k April (CWP) London: Department of Health.

Clinico-legal

In your report, you should set out the results of your assessment and your conclusions as to whether Roger has TBI, and, if so, the implications both for his potential for progress in prison, and his risk of further violence. The solicitor, in deciding whether to use your report, will weigh whether any advantage gained from your opinion on his disabilities is greater than any disadvantage from your opinion on his future risk of violence.

If you have established that Roger has significant neuropsychological impairment that limits his ability to participate, you should explain this to Roger and his OM. If he has, it is unlikely that any cognitive programme will be of benefit; you would then advise staff on how Roger's TBI limits his ability to adapt his behaviour and respond to consequences.

You may need to advise the OM that Roger needs a different sentence plan, with a different approach to risk management. His risk of future violence may be high, but may be better managed by giving him structure to his days and consistent meaningful activities.

When released he would need a high level of support, including in respect of accommodation, daily structure, and close monitoring of his intimate relationships, with oversight by MAPPA.

If Roger does not have TBI, and his refusal to engage is unrelated to cognitive impairment, then you may wish to consider a formal assessment for personality disorder, which could lead to referral to the OPD programme.

Ethical

The chief ethical issue here is justice. Many consider the detention of offenders long beyond their tariff, with no reasonable prospect of being able to meet the requirements for release by the Parole Board, to be unjust. Even if Roger still poses a risk to future partners, this does not distinguish him from other similar offenders who have been released after determinate sentences, despite their lack of insight and continuing risk.

If Roger has significant TBI then it is arguably unjust to detain him in prison at all. Rather, he should perhaps have been diverted from custody into a community mental health programme for offenders with cognitive impairment and/or learning disabilities. *The Bradley Report* highlighted the significant numbers of prisoners whose mental disorders and learning difficulties led them to repeatedly offend, and recommended that, where possible, they be diverted from prison into community services.

11 Risk assessment in sexual offending

Themes: *mental illness and sexual deviance (p.62) and sexual risk-assessment and management (pp.172, 246) [C]; hospital versus probation order (p.500) and child protection (p.510) [L]; sex offender treatment in prison (p.221) [CL]; and consent to risk assessment (p.342) and personal values influencing assessment and reporting (p.330) [E]*

Case description

Matthew is a thirty-six-year-old white British man. He was convicted of possessing indecent images of children, and then remanded to a forensic low secure ward for presentence assessment, having been found to be depressed and threatening self-harm.

Matthew was arrested after meeting in an internet chat room for teenagers someone he expected to be an eleven-year-old girl. In fact, the person he had contacted was an undercover police officer. The police alleged that he had been grooming the 'girl' and had set up the meeting for the purpose of having sex with her.

He normally lives with his wife and one son, aged twelve. His sister lives nearby, with her husband and two young daughters.

For several months before the alleged offence, Matthew's wife had been concerned about his odd behaviour. He went abroad without her and told her that he was on a special mission to do 'God's work'. He spent long hours on his laptop. His wife found magazines of his that contained bestial pornography. She told their GP, and Matthew was offered an appointment with a community psychiatrist, but he did not attend.

Matthew has a degree in history and a postgraduate teaching qualification. He worked at first in a prestigious girls' school, but was sacked after several years for reasons he will not disclose. He then worked as a history teacher in a less prestigious school until his arrest. In his early twenties, he was diagnosed with schizophrenia; he responded well to an oral antipsychotic, which he stopped after a year. He had several episodes of low mood over the next twelve years.

He has no prior forensic history and no significant history of alcohol or drug use. However, when arrested he had a bag containing flunitrazepam (Rohypnol) tablets, rope, duct tape, sweets, and biscuits. His computer was found to have several hundred indecent images of children on it, of both boys and girls, some depicting sexual acts with adults, including sexual violence.

You are the consultant on his current ward and are asked by the court to advise on sentencing, including offering a comprehensive risk-assessment.

Questions

1. What clinical, legal, clinico-legal, and ethical issues are presented by the case?

Clinical

The sexual-violence risk-assessment should include measures such as the RSVP, Static-99, SORAG, and SVR-20, and perhaps penile plethysmography (PPG) if available.[25] You may need a specialist clinical psychologist to assist you with this, if you and other team members do not have sufficient expertise. You will wish to consider in particular the future risk of acting out fantasies, and therefore of contact sexual offending, given his attempt to meet the eleven-year-old with a 'rape kit' in his possession.

Regarding historical risk factors, Matthew has no previous convictions and evidence of pro-social behaviour. The number of indecent images found, almost all of which featured children, suggests a high level of sexual interest in children (unless they were all downloaded simultaneously and rarely accessed since, for instance). There were also images of bestiality, indicating a range of deviant sexual interests.

You should take a detailed history of sexual fantasies and behaviour from Matthew, bearing in mind that he may not be honest, and explore his intentions for the meeting, and explanation for the 'rape kit'. You should also obtain collateral information from his wife and sister, regarding his behaviour with them and their children, and from his employers about his behaviour at their schools, particularly the reasons for his dismissal from the first school.

If you are satisfied that he suffers from schizophrenia and/or depression, you will need to consider its contribution (if any) to his sexual offending, either directly or by disinhibiting him to express underlying deviant sexual preferences.

He appears at first to have a number of protective factors, including pro-social attitudes, responding to psychiatric treatment, a stable family life, and long-term employment, but the latter are very likely to be lost if he is convicted (and perhaps even if he is not). At the same time, losing unsupervised contact with children at school, and perhaps at home as well, will reduce opportunities to offend and therefore perhaps the risk of offending.

You should go on to develop a risk-management plan based upon your assessment and risk scenarios, taking into account the possibility of Matthew receiving a hospital order, as well as the possibility of a community sentence.

Legal

The court will be concerned both to punish Matthew and to protect potential victims from him, and its sentence will reflect these dual aims. It will consider hospital, prison, and community mental health treatment, based on your recommendations; also restrictions on his behaviour in the community (possibly after a period of imprisonment) and on his access to his, his sister's, and other children.

Clinico-legal

If you find that Matthew is currently mentally ill, then a hospital order for treatment might be appropriate, and he could be offered therapy for sexual deviancy as part of his hospital treatment. The court is more likely to consider this if you report some causal link between his mental disorder and risk of offending.

If he does not require immediate hospital treatment, you should give advice about treatment options in prison, as well as in the community. You should liaise with the service that would provide the psychological treatment beforehand, so as to ensure he would be eligible. In conjunction with the probation officer and social worker, you may also recommend types of restrictions that would help manage his risk of future offending against children. This is likely to include a period of monitoring after release under MAPPA.[26]

---

[25] PPGs, which require specialist expertise in their use and interpretation, are mostly restricted to use in high secure hospitals.

[26] The Multi-Agency Public Protection Arrangements (MAPPA) in E&W and Scotland, and Public Protection Arrangements for Northern Ireland (PPANI).

Ethical

You will need to consider whether your expertise and experience are sufficient in regard to all aspects of the case, and whether there is a conflict of interest between your role as a treating clinician and your role as an expert (see ethical case 5). You maintain a clinical duty of care to Matthew, and the conviction and sentence may put him at risk of self-harm or suicide. But Matthew may need to be reminded of your duty to the court, and that you are providing an independent view of his risk.

You should also note your personal values and how to minimise any moral bias you may feel against sex offenders, especially paedophiles.

You will need to acknowledge, including to Matthew, the lack of a robust evidence base for sex offender treatment, as any treatment you recommend may result in him being deprived of his liberty beyond a penal sentence, and/or being coerced to accept that treatment.

12 Transcultural assessment in sexual offending

Themes: *psychosis and learning disability (pp.72, 110) and psychiatric and psychological assessment with different language and culture (p.148) [C]; sexual offending with a child (p.420) [L]; fitness to plead (p.602) and mitigation (p.638) [CL]; and assessor's cultural competence (p.330) [E]*

Case description

A solicitor has instructed you to prepare a report on Amir, a thirty-seven-year-old man charged with sexual assault on (touching) a thirteen-year-old girl. Your instructions include commenting upon any mental disorder, on whether Amir is fit to plead, and whether there are any mitigating factors were he to be found guilty.

Amir is from Bangladesh. He only recently moved to the UK following an arranged marriage. His wife found him employment in a local supermarket, stacking shelves at night. Amir has only limited English: he speaks Sylheti.

You are told that Amir's instructions to his solicitor are that he cannot understand why he has been charged since he believes he has not done anything wrong, in that it is entirely accepted in his country for men to have sexual relationships with girls who have reached puberty. However, he further instructed that sleeping with a virgin would cleanse him and make him pure.

Amir describes living with his family in Bangladesh, prior to coming to the UK, because he was unable to look after himself.

Questions

1. What are the clinical, legal, clinico-legal, and ethical issues in the case?

Clinical

Cultural experience and expectations influence various aspects of any clinical interview, beginning with the initial contact. For example, cultural beliefs and perceptions may influence how both you and Amir greet each other and understand gender differences and roles and how you each differently understand concepts such as consent and confidentiality.

Ideally Amir ought to be assessed by a clinician who shares his language, race, and culture. However, if that is not possible, a minimum requirement in a cross-cultural assessment is the ability to establish mutual understanding between you and the client. Assuming you do not speak Sylheti, you will need to work through an interpreter, who must be fluent, objective, and credible. You should meet him beforehand to check his understanding of the context and ability to relay to you any potentially psychiatrically relevant information (e.g. suggesting formal thought disorder), and to explore discreetly whether they might be biased because of Amir's caste, cultural identity, or values, or because of his alleged sexual offending. Likewise, when interpreting the data you will need to be aware of your own biases.

You should adapt your interview technique when operating through an interpreter (e.g. simplifying and shortening your questions and avoiding colloquial language), to minimise miscommunication or misinterpretation. The interpreter may assist beyond language per se, by being able to help you interpret nonverbal behaviours that may be culturally meaningful, such as body language, eye contact, and facial expressions. However, emphasise that he must interpret Amir's responses literally rather than try to explain them, unless you specifically request it.

Place the defendant in the normal position for an interview, with the interpreter behind or to his side, out of his line of sight, so that you maintain eye contact with Amir throughout. Encourage him to avoid turning to the interpreter, and do not do so yourself.

Where there are cultural issues you wish to ask the interpreter about, thereby going beyond pure verbal interpretation, make the status of your questions and their answers clear in your notes and report. It can be especially difficult to distinguish between delusional beliefs and culturally appropriate ones.

As regards cognitive abilities, the interpreter may be able to give some idea of Amir's comprehensibility, and to help in administering simple 'bedside' cognitive tests. You should obtain collateral information from his family about his usual behaviour and level of functioning, through any statements they may have given, and by contacting them directly if needed.

The use of psychological and psychometric assessments with non-English-speaking or non-Western-educated individuals may be unreliable because such tests are generally standardised using Anglo-European cultural norms and based upon Anglophone data (although there are culturally validated translations of some tests, such as the BDI2, WAIS-IV, and STAXI). The University of East London Test Set: Sylheti Version 2 might be most culturally appropriate for Amir.

Some of these difficulties can be avoided with nonverbal tests,[27] but cultural norms still have a strong influence on the ability to understand the test instructions, test-taking attitudes, and learned cognitive abilities, which may be compounded by mental illness or learning disability, and their symptom presentation within the defendant's culture.

The cultural influence on response bias should also be considered; although there are no published studies that have addressed the cross-cultural accuracy of measures that assess 'faking good', and only limited research on cultural influences on assessment of exaggeration.

Legal

Like other forms of law-breaking, the definition of sexual offences is influenced by cultural and ethnic norms. Sexual behaviours that are criminal in one society may be legitimate in another, and within one society the concept of what constitutes a sexual offence can change over time. However, these cultural influences are sociologically rather than legally relevant, and ignorance of the law, or dissent from it, is not a defence.

Assuming Amir has no mental condition defence to the charge he faces, which is likely unless he has quite severe mental disorder or intellectual impairment, his counsel may put forward his cultural attitudes in mitigation (i.e. as evidence that suggests the court might find his offending as worth of less severe punishment).

Clinico-legal

If you establish that Amir has a mental disorder, you will report on whether it has rendered him 'unfit to plead', and if so, what additional supports he may need during court proceedings (bearing in mind the difficulty of applying the Pritchard criteria to a defendant from a different culture).

Some symptoms of mental disorder may affect the offender's behaviour, and may explain criminal rule-breaking, no matter what the cultural background. However, it is unlikely that they would offer him any mental condition defence.

If you find that Amir has a mental disorder that warrants a hospital order then you should recommend that, even if the disorder is unrelated causally to the offence.

As regards the relevance of your clinical findings to mitigation, if it is your view that his attitudes towards the alleged offence likely arise from his cultural background then this *might* be discussed

---

[27] Such as Raven's Standard Progressive Matrices for intelligence and cognitive function.

in your report, but you may well not be competent to do so, and so may advise that a sociologist or anthropologist be appointed if expert evidence on the point is essential. Conversely, the prosecution may well argue that the offence was driven by culturally based misogyny, even if you have found a mental disorder or intellectual disability.

Ethical

The key ethical question is whether you should assess someone from a culture with which you are unfamiliar, particularly if you do not speak his language. It may be necessary, given the stakes for the defendant, that Amir be assessed by an expert who understands both his language and his culture. So you may wish to help the solicitor find such an expert. If they cannot find one, you should not be pressed to carry out a substandard assessment—though you may face a dilemma if the alternative is that Amir would have no expert evidence at all.

Four core elements of cultural competence have been identified:[28] 1) critical examination (i.e. the awareness of role, values, and beliefs); 2) cultural knowledge (i.e. understanding of the other's culture, history, and values); 3) ability to communicate effectively, incorporating cultural elements as appropriate; and 4) practice (i.e. continuing to hone one's skills). If you possess these and decide to take on the assessment you should seek advice from experts with language and cultural knowledge that matches the defendant, as well as use a suitable interpreter. Your report should explicitly address the boundaries of your expertise, and the impact of these upon your opinions.

---

[28] Balcazar et al (2009).

13

Community risk-management— sex offences, psychosis, and drug misuse

Themes: *formulation (p.146) and risk management (p.237) [C]; deferred conditional discharge (p.511) and right to discharge and psychiatrist as a 'public body' (p.512) [L]; continued inpatient care despite recommendation for conditional discharge [CL]; and disputed clinical decisions (pp.298, 304, 306) and values influencing decision (p.330) [E]*

Case description

Kevin from clinical case 8 was convicted of rape, and received a restricted hospital order to your MSU. His mental state improved further on medication; and with insight, he was distressed by what he had done. He agreed to extended psychological assessment and therapy, to understand his behaviour.

You arrange two personality disorder assessments (IPDE and Millon[29]) and an assessment for paraphilias. The former indicated clinically significant levels of avoidant, borderline, and compulsive traits, but not antisocial traits; the paraphilia assessment revealed no sexual deviation or rape-prone attitudes.

Kevin also participated in substance misuse. He accepts that his drinking had been a significant factor in the rape, and wants to stop. However, the thinks the skunk cannabis he has used since age thirteen years simply makes him 'mellow', and could not have contributed to the offence, because he had never previously been violent after using it; and he intends to use it after discharge to reduce anxiety. He sees himself as having been 'confused and unwell', and thanks to antipsychotic treatment, now back to his usual self. He has complied with all aspects of treatment over the past two years, and shown no antisocial behaviour or violence.

The team take the view that using cannabis after discharge will increase the risk of psychosis, and therefore of harm to others; Kevin disagrees.

In preparation for Kevin's forthcoming tribunal, you refer him to the local community psychiatrist[30] for follow-up after discharge from the MSU. She insists that Kevin is 'a psychopath', and adds that his willingness to use cannabis is evidence of this. She refuses to supervise him or take over his care.

---

[29] *International Personality Disorder Examination; Millon Clinical Multiaxial Inventory*, 4th ed. (MCMI-IV).

[30] Not all areas have a specialist forensic community mental health team.

Questions

1. What are the clinical, legal, clinico-legal, and ethical issues in the case?

Clinical

The community psychiatrist's clinical views have not so far been supported by detailed evidence or formulation, or been coherently argued. Rigidly held positions often indicate anxiety, but whatever its source, her professional opinion is likely to influence MoJ and tribunal decisions on leave and discharge, and must be addressed.

Your team needs to keep working with Kevin, as well as with the community psychiatrist. Making and maintaining relationships with offender patients is what relational security is all about, and this means that Kevin needs to be able to feel that he can trust his team, even if you do not always agree with him.

Co-working with the CMHT will involve making and maintaining relationships of a different sort. You could simply leave the community psychiatrist to defend her position at the tribunal, but this might only entrench her position, and could harm her relationship with Kevin if she is later forced to care for him. Instead, invite her to meet Kevin and get to know him, and politely explain the assessments showing that he does not exhibit psychopathy. A multiagency professionals' discussion, perhaps facilitated by a senior practitioner seen as neutral by both the community and forensic teams might also help. You could also offer support and advice on his management after discharge, perhaps even informal peer supervision with the community psychiatrist if she would find this useful.[31]

If she cannot be persuaded, then the disagreement will be resolved by the tribunal. If it agrees with your view, it will order deferred conditional discharge[32]; the deferment allowing time to find a supervising consultant and team, and accommodation (e.g. in a hostel). To satisfy the criteria for this order, Kevin must be medically ready for discharge, not just predicted to be ready at some future date, or after some change in circumstances. The tribunal cannot direct the community psychiatrist to manage the patient, although it may adjourn to allow her to reconsider her position, and may direct her to attend a further hearing to explain her views.

One option for discharge is that Kevin could be placed in a community setting with the inpatient forensic team supporting him, although this would be a drain on your resources and might contravene local hospital policies.

Legal

In IH,[33] the House of Lords addressed a similar conflict between a patient's right to liberty, and their perceived risk of harm to others. IH had argued at a tribunal that he should be conditionally discharged because he no longer suffered from a mental disorder of a nature and degree that made it appropriate for him to be liable to be detained in hospital. The balance of medical evidence supported this, and the tribunal ordered a deferred conditional discharge, with a condition that he be supervised by a forensic psychiatrist. No forensic psychiatrist could be found to take on this duty, so the patient applied for judicial review of the hospital's failure to discharge him. It was argued that in such situations a psychiatrist is a 'hybrid public authority',[34] which required them to take explicitly into account the patient's right to liberty under article 5 of the ECHR, which was being violated by the refusal to supervise him in the community. The respondents argued that article 5 could not require psychiatrists to administer treatment or supervision against their professional judgment made in good faith, and that, because no responsible body of psychiatrists considered him to be safely manageable in the community, an individual doctor who did so could be liable in negligence if an adverse event occurred.[35] However,

---

[31] Another factor in her anxiety might be the likelihood of blame were there to be a serious incident after discharge, when she is responsible for his care. Your continued involvement (on an informal, consultative or peer-supervisory basis) after discharge might help reduce this fear.

[32] Except in RoI.

[33] *R(IH) v SSHD* [2003] UKHL 59; an appeal to the European Court of Human Rights was ruled inadmissible as he had had access to sufficient legal remedies in the UK: *IH v UK* 17111/04 [2005] ECHR 934.

[34] For instance carrying out functions of a public nature when deciding whether or not to offer to treat or supervise a patient, or by extension, to admit them for example.

[35] *Bolam v Friern Hospital Management Committee* [1957] 1 WLR 583.

the House of Lords left undecided whether or not psychiatrists are hybrid public authorities in such situations.[36]

Clinico-legal

The tribunal could be asked to set conditions of discharge that include a requirement not to smoke cannabis, although this would be unlikely to be effective without his acquiescence and proper community support (and could be opposed at the hearing on the ground that no link between cannabis use and offending has been established).

If no community supervisor can be identified, then Kevin may stay in hospital indefinitely, provided he still suffers from mental disorder of a nature or degree warranting follow-up after discharge. This would be the case even though it violates the principle of treatment in least-restrictive conditions, and even if the team believed that there were no inpatient therapeutic interventions capable of offering further benefit. The tribunal would then be in the position of allowing detention to continue whilst a conditional discharge remains deferred indefinitely for a supervisor to be found.[37]

Ethical

A psychiatrist's decision whether or not to accept a patient for supervision should be evidenced-based. So any refusal to supervise should not be based solely on negative emotions, or anxieties arising from their own value judgment about a patient or their offence. Although the community psychiatrist's view may be honest and genuine, like any clinical view, it must meet professional standards. In this case, the claim that use of cannabis is evidence of psychopathy is simply false; to claim that Kevin is a 'psychopath' on such a basis is like saying that a patient has Ebola virus because they have a cough.

If the quality of a clinical opinion is poor enough, or the evidence for it weak enough, it becomes unjust to make a decision affecting liberty on the basis of that opinion. Offenders who have committed odd and unusual offences, especially sexual offences, are particularly at risk of this since there is often professional anxiety when there is no easy formulation to link their mental disorder and their odd or sexual offending. A study of people sent to hospital instead of prison found that sex offenders were likely to be detained for longer in hospital than in prison, especially if their offence was puzzling to professionals.[38] It may be ethically justifiable for well-founded professional anxiety about future risk to prevent discharge; it cannot be justifiable for Kevin's detention to be extended on the basis of unfounded professional anxiety, lacking clinical evidence.

As Kevin's inpatient consultant, you have a duty to try to implement the discharge you believe is warranted. The duty of the community psychiatrist is more limited, as she is not currently responsible for his treatment, and only needs to respond to the referral. However, you both have a duty of care towards him, and to ensure that NHS resources are used fairly and justly; an extended stay in a secure setting would be costly, and prevent another patient being admitted.

---

[36] The patient went on to appeal to another tribunal hearing once sufficient time had passed; the tribunal cited 'new clinical evidence' and ordered continued detention.

[37] Such indefinite deferred conditional discharge can also be brought about by the MoJ refusing to allow leave prior to discharge, unless the tribunal can be persuaded that the risk of discharge without testing on leave is sufficiently low.

[38] Dell S and Robertson G (1988) *Sentenced to Hospital: Offenders in Broadmoor*, Oxford University Press.

14

Psychosis and PD–complex violence, step down in security

Themes: *comorbid PD (p.78), transfer from high to medium security (p.190), and explanations of homicide (pp.26-37) [C]; appropriate treatment (p.471) and tribunal recommending transfer (p.512) [L]; and risk reduction as 'beneficence' (p.287), refusal of treatment (pp.322, 332), and the value of truth (p.290) [E]*

Case description

Michael from clinical case 9 was admitted to a high secure hospital after his conviction for manslaughter on the grounds of diminished responsibility when psychotic. As set out in clinical case 9, he has paranoid schizophrenia and psychopathy, and a long history of violent offending.

Michael claims that he only killed his neighbour in self-defence, because he was involved in a conspiracy to get Michael evicted. There is some truth in this: since the victim was one of a group who had contacted the council with complaints about Michael, including his hostile behaviour, the smell from his flat, and his cruelty to his dogs. Michael does not accept that he was mentally unwell at the time of the offence, and his compliance with his antipsychotic medication has fluctuated.

After five years in high security, Michael is on an assertive rehabilitation ward, where he rarely gets into disputes with staff or fellow patients. He has engaged in psychological therapies, including individual psychotherapy, behavioural therapy for what he calls 'my OCD', a 'hearing voices' group, and other recovery-focused sessions. However, he has refused to attend groups that focus on past violence, although he has been keen to engage in individual therapy. He thinks he may be on the autistic spectrum and have PTSD from some unspecified past trauma.

You are a consultant in the local MSU, and the high secure service has referred Michael to you. He and his solicitor want to know whether you will support transfer at his forthcoming tribunal.

You assess Michael, as do a senior nurse and a senior clinical psychologist from your service. You all differ in your view about insight, treatment and security needs, and future risk.

Questions

1. What clinical, legal, clinico-legal, and ethical issues arise in this case?

Clinical

High secure hospitals admit patients with complex, often treatment-resistant, mental disorder and high risks of harm to others; many, like Michael, have psychosis and severe personality disorder, making it difficult to tease out which aspects of mental disorder are most relevant to their risk of violence.

The patient's viewpoint is not only important to the therapeutic alliance and shared decision-making, but is also relevant to risk assessment and management. Insight affects the formulation of risk, and whether that formulation is agreed between the patient and the team. Here, the team's formulation of the offence is rather different from Michael's.

In the past forensic patients were often admitted to secure care for behavioural stabilisation, so that, when their behaviour was settled, they could move to lower levels of security. Now it is more common to undergo psychological treatment addressing long-term risk while in secure conditions, as this may uncover issues that temporarily increase the risk of harm while the patient works through them.

It will be helpful to set out the areas of agreement and disagreement between your view and the views of your colleagues (and that of the high secure team), and to list the evidence for each, and the implications for Michael's treatment plan. For example, you may think that Michael needs to work on his index offence and his resistance to understanding why others have a different view from him.

There is a range of views on whether denial of an offence and lack of insight is a bar to treatment and risk reduction, and on whether and how to treat individuals like Michael with high PCL-R scores (it used to be accepted that psychological treatment was counterproductive, but this position is now disputed). There is also uncertainty about whether offence-based work should take place early in an admission, or should wait until the patient's mental state is stable.

Legal

The tribunal will focus upon diagnosis, treatment availability and completion, and the feasibility of future plans. However, tribunals can only make decisions about continued detention or discharge. Beyond this they can merely make recommendations, for example, that a patient move to a lower security unit; although such recommendations can sometimes influence the decision of the MoJ, or the MSU.

Clinico-legal

You do not have a right to attend the tribunal, but you may be invited to do so, and if not, the panel will still consider your assessment report in detail. It will be helpful to offer a nuanced and evidence-based view that sets out clearly your concerns and recommendations.

Ethical

This case raises questions about whether secure services have a duty to help offender patients to take their violence risk seriously, beyond their *usual* duty of 'beneficence'. It is arguably in Michael's interest to understand the reality of what he has done and its impact upon others, and it seems both unjust and disrespectful to collude with his view of himself and his history, leaving him unprepared to face the conflicting social and legal truths about his behaviour.

Respect for truth is a part of respect for justice and autonomy; failure to respect truth risks doing harm to patients. It can nevertheless be difficult to hold complex conversations about truth and respect with people in psychotically disordered states of mind, or with those who have long standing antisocial views and values. Communication and reflective skills are keys to having the kind of conversations with Michael that will be needed for him to recover.

It might be argued that Michael ought to have to gone to prison, where he could have accessed the OPD pathway for high-risk offenders with personality disorder—either directly from court, or after a period of treatment in hospital for psychosis. This might have been more legally and ethically truthful to Michael's conviction for manslaughter (still a very serious offence), and to his belief that he was justified in what he did. It also might have helped him develop a narrative of himself as an offender with some responsibility for changing his mind and behaviour. Arguably it would also have a freed a high secure bed for someone who could have made better use of it; although this invites another question, about what 'better use' amounts to in secure services.

15

Patient threats against staff, request for transfer to higher security

Themes: *borderline personality disorder (p.84), use of security (p.190), and objectivity in risk assessment (p.166) [C]; 'treatability' test (p.471) and confidentiality of psychological notes (p.320) [L]; 'least-restrictive principle' (p.471) [CL]; and impact of staff anxiety on clinical opinion (p.674) [E]*

Case description

You are a consultant in a high secure hospital. You assess Max, a thirty-year-old man detained in a medium secure unit following transfer from an open acute ward.

Max has been diagnosed with emotionally unstable personality disorder, with some antisocial traits. He was first admitted to adult services six months ago because of extreme self-harming. In hospital he became increasingly hostile and aggressive; he threatened staff, stating he would find out where they lived and burn down their houses. His admission to the MSU was precipitated by this and the discovery that his family were smuggling in sharps, for him to cut himself.

The MSU team express anxiety that he may make and conceal weapons either to kill himself or to injure staff. They are also concerned that he has encouraged other vulnerable patients to self-harm, and to complain about their care. He is therefore nursed on constant 1:1 observation, but has nevertheless managed to cut himself repeatedly, requiring frequent escorted trips to A&E for suturing. He has also been secluded on several occasions.

He sees a female psychologist twice a week for trauma-related therapy. She refuses to discuss session content with the rest of the team because, she says, the sessions are confidential, although she has provided summary Care Programme Approach (CPA) reports.

You interview Max. He is dismissive, truculent, and hostile. He calls you 'a stooge with no skills', and says your job is 'to take [him] off to Broadmoor'. He says he has committed no crime and should be released immediately, denies he has been aggressive, and calls staff 'pathetic pussies' who care only for themselves. He threatens that, if you recommend transfer, he will 'sue your ass off'.

As you leave the MSU, the consultant and service manager try to impress upon you how great a risk Max poses to their staff and other patients, and to persuade you to admit him.

Questions

1. What are the alternative courses of action that might be pursued, and how might each be justified?

2. How should you approach the question of potential transfer to high security?
3. What other clinical, legal, clinico-legal, and ethical issues arise in the case?

Clinical

This case raises questions about the functions of the different types of secure service. Their roles are defined in national guidance: for high security, it is 'to provide a therapeutic psychiatric service for individuals with a mental disorder ... who present a grave risk of harm to others'.[39] Hence, secure services are not intended primarily to manage patients' risk of harm to themselves.

Security has three aspects: 'physical' (e.g. walls, doors, and locks), 'procedural' (e.g. searches, leave rules, and urine testing), and 'relational' (e.g. knowing your patient, spotting signs of change, reflective practice, and managing professional boundaries). The level of security required is determined by clinical assessment and consultation, risk formulation, and risk-management planning.

Most people who frequently self-harm exhibit traits of personality disorder. The majority do not need inpatient treatment and do not attack the people trying to help. Max is therefore unusual, and his complex psychopathology should make you cautious in risk management, and vigilant for dysfunctional team dynamics arising from his projection of intolerable thoughts and feelings. The people most obviously at risk are the MSU staff, who are experiencing unusually high levels of fear and anxiety about the patient.

In risk assessment, what weight should be given to professional anxiety? Some argue that staff anxiety is useful information; others that there are too many confounding factors for it to be informative. For example, if the MSU were willing and able to recruit and pay for extra staff to work with Max, this might reduce anxiety, and transfer might not be requested.

In a case such as Max's, good advice is to do nothing in haste. Make an extended multiprofessional assessment, as part of which members of your team offer consultation and advice to the treating team, and the different professionals involved. To facilitate this, meet Max more than once, even if you do not expect the second assessment to yield any new information.

It may also assist to review with the team the patient's grounds for detention under the MHA, the diagnosis and formulation of his mental disorder, the genesis of both his self-harm and his aggression, and his risk assessments to date—all of this being aimed at increasing objectivity and potentially reducing anxiety.

In risk assessments, some professionals like to use security-assessment instruments such the SNAP[40], and it may help to complete this jointly with the team. (Having said this, neither the HCR20v3 nor the SNAP has been standardised on cases such as Max's, and both may be influenced by staff anxiety.) Such discussions can also provide a reflective space within which staff can discuss their anxiety about Max, any hostility they may feel towards him, and their understanding of how this may have affected their behaviour and generated splits within the team.

Cases like Max's, in which the patient has a 'hostile/helpless' state of mind, often generate such splits, and increase the risk of professional boundary violations. For example, the psychologist may already have crossed a professional boundary by withholding information from the rest of the clinical team. Although there may be some discretion in how much detail a professional should share with the team, the psychologist's position is both unusual and arguably disproportionate, and may suggest emotional over-involvement with Max. The consultant or team manager should therefore discuss this issue calmly and nonjudgmentally with the psychologist and his line manager (if he is separately managed).

Note that NICE guidelines on the management of self-harm in borderline personality disorder[41] do not recommend long admissions since reduced personal responsibility can lead to dependency that neither contains nor empowers.

Here the only argument for transfer to high security is that the greater physical security could allow a relaxation of some aspects of day-to-day procedural and relational security (less use of seclusion e.g.) and allow Max to take more responsibility for his behaviour.

---

[39] NHS Standard Contract for High Secure Mental Health Services (Adults), 2014. This defines *mental disorder* as mental illness, personality disorders, and neuro-developmental disorders. Previously the working criterion for admission to high security had, for decades, been that the patient should be 'a grave and immediate danger to the public'.

[40] Collins M and Davies S. *The Security Needs Assessment Profile: A multidimensional approach to measuring security needs*, International Journal of Forensic Mental Health 2005 4(1): 39–52.

[41] CG78, *Borderline Personality Disorder: Recognition and Management: Guidance* (2009) NICE, section 1.4.1.2.

Legal

Increased security for the staff implies reduced liberty for Max. The law in the E&W and NI permits detention of capacitous people with personality disorder (or any other mental disorder) without prior conviction, even if successful treatment is unlikely[42]; and its use therefore requires careful ethical reflection (see below).

The psychologist's assertion that her clinical notes are confidential *from the rest of the multidisciplinary team* is not consistent with either data-protection law or the law on confidentiality and disclosure.

Clinico-legal

Max can be transferred to high secure care without a change of legal status, although codes of practice state that patients should be detained in the least-restrictive conditions possible, so the case for high security will have to be made out clearly.

As part of the discussion with the psychologist, he should be asked to place his notes of therapy into the clinical record, after informing Max and receiving assurances that other MDT members will not discuss them with Max without their prior agreement.

Ethical

The reduction of risk of harm to oneself or others can be an ethical justification for deprivation of liberty and compulsory treatment. However, the risk must be assessed objectively.

Human beings are risk-averse. The culture and structure of the NHS, plus the sometimes punitive nature of serious incident reviews and inquiries, makes NHS staff in mental health services the more so, and therefore more likely to allow their anxiety to affect clinical decisions. If this is not countervailed by careful ethical reflection and objective risk-assessment, the patient pays the price, in loss of liberty, therapeutic disadvantage, and stigmatisation.

---

[42] In E&W, all that need be demonstrated is that 'appropriate treatment is available', not that there be a likelihood of patient benefit. In NI there is no treatability test at all. However, in Scotland it is required that detention 'is likely to prevent worsening of the disorder'. RoI has a slightly stronger test, that treatment 'is likely to benefit the condition to a material extent'.

16

Deciding on unescorted leave outside medium secure perimeter

Themes: *schizophrenia (p.73), PD and antisocial behaviour (p.78), and individual risk formulation (p.146) [C]; authorisation for leave (p.510) [L]; what counts as 'leave' (p.486) [CL]; and conflicting opinions in MDT (p.312) and values-based practice (p.288) [E]*

Case description

You are a consultant on a medium secure ward preparing for a CPA review for Anderson, a twenty-four-year-old transferred recently from prison. He had served nearly all of a four-year sentence for GBH with intent when he then suffered his first psychotic episode. You diagnosed paranoid schizophrenia. Treatment has gone well: Anderson's delusions of reference, thought broadcasting and auditory hallucinations have resolved, and he has used escorted community leave successfully for several months.

An aim of the review is to plan Anderson's rehabilitation, after which he would be discharged to the community because he will have passed his earliest date of release (EDR). You also need to decide whether to trial unescorted ground leave.

As his psychosis has waned, you have received reports from nurses and the OT of 'bad behaviour', such as denying borrowing cigarettes and refusing to repay; making inappropriate sexual comments to a young female nurse, who had to move wards; and attempting to persuade other patients to refuse to return to the ward at the end of a smoking break.

You suspect Anderson may also have antisocial personality disorder (ASPD), and intend to ask the team psychologist to undertake a formal personality assessment. You would regard ASPD as increasing his risk of violence, and meaning risk management must go beyond preventing a relapse of psychosis.

You review relevant literature on the risk of absconding. One article states 'up to one patient in 30 will abscond at least once during their admission' (with other studies putting the risk no lower than 1 in 100). You worry about the risk of Anderson absconding from unescorted leave and assaulting someone in the community, and the inquiry into your decisions that would follow.

Questions

1. Are you adequately prepared for the CPA review?
2. What further could you consider in order to make a good decision?
3. What legal constraints are relevant to deciding on unescorted ground leave?
4. What could you or others do in the review to improve the chances of a good decision?
5. What other clinical, legal, clinico-legal, and ethical issues are there in the case?

Clinical

Leave is a part of rehabilitation, and behaviour on leave can assist in understanding current risks—but this does not justify exposing others, including previous victims, to unacceptable risk. There are no accepted structured clinical approaches to considering leave; most leave decisions are made by discussion in multidisciplinary meetings.

You appear to have already spent more time preparing for the CPA review than is often available to busy consultants. However, if time allows, you should give further thought to the impact of the emotive research statement 'one patient in every 30 will abscond at least once during their admission' on your thought processes. This appears to have been associated in your mind with concern with avoiding the possible negative consequences of granting unescorted ground leave. Consider the denominator[43] in this statistic, which was 'every 100 beds in a general psychiatric ward'—not a comparable environment to a medium secure ward, where the rate of absconding from leave is much lower. You should also consider the effect upon your judgment of the way the statistic was presented: had it been 'the risk of absconding is 0.11% per patient on any given day', it would have seemed far lower. You could then have gone on to extrapolate from this baseline rate to an individualised estimated probability of absconding for Anderson using the BSCM procedure. You should also bear in mind that, even if Anderson were to abscond from unescorted leave, harm to others might still be relatively unlikely, and certainly not inevitable.

Your job is to rehabilitate patients *and* to protect others; over-reacting to risk to others will prevent rehabilitation. You should aim to achieve a 'safe balance' between the two.

Legal

Leave outside the hospital and its grounds specified in the transfer warrant can only be granted to restricted patients if first authorised by the MoJ.

Clinico-legal

After the EDR, permission of the MoJ will no longer required. You should check this date, and the wording of the transfer warrant, as it may allow you to give the patient leave within an area of hospital grounds without prior permission, if you think that appropriate (it may be unwise to grant such leave without approval if there would be nothing to stop the patient walking outside the unit or the hospital grounds whilst on leave from the ward).

Ethical

The decision involves weighing the risk of absconding, and the harm to others that might result, against the rehabilitation benefit to Anderson. The chances of a good decision being made would increase if the team did not experience time pressure during the meeting (e.g. arising from the need to complete certain check-box exercises or to document the meeting and still to finish within a certain short time).

It would help if all team members, including you, were aware of the various personal and professional values they each brought to the discussion and decision, within the approach of 'values-based practice'; this also would reveal conflicting interpretations of the same information, and related misunderstandings. Lastly, it might assist the process to have the meeting chaired by a competent team member who does not have a strong personal interest in the decision in the way that you and the ward manager may do.

[43] See prospect theory, denominator neglect, and framing in Part A, and its explanation of the BSCM (Baseline, Subjective, Correlate, Multiply) procedure.

17

Coercion in hospital and the community

Themes: *schizophrenia (p.73) and substance misuse (p.76) [C]; prison transfer (p.506) compulsory community treatment (p.488) [L]; least-restrictive principle (p.471) and coercion by threat of recall (p.589) [CL]; and ethics of coercion, objective and perceived (p.324) [E]*

Case description

You are the RC for Billy, a twenty-four-year-old man with paranoid schizophrenia given a short prison sentence for shoplifting, who has been transferred to your forensic low secure unit. He was neglected as a child. He has several convictions for assault, possession of cannabis, and being drunk and disorderly. He failed to comply with treatment in the community; he has never previously been an inpatient. His sentence expired a year ago, but he remains detained in hospital.[44]

He has complied with medication, knowing it could be imposed upon him, and with restrictions such as graded leave, searches of his room and property, plus testing of his breath and urine for alcohol or drug metabolites, all of which you consider necessary to prevent relapse and further violence.

Billy appealed to a tribunal previously but was unsuccessful, the tribunal accepting your opinion that continued detention was necessary 'for his safe rehabilitation'. However, at a more recent hearing you were closely questioned about the possibility of safe management in the community, and the tribunal decided to adjourn, with a formal recommendation[45] that you consider a community treatment order (CTO) before it reconvenes. Billy says that he would be happy to receive a CTO. However, you and the team think community treatment would be premature.

Questions

1. What is the nature of, and the justification for, coercing Billy to accept treatment in hospital or the community?
2. What other clinical, legal, clinico-legal, and ethical issues arise in the case?

---

[44] In E&W and NI, this would be under a 'notional' hospital order. Assuming Billy will not consent to voluntary treatment and/or it would be considered inappropriate in the low secure setting, a new admission order (in RoI) or a new compulsory treatment order (in Scotland) would be necessary.

[45] This is a specific power of tribunals in E&W, falling short of a power directly to impose the CTO itself. There is no equivalent in the MHNIO (even after the MCANI comes into force). In Scotland, assuming a new compulsory treatment order had been made, the tribunal could vary that order so that it authorised compulsory community treatment instead of compulsory inpatient treatment. There is no power to compel civil community treatment in RoI.

Clinical

Patients like Billy are often glad to be out of prison and therefore accept suggested treatment. However, they are clearly detained patients subject to coercion. If Billy is discharged under a CTO he will still be coerced: not by daily impositions, but through his knowledge of the threat of recall if he fails to comply.

The tribunal's decision means you must now reconsider[46] a CTO, and how to manage him safely were such an order to be made. You should take account of Billy's views and attempt to negotiate a package of treatment and care that you deem adequate, even if not ideal.

Legal

A convicted prisoner can be transferred to hospital for treatment of mental disorder if they do not accept treatment in prison, which cannot be compelled within the prison itself.[47] Once in hospital, mental health law provides for various procedures to authorise compulsory treatment, depending upon its perceived benefits, plus its risks and its reversibility.

When reconsidering community treatment, under a CTO in E&W or Scotland[48] you may specify conditions,[49] or apply for measures or recorded matters,[50] that in your view would facilitate safe management. These might include, for instance, attendance at appointments for examination or treatment or participating in psychotherapy; residence at certain accommodation; or allowing staff access for home visits. If Billy were to refuse to comply, he could be forced[51] in certain circumstances, or returned to hospital[52] to resume treatment.

Clinico-legal

Compulsory community treatment is a substantial infringement on liberty, needing careful ethical decision-making. The least-restrictive principle means that coercion must be limited to the minimum necessary for safe management in relevant scenarios.

Further, if Billy breaches a condition or a measure you should not automatically seek immediate enforcement, but balance what you believe to be in his best interests against what *he* deems in his best interests.

If Billy is unhappy with the coercion he experiences after discharge, he can appeal to another tribunal. However, it can be difficult for patients to challenge their clinical teams in this way; they may fear antagonising the professionals on whom they depend, and who exercise power over them (who can e.g. return them to hospital). Patients may also doubt that the tribunal would support their view against professionals, even if legally represented; and there is evidence that tribunals are sometimes ineffective protectors of civil rights.[53] All these anxieties may reflect Billy's early childhood experiences of feeling helpless with powerful caregivers.

---

[46] In E&W, you have several weeks to do this before the tribunal reconvenes. In Scotland, the only reconsideration you could do would be during the hearing, once it became clear that the tribunal was considering compulsory community treatment, but before it issued its decision, you might have the opportunity, if you thought it appropriate, to give an updated opinion during the hearing on community treatment and the conditions you thought necessary to manage Billy. Neither scenario is possible in NI or RoI.

[47] Treatment cannot be compelled in prison under mental health law, but if the patient lacks capacity, it may be possible to compel it under mental capacity law. This is only likely to be justifiable in short-term emergency situations, while transfer to hospital is arranged.

[48] In this case a CTO.

[49] In E&W only, if patients fail to adhere to CTO conditions, they may form part of the grounds for recall, provided the patients require treatment in hospital and there would otherwise be a risk of harm to the patients or others.

[50] In Scotland only, measures are forms of compulsion (e.g. detention in hospital or a requirement to reside at a particular place), whereas recorded matters are services that should be provided to the patient.

[51] Only in Scotland, and only for breach of an attendance requirement.

[52] Recalled under the CTO in E&W, or taken into custody in hospital for breach in Scotland, provided (other than for attendance) that there is a risk of significant deterioration, and the patient has had a reasonable opportunity to comply, or the situation is urgent.

[53] For example Peay J (1989) *Tribunals on Trial: A Study of Decision-Making under the Mental Health Act*, Clarendon Press, which described tribunals as 'glorified case conferences'.

This power imbalance, and Billy's comparative vulnerability, makes it particularly important that there should be careful thought about Billy's needs and values, and an unhurried shared dialogue with him.

Conversely, clinical teams may feel ambivalent about commenting on a patient's appeal, especially if it seems unwise and unlikely to succeed. Clinical teams may also be aware that the tribunal process could harm the relationship with Billy. You should respect Billy's values, and recognise that dissonance is an inevitable part of forensic psychiatric practice, which can be an opportunity for patients to learn about tolerating difference and managing conflict pro-socially.

Ethical

Psychiatric practice, especially forensic, utilises a range of legally sanctioned coercive frameworks; the question is to what extent they are ethically justifiable?

Billy's previous loss of liberty as a sentenced prisoner was ethically justified by the due process that found him to have broken accepted social and legal rules, and by the proportionate nature of his sentence,[54] and many sentenced prisoners accept the justice of 'doing time for a crime'. Typically, the loss of liberty is a combination of imprisonment and subsequent community supervision, with an emphasis on prevention of future harm to others.

In hospital, Billy's loss of liberty was initially justified by the sentence and then by his need for treatment. Once his sentence expired, the only justification was his need for treatment, and once he was ready for discharge, that too fell away. A clinical need for community treatment would be required to justify further compulsion.

Detained patients do not always dislike detention, especially transferred prisoners who have been very unwell in prison. And their lack of resistance places an extra duty on clinical teams not to exploit their compliance. Respect for autonomy includes dialogue with patients about treatment, even if their consent is not legally required, and allowing discussion about the limits to freedom (e.g. to refuse treatment, as they could have done in prison).

Many aspects of long-stay residential secure care convey to detainees a message that staff have authority over them, whatever actual powers staff have, and that they should comply with what is asked of, or imposed upon them. That is, beyond 'objective coercion' there is 'perceived coercion',[55] meaning that residents do not feel free to say what they want, or to refuse activities or advice, at least not without there being a perceived cost.

Hence, some philosophers[56] have argued for a more relational understanding of autonomy that takes account of our dependence on each other at times of illness and distress, and challenges the absolute right to be left to make one's own choices, no matter how foolish.[57] This allows restraints on liberty by reference to pro-social values and communities. This can be argued as a justification for people like Billy being detained in secure psychiatric hospitals: in that, through compliance with the regime and with treatment, Billy may come to adopt more pro-social attitudes and behaviours and be rewarded with increased freedom.

[54] Imprisonment beyond 'punishment that fits the crime', such as extended or indefinite sentences on grounds of risk, may be lawful but is more ethically problematic.

[55] There is a substantial body of research literature that many of those subject to legal coercion do not feel coerced, whilst many who are not legally coerced feel as if they are.

[56] For example Gilligan C (1982) *In a Different Voice: Psychological Theory and Women's Development*, Harvard University Press; Agich G (1993) *Autonomy and Long-Term Care*, Oxford University Press.

[57] Such as Berlin's concept of 'negative liberty': the freedom of the individual from coercion or interference with their private actions. See Berlin I (1969) *Four Essays on Liberty*, Oxford University Press.

18 | Management of violent behaviour absent current mental illness

Themes: *antisocial personality disorder (p.82), violence (pp.26-37), use of security (p.190), and rapid tranquilisation (p.200) [C]; seclusion as treatment (p.196) [L]; and balancing patient and staff interests (p.298) and values-based practice (p.288) [E]*

Case description

Andy has schizophrenia and ASPD, plus intellectual impairment. He was admitted under section to a general psychiatric ward, where he assaulted nurses and was restrained and given rapid tranquilisation. He has since been transferred to a PICU, and thence to your medium secure ward, because of his violent behaviour. The frequency of assaults has increased in the MSU.

Andy accepts a regular long-acting antipsychotic, and is now free of psychosis. At one point he took a second antipsychotic in combination, and this may have reduced the frequency of violence, but it over-sedated him and was stopped.

His anger and violence are often precipitated by frustration at being in hospital, and long waits for his requests to be met. Nevertheless, he has a good relationship with some staff.

Some in the team favour additional medication, long-term seclusion, and referral to high security. Others believe this will increase the risk of violence, and instead he should be discharged now that his psychosis has been treated.

Questions

1. What should you do?
2. Are there justifiable alternative courses of action?
3. What other clinical, legal, clinico-legal, and ethical issues are there?

Clinical

Andy's illness, personality, and learned patterns of behaviour are all relevant to the assessment and management of his risk of violence, as are the attitudes and behaviour of staff, and the environment in which he is treated. Some proposed treatments involve greater restriction, and its predicted impact will affect the risk-management plan, informed by clinical guidance.[58]

---

[58] For exampleNICE (2015) *Violence and Aggression: Short-Term Management in Mental Health, Health and Community Settings*, NICE guideline NG10, 28 May.

Andy's violence should be analysed to identify antecedents and triggers. Tactics for de-escalation should be discussed, including with him, as should the criteria for deciding that de-escalation has failed and rapid tranquilisation or other coercive means are necessary.

Seclusion is only recommended to prevent prolonged physical intervention or restraint; it does not necessarily reduce risks to the patient or others. It can worsen a person's mental health and increase the risk of assault (e.g. during seclusion reviews). Secluding a patient is therefore a measure of last resort; it should be used rarely, with a plan from the outset of how to stop using it. At reviews, the emphasis should be on staff finding an alternative safe way to manage the current risk outside of seclusion, rather than on the patient showing that they are now safe to be released.

Legal

Mental health legislation and accompanying codes of practice provide the legal basis for applying seclusion, which in this context is included within the broad definition of *treatment*.

However 'treatments' such as seclusion have the potential to infringe human rights. It may be argued that they are inhuman or degrading under article 3 of the ECHR, or (more commonly) that they breach the patient's rights to a private and family life under article 8, or to liberty under article 5. A restrictive intervention can be held to breach article 5 even if the patient is already (lawfully) deprived of liberty by detention in hospital.

Clinico-legal

The proposed restrictive treatment will only comply with human rights law if it is both necessary[59] and proportionate (i.e. the degree of restriction is justified by a sufficiently high risk of a sufficiently severe harm).

Ethical

Deciding on treatment for Andy is ethically challenging because it is clinically disputed what will benefit him or others, and what will cause him harm. Taking into account this uncertainty, you must balance the risks and possible benefits to him and to other people when deciding what the approach, including seclusion, should be. A 'values-based' discussion (see part A) may assist the team in resolving the dispute about the best way forward.

---

[59] *Herczegfalvy v Austria* (1993) 15 EHRR 437.

19

Management of self-harm and threats to others in borderline PD

> **Themes:** *treatment of BPD (pp.200-219) and risk of self-harm, suicide and harm to others (p.176) [C]; grounds for detention (p.510) and right to life (p.516) [L]; psychological dependence fostered by detention (p.338) [CL]; and availability of services (p.316) [E]*

Case description

Mary is a thirty-five-year-old woman who has experienced poor affect and arousal regulation since her early teenage years. She was referred to CAMHS aged twelve, and diagnosed with anorexia nervosa and bulimia, and some years later with borderline personality disorder.

She frequently ties ligatures around her neck and cuts her arms and thighs. She has taken numerous overdoses of paracetamol: she seeks medical advice each time, and the self-harm has not been life-threatening, although one overdose caused temporary impairment of liver function.

Her psychiatrist has asked you for a forensic opinion on whether Mary now needs secure care. She was admitted after another large overdose, and continues to self-harm whenever she is not observed. She states that she will kill herself as soon as she has the chance. She has also made threats to nursing staff, such as, 'When I get out of here, I will find out where you live and torch your house'. When last given community leave, she returned with a lighter, which she gave to staff, saying she did not feel safe with it.

An earlier funding request for psychological treatment by a specialist service at another hospital has been refused by commissioners, on the basis that all locally available treatments have not yet been considered. The general psychiatrist feels unable to manage Mary's risk to herself or others, and recommends psychological treatments that they cannot provide, but would be available in your care.

Questions

1. What should you do?
2. What other clinical, legal, clinico-legal, and ethical issues in the case?

Clinical

Forensic services exist primarily to manage the risk of harm to others, and to advise other services about risk management that goes beyond their expertise.

Mary's presentation will be familiar to many psychiatrists, and is troubling for two main reasons. First, understanding of the meaning and function of such behaviour is limited, despite good descriptions of repetitive self-harm since the 1960s. It appears commoner in women than men, and is associated with various diagnoses, including depression and borderline PD. Second, it is associated with a higher risk of suicide, if, like Mary, patients are reckless about the consequences of their self-harm and deceive people who try to help.

In Mary's case her wish to harm herself may not be an authentic choice, but a consequence of fear, distress, anger, and hopelessness. She appears ambivalent about harming herself (e.g. because she seeks help), and staff should support that part of her mind that wants to live. If services take sole responsibility for keeping Mary alive, she then has no need to care for herself and can instead enact the struggle in her mind with the clinical team on the ward, resulting in total dependence on the staff to remain alive.

You can help Mary's clinical team by formulating her risk to herself and others in the context of her affective instability and impulsivity, and identifying the risk factors (and meaning) of her threats to others (e.g. an attempt to force others to contain her behaviour for her). You might recommend reflective practice and supervision to help staff understand and manage Mary's behaviour.

The best evidence to date shows that admissions, especially if longer than a couple of days, are rarely helpful for people like Mary[60]; and may also enhance risk to self and others. Instead they are most likely to benefit from long-term community psychosocial interventions that enable them to live with their own self-directed hostility and destructiveness, and develop better methods of self-soothing and affect management. A range of clinical interventions have been shown to be helpful, including dialectical behaviour therapy and mentalisation-based treatment; you should recommend these.

You should not usually offer to take over care of patients whose main risk is to themselves, or simply because a treatment is funded within your service that is not funded elsewhere. It would be more appropriate to support the general psychiatrist to challenge the commissioners' decision.

Legal

Adults are assumed to have capacity to make treatment decisions, including refusing treatment; they may lawfully refuse lifesaving treatment, or harm themselves.[61] However, mental health law largely ignores mental capacity, provided there is sufficient mental disorder and a risk to the patient or others. Mary can legally be detained in hospital provided appropriate treatment is available,[62] including treatment for the consequences of the mental disorder (e.g. self-harm).[63]

The courts have sometimes been reluctant to accept that mentally disordered patients have capacity if the likely outcome of their decision is their death. For example, Ian Brady, who had a severe personality disorder, was prevented from starving himself to death in a high-security hospital.[64] They have also found that a failure to prevent the suicide of patients known to be at high risk may breach their right to life under article 2 of the ECHR.[65]

Clinico-legal

Staff often consider admitting people like Mary in order to manage their anxiety about the risk to life (and of being found to blame by a court or inquiry), especially if the patient is young. Yet detention can worsen a patient's psychological dependence on staff.

An underlying issue is that the legal tests of mental capacity currently fail to account adequately for the affective instability seen in some personality disorders, and how it causes rapid shifts in beliefs and intent, as well as for associated cognitive distortion.

[60] NICE (2015) *Personality Disorders: Borderline and Antisocial.* NICE quality standard QS88, June.
[61] Though it may be illegal for another person to harm them at their request: *R v Brown* (p.VI.19).
[62] In Scotland & NI there must be some likelihood of treatment improving the patient's disorder.
[63] *B v Croydon Health Authority* (p.VI.19).
[64] *Brady v Ashworth* (p.VI.19).
[65] See the cases of *Rabone* (allowing a suicidal patient to leave hospital) and *Savage* (failing to prevent a suicidal patient absconding) (p.VI.19).

Ethical

You should offer Mary the best treatment for her condition, based upon the best-quality evidence. However, in Mary's case, this may not be available because of limited resource allocation. There is often a public tolerance of failure to provide mental health services where a similar failure of, say, cancer services would be unacceptable.

Forensic services have in the past sometimes admitted women like Mary for want of an alternative. However, Mary is not an offender, and detaining her 'unnecessarily' in secure conditions so that she can obtain the right treatment is discriminatory. It also indirectly supports poor-quality resource allocation decisions in that it would have been cheaper and fairer to fund specialist community psychological treatment. There is no ethical argument that justifies a citizen losing their liberty so that they can gain the clinical treatment to which they are entitled.

20

Covert treatment of violence in psychosis, LD, and epilepsy

Themes: *learning disability (p.110) and epilepsy (p.114) [C]; treatment without consent (p.482) [L, CL]; and autonomy in consent (pp.331, 332) and utilitarian and values-based ethical approaches (pp.286, 288) [E]*

Case description

Aaron is a forty-two-year-old man with severe disabilities arising from schizophrenia, learning disability, and epilepsy. He is detained in a long-term low secure unit. Aaron hates hospitals, and does not accept he has mental illness, although he has mental capacity to make treatment decisions. He wants to be free to live on his own, and regularly appeals against detention. He does not accept that he cannot function on his own, nor that his family are scared of him.

An experienced senior nurse who knew Aaron well has recently left the ward, which is now often staffed with agency nurses. Aaron has recently become much more paranoid about staff, and more verbally aggressive. Many staff avoid him.

You are unsure what to do for the best. Some nurses want Aaron moved to a more secure ward; others would prefer to try medication, but he refuses to take this. Although Aaron could be medicated involuntarily, all agree this would further damage any therapeutic relationship with him.

After much deliberation, you and the team decide covertly to administer a liquid antipsychotic in his drinks. This has an immediate positive effect: Aaron becomes much more settled, and more engaged with staff. He says he feels much better in himself, and states he will apply for a tribunal, on the ground that he clearly does not have a mental illness, because he is well on no medication.

Questions

1. Is the covert medication ethical?
2. Should it continue?
3. If so, will you disclose it to Aaron at the hearing?
4. What other clinical, legal, and ethical implications are there?

Clinical

This scenario is based on a real case, and demonstrates the complexities of long-stay secure care, where relationships between staff and patients are the main clinical framework for treatment, and 'recovery' may entail long-term dependency and limits on autonomy. This is quite unlike the archetype of illness, in which the patient recovers quickly to regain full autonomy with the right treatment.

The staff are frightened of Aaron, do not want to engage with him, and are reluctant to treat him against his will, although they have the legal power to do so. Continued covert medication might be the only way to improve Aaron's mental state and to reduce his hostility and paranoia.

There is some literature reporting good outcomes with covert medication in elderly patients with dementia (e.g. given by their carers), in A&E, when used very briefly during emergency treatment, and in patients with severe LD and other chronic conditions who lack capacity. There is virtually no modern clinical literature supporting the use of covert medication in patients with capacity.

Legal

The case of RM[66] involved very similar facts to Aaron's. RM had epilepsy, organic personality disorder, and organic delusional disorder, and he refused to accept anticonvulsants or other medication voluntarily. His condition improved with covert medication, but after this was disclosed at a tribunal hearing, he angrily stopped it and deteriorated, to the extent that he required restraint and seclusion (and was at risk of sudden death from a seizure). He improved again after covert medication was reinstated a few months later. He subsequently appealed for release from detention, and in advance of the hearing the hospital applied to prevent the disclosure of the covert medication to him at the hearing (it was mentioned only in an addendum to the medical report, which was given only to the judge and RM's solicitor). The tribunal judge held that disclosure would cause serious harm, and that prohibition was proportionate[67]; and that RM's solicitor could still 'take instructions on the themes' of the appeal.

RM's solicitor appealed against this prohibition order, and the Upper Tribunal set it aside on the ground that not knowing a crucial fact meant that the patient was unable to 'make an effective challenge to the decision to continue to detain him', as his misunderstanding that he was well without medication was a central element of his case for release. It went on trenchantly: 'His legal team will not be able to present the real case. They cannot disclose the covert medication. Nor can the medical witnesses or the tribunal. Everyone in the room will know what the patient does not. They will be reduced to performing a mere mummery. Justice will not be done at the hearing; it will only seem to be done. The real proceedings will have to be conducted out of the patient's sight and knowledge.'

Clinico-legal

The benefits in terms of improved patient state and staff safety, as well as avoidance of other measures, are clear. Although covert medication is not unlawful, it will only be practical to give it in scenarios where an incapacitous patient is expected to regain capacity and come to accept the medication voluntarily or to remain incapable but not to object to it (and by extension not to participate in any appeal hearing).

Ethical

The ethical argument for the use of covert medication is utilitarian: there will be a benefit to covertly medicating Aaron (his behaviour will improve) that outweighs the cost (deceiving Aaron and involving staff in the deception). Other benefits include reducing the risk of harm to others, avoiding greater restrictions on Aaron, and avoiding the use of force to medicate him.

Utilitarian reasoning is common in medicine and works well for short-term clinical encounters. It is problematic in longer-term treatment: what about the future cost to Aaron's care when Aaron finds out that he has been deceived? Cost-benefit analysis is also hampered by a lack of relevant information, particularly about unknown and unintended consequences. In this case, the team might never have proceeded had they anticipated that his lawyer might not support deception within a legal process.

Cost-benefit calculus is subject to the tendency to overlook costs that are uncomfortable to think about, such as treating Aaron as less than fully human, despite having capacity. Similarly, the

---

[66] *RM v St Andrew's Healthcare* [2010] UKUT 119.

[67] The relevant tests under Rule 14(2) of the *Tribunal Procedure (First-Tier Tribunal) (Health, Education and Social Care Chamber) Rules 2008* in E&W.

immediate benefit of not feeling afraid of Aaron may cause you to jump to the conclusion that covert medication is right.[68]

What is missing is Aaron's perspective, beyond his lack of insight and noncompliance. The cost of deceiving Aaron includes the indignity of being treated as a lesser person, who does not deserve the truth. People who are vulnerable, powerless, or low in status because of disability are most at risk of such deceit.[69]

A different ethical analysis might start with discussing the different values at play, including Aaron's. If Aaron would not engage, then a patient advocate, or a lawyer, could speak for him (which may also reduce his fear). Aaron needs to understand that staff are frightened of him, that his hostility must change, and that alternative interventions (e.g. a ward move or forced medication) can be legally imposed on him. He does not have to like this, but threatening people will not help him.

Conversations about values take time and may be personally difficult. Mental health professionals require training to help them to have difficult discussions with patients that involve conflict and anger, given that many 'ethical' tensions arise from a deep discomfort amongst staff with conflict, and a reluctance to accept that there may be no options for action that do not involve distress or disappointment.

It may be more respectful to forcibly medicate Aaron, rather than deceive him, even if this does infer short-term costs in terms of anger and distress, or even a ward move. These costs are significant, but the value to Aaron of being treated as a fully informed citizen is likely to cohere best with his sense of himself as a person who wants to make his own choices. There is a value to staff morale too in carrying out a difficult duty well.

---

[68] An example of an affect heuristic: see page 24.

[69] That is, deceit by others. In contrast, the powerful often deceive themselves to avoid awareness of the consequences of their actions—hence the importance (and danger) of 'speaking truth to power'.

21 Life-sentence prisoner– remission from hospital back to prison

Themes: *learning disability (p.110) and psychotic depression (p.72) [C]; prison transfer (p.506) and tribunal and parole hearing (p.512) [L]; decision on remission (p.588) [CL]; and prisoner patients (p.338) [E]*

Case description

Zack is a thirty-four-year-old man who has been transferred from prison for treatment in hospital; eight years into the fifteen-year-minimum term of a life sentence for the murder of his girlfriend. No psychiatric defence was raised at trial. In prison, Zack developed severe depression; he stopped eating and drinking, and had nihilistic delusions about his body rotting away; he also expressed suicidal ideation and self-harmed seriously.

Zack has previous convictions for common assault, indecent assault, and drug-related offences, but this is his first long sentence. On remand, a cognitive assessment found he had mild learning disability and he had special educational needs as a child. He struggles with reading and writing.

Zack complied with treatment and made a good recovery. He completed a variety of personality assessments: he scores only sixteen on the PCL-R, but his MMPI scores suggest significant borderline, dependent, and obsessional traits.

As the first CPA review meeting approaches, you and the team need to plan Zack's treatment and security needs.

Questions

1. What legal, clinico-legal, and ethical issues do his treatment options raise?
2. What treatment should you recommend at the CPA meeting?

Clinical

This case exemplifies the dual nature of forensic care: Zack needs both treatment for his mental disorder and interventions to reduce his risk of harm to others. You will need to formulate how his mild learning disability, likely personality disorder, and vulnerability to serious mood disorder contribute to the risk of violence. You will probably recommend psychological treatment to minimise expression of PD and LD, and the risk of another depressive episode.

Most psychological treatment planning starts with treating mental disorders, reducing distress, and improving general psychological function. In this case, it would be sensible to combine medication for depression with adjunctive cognitive therapy, to address depressive cognitions and persisting delusions.

Once Zack's mental state is settled and he has developed some insight into his depression, you can address his personality. NICE guidelines recommend both dialectical behaviour therapy (DBT) and mentalisation-based treatment (MBT) for borderline personality; many services offer the emotional coping skills module of DBT, followed by an MBT group. If Zack can learn emotional coping skills and the ability to self-reflect, this will enable him to make good use of (and cope with the stress of) offence-based work, which is also pursued in groups.

Offence-based work depends upon the formulation of the offences. Some clinicians would see his indecent assaults as distinct from other offending; some as linked and influenced by his LD. As significant is the meaning of the murder, motivated by sexual desire or jealousy or otherwise, since no mental disorder was put forward at the trial.

Cognitive-based interventions adapted for individuals with LD include pictorial information, tasks broken down, and simplified vocabulary. Treatment has to be individualised to meet Zack's needs; he may need more creative and skilled staff to deliver shorter sessions at a level he can comprehend over a longer timescale if risk reduction is to be achieved.

If he is able to cope in the prison environment, the later stages of rehabilitation can be carried out in prison.

Legal

Zack's mental illness was the basis for his transfer to hospital from prison; the law assumes he will return to prison as soon as mentally well. The time he has spent in secure hospital will count towards his sentence, although the therapies may not be accredited for risk reduction by the Prison Service.

In theory Zack could apply to be discharged from his section by a tribunal and request that he stay in hospital to await a parole hearing. However, this is only usually attempted if his minimum term is complete or nearly complete, there are clear plans for community rehabilitation, and the OM supports parole. As Zack has seven years of his minimum term remaining, he will almost certainly be remitted to prison.

Clinico-legal

Most psychological programmes have been developed in outpatient settings with nonforensic populations, and adapted for prison or secure hospital settings. There are varying degrees of standardisation and validation of these programmes.

Cognitive interventions have only recently been adapted for LD populations, and those available are not yet standardised or validated. Sex offender treatments are usually adapted versions of the mainstream programme, but it is unclear which components are most effective in reducing sexual recidivism in people with LD.

Ultimately the key decision clinico-legally is whether to recommend remission to prison, where Zack's mental disabilities may not receive adequate attention, or remaining in hospital, where he will not have access to some of the accredited programmes required for parole.

Ethical

Given the constraints on funding in the NHS and HSE, there is debate about how to ensure that prisoners gain treatment for mental disorders in ways that address their welfare needs (beneficence), prevent risky situations like suicide in prison (do no harm), and give fair access to secure psychiatric services.

Serving prisoners need expensive secure beds, but may occupy them for longer if the prison is reluctant to readmit them. Do they deserve those beds more than general psychiatric patients presenting high-risk behaviours?

It is sometimes argued that it is cruel, distressing, and unethical to remit a prisoner after recovery in hospital if he could benefit from longer-term rehabilitation in hospital. The counter-argument is that it is unjust effectively to given him better care than nonoffenders. Forensic services should have clinical ethics fora in which these issues can be discussed, and the underlying values explored.

This case also raises ethical questions about the provision of intensive and complex therapies which can only be offered effectively by highly trained and experienced therapists, who are not cheap to employ. Cheaper therapists might cause harm, and the evidence base for such other therapies is weak.

22

Use of social and occupational therapies in forensic psychiatry

Themes: *schizophrenia and violence (p.44) and occupational and social therapies (pp.226-229) [C]; consent to such treatment (p.482) [L, CL]; and coercion and encouragement (p.324) and fairness in the standard of expected behaviour (p.330) [E]*

Case description

Bob is a patient in a low secure service. He developed schizophrenia in his twenties when at college, and has had repeated relapses in the subsequent twenty years. These have been triggered by alcohol abuse, but more often by family rows and high expressed emotion. Bob lives with his mother who is supportive but also highly anxious. She misuses alcohol sometimes, and takes overdoses, which upsets Bob and can trigger a relapse. There have also been long periods when both Bob and his mother are well and able to enjoy life together.

Bob's secure admission followed a relapse during which he attacked his mother, causing multiple cuts and bruises; he was also very aggressive to the police and ambulance staff. He had never done anything like this before. He eventually pleaded guilty to assault, and received an unrestricted hospital order.

Bob's treatment has gone well, and he has complied throughout with medication and ward regimes. He has a particularly good relationship with the OT assistant, and has developed a keen interest in vegetable gardening. However, he refuses to take part in ward social activities, or psycho-educational courses. Recently he refused to participate in an alcohol misuse group, arguing that it is his mother, not he, who has the problem with alcohol.

Questions

1. What clinical, legal, clinico-legal, and ethical issues are raised by the case?

> **Clinical**
>
> Developing pro-social skills is a key part of rehabilitating offenders; social and occupational therapies are just as important as medical and psychological therapies for recovery and risk reduction.
>
> By working well with the ward OTA, Bob effectively interacts pro-socially with another person based upon his strengths, not his vulnerabilities. The OTA can help Bob recognise his risk to others and understand his recovery, and perhaps informally cover some social and educational topics, which should be fed back to the team regularly.

Try to understand the reasons for Bob's refusal of other forms of treatment. It might reflect social phobia and anxiety. In the case of the substance misuse group, it may represent unresolved distress about his mother's alcohol use, which could be a useful starting point for a discussion about their relationship. In short, the refusal should be a point for reflection and discussion, not simply a reason to be coercive.

Occupational therapies can sometimes be overlooked in the treatment of forensic patients, who often have good self-care skills, and where the offence was not casually related to occupational issues. Nevertheless, OT is a holistic, person-centred and strengths-based approach to rehabilitation that can sidestep much of the resistance and anxiety often associated with other forms of treatment.

Legal and clinico-legal

Although Bob cannot be compelled to participate meaningfully in other treatments, you may want to talk frankly with him about how refusal may be regarded by the MoJ and tribunal. It is widely believed that noncompliant patients recover slower and are more likely to relapse, although there is little evidence for this, and some tribunals will insist certain work is completed before considering release.

Bob's OT is part of the multidisciplinary care plan, not separate from it. The OTA's views should be incorporated into CPA reports, and into psychiatric reports for hearings.

Ethical

Bob has consented to the gardening project; he may need reminding that the OTA is part of the team, and feeds back to them. Supporting Bob's interest in gardening is respectful of his choices and autonomy. Likewise, his reasons for refusal to undertake other treatments should be understood and respected, while advising him of the likely consequences.

Patients like Bob may face injustice by being held to a higher standard of 'good behaviour' than others, with any hint of antisocial behaviour or attitudes being given undue weight. The OTA, seen as less of an authority figure, may be in the best place to explain this and to help Bob make sensible yet authentic choices.

23

Working with public protection arrangements

Themes: *restricted patient and recall decisions (p.588) and public protection arrangements (p.592) [C]; duties to co-operate and right to disclose (p.588-593) [L]; veracity of information in risk assessment (p.356) [CL]; and conflicting duties (p.298) and ethics of disclosure (p.320) [E]*

Case description

James made good progress in your MSU after receiving a restriction order for GBH. He complied with depot medication and has been conditionally discharged to a hostel for ex-offenders with mental illness. A level 2 MAPP meeting has been called. James consents to you disclosing his diagnosis, his care plan including the hostel location, and a few details of his history.

A police officer at the meeting says, 'He sounds like a James we interviewed several times three years ago about the murders of two women. They have not been solved. If this is the same guy, he also has a long history of domestic violence, but his ex-partner wouldn't press charges. We might come and interview him again.'

James's social worker is also at the meeting. She suggests that his latest risk-assessment should be shared, to assist in deliberations. She also expresses the view that, on the basis of the police officer's information, you should contact the MoJ and recommend recalling James to hospital.

Questions

1. What are the clinical, legal, clinico-legal, and ethical issues in the case?
2. Should you agree to the police officer's request and the social worker's suggestions?
3. Are there any justifiable alternative courses of action?

Clinical

You have responsibility for James' treatment and welfare, but also for public protection. If it concerns the same man, the information from the police would significantly alter your risk assessment. However, until the uncertainty over whether it is the same James is resolved, there is no clinical rationale for sharing information other than based upon your prior assessment of James and his consent.

As regards the police interviewing James, you may give an opinion on his fitness for interview (and any safeguards you might recommend) in the usual way.

Legal

The statutes that established the MAPPA and PPANI require NHS bodies to co-operate with other relevant agencies, and trusts delegate this duty to the employees they designate to represent them. However, this is not a duty to accede to all requests by MAPPA partners, or a duty to share information (or make disclosures) beyond the ordinary rules of confidentiality that apply in other situations.

Clinico-legal

To share the risk assessment without James' consent, you would need evidence that disclosing this additional information was the minimum necessary to protect others from a significant risk of serious harm (e.g. by facilitating prosecution for a serious crime). Given the uncertainty about the identity of the police suspect, this threshold is not currently met. You therefore have time to seek James' consent while the suspect's identity is confirmed.

If it is confirmed, your updated risk-assessment might lead you to decide to recommend recall, if the risk cannot be safely managed in the community (assuming he is not arrested and charged, which would take the matter out of your hands). Until then, however, there is not enough to justify even a discussion with the MoJ. Its own guidance[70] makes clear that, while clinical supervisors should never overlook problems or information for fear of jeopardising the patient's progress, the threshold for an immediate report is 'being accused of, charged with, or convicted of a serious offence or an offence similar to the index offence', which has not yet occurred.

You should inform the MAPP meeting that you and your team will review your position on recall once you have confirmation of identity. If the police or others are unhappy with this, you can remind them that they are free to contact the MoJ themselves.

Ethical

Your duties towards James as his doctor may conflict with your duties to others. There may also be conflict between your duties and those of the police and probation.

One principle of information-sharing is to share only the minimum necessary for the issue in question. You have decided what it is currently appropriate to share, and obtained James' consent to this. Even if you now believe (because you are sufficiently sure that he is the same James even without formal confirmation) that the risk of harm he poses is substantially higher than you had previously thought, does the management of that risk require further information to be shared with the police?

It may not, in that the police may already have enough to be able to take their own actions, such as circulating his details and address to the local neighbourhood police team, liaising with hostel staff on a regular basis, or even arranging surveillance. Even if it does, is the urgency sufficiently great to justify disclosing before first seeking James' consent to whatever additional disclosure you now propose?

If you do decide to make further disclosures to the meeting, it is very unlikely that you could justify sharing the entire risk-assessment document, as opposed to sharing selected relevant facts and the overall summary and conclusions.

The police do not need your agreement to interview James again; they now know his address, as you have shared this with his consent, and can contact him directly. Your duty to co-operate does not extend to facilitating an interview when there is no obstacle to the police doing this themselves.

[70] MoJ (2009) *Guidance for Clinical Supervisors*, May.

24 Relationship with justice ministry—partnership or productive tension?

Themes: *patient conditionally discharged (p.589) and borderline personality disorder and drug use (pp.76, 84) [C]; recall to hospital (p.589) [L]; information disclosure and timing (p.592) [CL]; and conflicting values of patient welfare and public protection (p.314; p.352) [E]*

Case description

You are the clinician responsible for treating John, who was conditionally discharged a year ago. His conditions include living in a twenty-four-hour-staffed hostel, complying with medication, abstaining from drugs, and providing urine samples for testing. He has borderline PD, with labile mood and transient psychotic episodes, plus a chaotic pattern of drug use. The care plan has reduced his disorganisation and improved his nutrition and his ability to look after himself, but has not stopped his drug use altogether.

He left the hostel without staff agreement three days ago, and has not answered his mobile phone. None of his known acquaintances can say where he is. You reported him missing after twenty-four hours, but the police have not located him and will take no further action without more information.

John has absconded many times before, and has usually been incommunicado. However, this is the longest absence since discharge. You suspect that one of the triggers was an argument with his girlfriend that led to her leaving him the day before he disappeared.

Your practice up to now has been to inform the MoJ a day or two after he has left the hostel, once he has made contact; you understand the situation; and you have a plan for managing it. His care co-ordinator thinks you should inform the MoJ now, but you are concerned that he will then be recalled to hospital for breaching his conditions of discharge, and you do not want this to happen because you do not think his behaviour is the direct result of a medical condition that could be successfully treated through further care in hospital.

Questions

1. What are the clinical, legal, clinico-legal, and ethical issues in the case?
2. What will you do?

Clinical

Your clinical opinion is informed by your prior knowledge of John. However, you lack information about his current mental state, beyond your hypothesis about him being distressed by his girlfriend leaving him. Clearly you need to see John, or at least hear from someone who has seen him, to form an opinion on his current condition, and therefore the need (or not) for readmission to hospital.

Legal

The only relevant issue at this stage is the legal power of recall of the MoJ. Although this is usually initiated on the recommendation of a clinician, this is not essential. The MoJ has wide discretion to decide whether or when to recall, and can take into account evidence of risk unconnected with mental disorder.[71]

Clinico-legal

Considered as a binary decision, there is no question that you must inform the MoJ of John's absence. You might delay further, but as more time has already passed than John has been absent for before, this would be difficult to justify.

You could inform the MoJ while asking them to wait for further information before making a decision. If you do so, be prepared to explain what the scenario could be in which recall would not be necessary, and why you think such scenarios are more likely than ones involving significant risk to others. Ultimately, though, the decision is not yours.

In the longer-term, this is an opportunity to build a stronger working relationship with the relevant caseworkers and managers at the ministry. You can demonstrate to them that you are open and trustworthy, and that you are aware of, and respect, their perspective and their primary duty, even though it may sometimes conflict with your own. This should make it more likely that, even if they do not accept your argument not to recall the patient on this occasion, they will do so in future.

Ethical

The proposition that clinicians and the MoJ work 'in partnership' in respect of patients is at best overstated, since partnership requires common values and goals. Most MoJ staff and most clinicians operate according to quite different models: the primary concern of the former is public safety; that of clinicians, their patient's welfare. Hence the relationship is characterised by productive tension as much as by partnership.[72]

Clinicians have a duty to be honest and truthful, which can at times conflict with acting in the patient's best interest if there are concerns that shared information will cause the MoJ or others to act counter-therapeutically. The solution is not to conceal information unethically, but to build relationships with the MoJ caseworkers that enable you to influence their decision-making so as to make it more therapeutic.

[71] *R(MM) v Secretary of State for the Home Department* [2007] EWCA Civ 687 at paragraph 50; the judgment, only binding in E&W, refers to a belief 'on reasonable grounds that something has happened, or information has emerged, of sufficient significance to justify recalling the patient'.

[72] Eastman N (2006) Can there be true partnership between clinicians and the Home Office in managing 'restricted' patients?, *Advances in Psychiatric Treatment* (12): 459–461.

Themes: *borderline personality disorder with transient psychoses (p.84) and formulation of behaviour (p.146) [C]; power to enforce community treatment (p.488) [L]; differences from recall under restriction order (p.589) [CL]; and tension with patient autonomy (p.331) [E]*

Case description

Rachelle is a nineteen-year-old woman with severe borderline personality disorder who frequently experiences transient psychotic episodes when under stress and/or when using cannabis. After treatment in a low secure ward, including quetiapine and a year-long course of DBT, she is discharged to your care at a local hostel, under a CTO[73]). One of the conditions of the CTO is that she must reside at the hostel and abide by its rules.

Within the first two weeks, her relationship with hostel staff begins to break down. She misses sessions with her hostel keyworker, stays out after her agreed 'curfew' time, and does not attend follow-up DBT sessions at the hospital. She turns up late (or not at all) to collect quetiapine from hostel staff; and they think she often throws it away. She also alleged that a hostel staff member assaulted her: he was suspended during police interviews and an internal investigation, then returned to work once he had been exonerated after a few days.

You and Rachelle's Community Psychiatric Nurse (CPN) review her at the hostel; you are both sure that she is mentally well, despite the suspected noncompliance with quetiapine.

The hostel manager tells you that, in her view, the placement is failing; and, if Rachelle's behaviour does not change, she will evict her. She and the CPN urge you to recall her to hospital whilst an alternative placement is sought.

Questions

1. What justifiable alternative courses of action are there?
2. What should you do?
3. Would your answer differ if she were instead conditionally discharged under a restriction order?
4. What other the clinical, legal, clinico-legal, and ethical issues in the case?

Clinical

One possible formulation of Rachelle's behaviour is that she does not have a trusting relationship with hostel staff (or you), does not feel safe or psychologically contained there, and is trying to force a return to hospital because she has felt safe there in the past. It might also be that recalling her would replicate past instances of her being punished for misbehaviour by detention in an institution.

---

[73] Or in Scotland, a Compulsory Treatment Order (CTO) covering treatment in the community as well as (or instead of) in hospital. Neither type of CTO is available in Northern Ireland; the closest equivalent, guardianship, is not applicable to patients with personality disorder alone.

If it is safe to do so, respond to her behaviour by assisting her to deal with the consequences of her actions, rather than taking over responsibility. This could include, for example, the CPN helping her arrange for storage of her belongings before eviction, going with her to the local housing department or homeless persons' unit to help her apply for emergency accommodation, or helping her to negotiate a temporary stay with a friend or family member.

Legal

In E&W, recall is the only way to enforce medication, except in an emergency.[74] In Scotland, a CTO covering community treatment allows reasonable force to be used to administer it: for example, by taking Rachelle to hospital for up to six hours for medication to be administered, or for her to attend a DBT follow-up session, provided that the CTO explicitly authorises this.

Clinico-legal

Rachelle's case highlights the dual nature of the CTO: it is simultaneously a device to ensure she receives appropriate treatment, and that she does not harm others. Imposing conditions that can lead to a clinical response (e.g. readmission to hospital) because of behaviour that might not be directly related to mental disorder could, however, result in a legal challenge, either at a tribunal or by judicial review.

In addressing recall, it is important to consider whether the issues of concern relate to mental disorder and the need for inpatient treatment (which may be needed even if they are not yet symptomatic). If there is evidence that poor compliance with quetiapine has usually led to Rachelle experiencing another transient psychotic episode, that could justify a decision to recall her. Similarly, if the hostel manager gives notice of eviction, and such stress has in the past caused a psychotic episode, then recall might be warranted. In Scotland, depending upon the formulation of Rachelle's behaviour, and the relevance of her taking responsibility for her own behaviour, the exercise of reasonable force might be an appropriate option.

The complication where the patient is under a restriction order is that the decision to recall is made by the relevant Minister, not by you alone, using subtly different criteria. While there must still be evidence of mental disorder of a nature or degree warranting detention,[75] there does not need to have been a change in the patient's mental state in order to justify recall. An elevation of the risk of harm to others is sufficient, provided the risk is linked to mental disorder, even if the reason for the elevation is not (e.g. an external stressful event, or the use of illicit drugs).

Ethical

The tension here may be between what you suspect Rachelle's wishes to be, her expressed wishes, and what you believe is in her best interest. Rachelle may, for example, benefit in the short-term from being recalled, but it may have a longer-term negative impact upon her recovery and exercise of autonomy. Developing and sharing a clinical formulation should be the starting point for considering the competing issues.

[74] Where the patient lacks capacity and enforced treatment is proportionate and immediately necessary to prevent harm.
[75] *Winterwerp v Netherlands* (1979), which must include up-to-date evidence that the legal criteria for detention are met: *R(B) v MHRT* [2002] All ER 304—except in an emergency: *K v UK* (1998).

Supporting a court diversion scheme via consultation

Case description

You are the psychiatrist for the liaison and diversion service at a local Sheriff Court. A nurse specialist calls you to explain that they have seen and given evidence about a young man charged with ABH who has been behaving oddly in the cells. His electronic NHS records show he was admitted briefly to hospital last year for a suspected psychotic episode, but his behaviour returned rapidly to normal without treatment and there was no evidence of drug use.

He appears to misunderstand basic questions, often ignores the questioner, appears disorientated and nonchalant about the serious charge he faces, and misunderstands the court process. The nurse thinks he is unfit to plead, even without any clear symptoms of psychosis, mood disorder, or other mental illness. They told the court that they could not make a diagnosis or explain his behaviour at this stage; the Sheriff's response was to dismiss their opinion and to insist that he be reassessed by a psychiatrist (you) who 'should complete a full report on his fitness to plead and his behaviour in relation to the alleged assault, including giving any a diagnosis and recommendation for disposal'.

Questions

1. Will you see the defendant?
2. What advice would you give to the court, either having or not having seen the defendant?
3. What other clinical, legal, clinico-legal, and ethical issues in the case?

Clinical

You should go through the information available from the nurse, and their reasoning, particularly if you are not already familiar with their work. Unless you and they uncover a mistake or oversight, however, you should reaffirm their professional opinion. You do not need to see the patient yourself to do this, provided you are confident of their opinion.

Legal

The procedure for determining fitness to plead in the High Court or Crown Court is that medical practitioners provide written or oral evidence. In lower courts, the procedure may be less formal, but evidence from a medical practitioner will still be needed if hospital treatment is recommended. Even if the court accepts the nurse's opinion on unfitness, it will need medical evidence to act on.

In E&W, confusingly, Magistrates' Courts do not have a proper procedure for determining fitness to plead, but if the court is satisfied the defendant is unfit to plead, in some circumstances, it can make a hospital order (absent conviction).

Clinico-legal and ethical

Although clinically there is no need to reassess, it may allay the Sheriff's concerns (however ill-founded) if you choose to see the defendant and give a second opinion. However, establishing firmly a new diagnosis, or explaining behaviour at a material time, will require the court to commission formally a forensic psychiatric report; a court diversion team cannot usually provide this. You should advise the Sheriff how to request it.

More generally, your role as a consultant or supervisor to court diversion colleagues should be explicitly agreed (e.g. within the service operational policy and at the start of supervision). You should ensure that the author of any report uses an agreed form of words detailing your involvement. You should also keep a record of the advice you give.

It is laudable that the Sheriff wants to understand the defendant's odd behaviour, in case it represents something that would make trial or conviction unjust. However, it is wrong to leap to the assumption that it must be related to mental disorder. Moreover, the Sheriff may conflate fitness to plead (which relates to the defendant's functional ability on the day) with diagnosis and its impact on behaviour (which requires a longitudinal perspective and a more thorough assessment).

Your role here is not as either a professional or an expert witness. It is not your opinion that is offered to the court, but you can express your support for your colleague's opinion and the method by which they have reached that opinion (if this accords with your view). If you were required to give evidence about your own opinion, you would need to be clear about the nature of your role and avoid giving definite opinions about diagnosis or formulation, as you have not personally assessed the defendant. If under pressure you do give opinions, then you should explain the limits placed on your opinion by not directly assessing the defendant, and be able to justify your view.

27 | Borderline PD and severe self-harm—prison or hospital?

Themes: *borderline PD (p.84), high-risk self-harm or suicide (p.176), prison unable to manage (p.270), and specialist PD services (p.260) [C]; prison transfer (p.506), right to life (p.516), and negligence (p.548) [L]; the least-restrictive principle in practice (p.471) [CL]; and equivalence in prison services (p.314) [E]*

Case description

Lucas is a twenty-seven-year-old man serving an indeterminate sentence for public protection, for wounding with intent, his twenty-first conviction. He is three years over his minimum term but remains in a category B prison. He is diagnosed with borderline personality disorder and substance-induced psychotic episodes. During his sentence, he has repeatedly tried to hang himself, and twice been transferred to psychiatric hospital; both times, he then tried to escape, once climbing onto the roof of the secure hospital. He is currently prescribed the maximum dose of a long-acting antipsychotic injection, which he accepts.

He has attempted hanging twice in the last week; last time, he was cyanotic when officers entered in his cell. He intends to keep trying until he is released from prison. He has also cut himself with plastic shards, and swallowed his toothbrush.

You are the psychiatrist in the prison's mental health in-reach team. You have transferred him to the hospital wing, and adopted a suicide prevention care plan. You rereferred him to the MSU two months ago, which assessed him and concluded he would not benefit from further hospital treatment, citing NICE guidelines, while noting he was accepting treatment in prison.

You are under pressure from healthcare and prison colleagues to refer him again. They believe that his behaviour cannot be adequately managed in prison, and that he is vulnerable to bullying by other inmates. His mother has contacted the local press to complain about the prison's care of her son.

Questions

1. What are the clinical, legal, clinico-legal, and ethical issues in this case?
2. How do you manage the disagreement with the hospital?
3. What can you do if agreement cannot be reached?

Clinical

Self-harm in prison is a common manifestation of poor distress tolerance and emotional dysregulation, and prisons often find it difficult to manage, especially if it is repetitive and severe.

Look at information about the OPD pathway in prisons, and consider whether Lucas would benefit from some of the prison services for BPD, if available locally. There are two MSUs in the OPD pathways that specialise in working with offenders with PD (unlike the local MSUs from which he tried to escape).

Convening a case discussion with relevant professionals and officers from the prison, local MSU, and the OPD pathway should assist in clarifying the options available, and the benefits and risks of each, and then agreeing which to pursue and when to review its effectiveness.

Legal

Transfer to hospital is of course possible, if the hospital agrees that appropriate treatment is available (with some likelihood of benefit in Scotland and RoI).

The main risk for Lucas is suicide. Failing to prevent persons dying in custody may be a breach of their right to life under article 2 ECHR: this imposes a positive obligation on the prison, prison healthcare, and hospital to protect him while in their care. Each must take appropriate steps to safeguard any persons they know (or should have known) faces a 'real and immediate' risk to their life (see case 5.1 concerning negligence).

Clinico-legal

In this scenario, applying the principle of least-restrictive treatment is complex, because informal treatment in prison may involve more restrictions than treatment under section in hospital. On the other hand, spending time in hospital whilst on an indeterminate sentence can lengthen the overall sentence because it delays participation in the prison programmes necessary to progress and be considered for parole.

Ethical

Your duty as a doctor is to provide the most appropriate care, and to arrange care elsewhere if it cannot be provided in prison. As a senior professional, you will also be expected to manage conflict between different professional groups and services, and to act in Lucas's best interests whilst minimising the impact of your and others' personal values.

The manifestations of Lucas's mental disorder (in the form of suicide attempts) are closely related to the detention itself, and to experiences of setback, disappointment, and rejection. Some may perceive this as conscious manipulation on his part, or even as evidence that there is not a 'genuine' mental disorder. It is not easy to manage this in a way that allows people to think and reflect, and avoid acting on their emotional reaction to his behaviour.

If, after discussion, you believe that transfer to hospital is necessary, but the relevant local or specialist MSU declines him, you will need to manage your response carefully. Your duty of care does not end because you sent the referral. You may need to have further discussion with more senior clinicians and managers at the hospital, whilst continuing to coordinate care in prison.

B.2
Ethical cases

Right or duty to disclose defence report in criminal law context

Themes: *assessment for defence (p.666), memory impairment in depression (p.636), malingering (p.118), and psychopathy (p.90) [C]; fraud (p.427) and breach of professional confidence (p.320) [L, CL]; and impartiality (p.674) and disclosing defence report (p.660) [E]*

Case description

Louis is a sixty-two-year-old man charged with fraud. He has three previous fraud convictions, and received an eight-year sentence for the last of them. His solicitors become concerned that he is depressed and has memory impairment, and ask you to provide an opinion on his ability to give instructions, and on any mental disorder that might be relevant in mitigation if convicted.

You assess Louis, who is affable, warm, co-operative, and in good physical health. He describes mild memory loss, weight loss, and early morning wakening, and occasional thoughts of suicide relating to his fear of renewed imprisonment. He says he was married but is no longer in touch with his wife and adult children.

You are an older male psychiatrist. You ask a psychologist colleague, Dr Friedan, who happens to be a young woman, to assess Louis's memory and executive function to rule out organic disorder. Dr Friedan sees him twice, then tells you that Louis's tests do not suggest that he has a dementing illness, or any other organic brain disorder. She also says they suggest he may be malingering. She adds that he was sexually intimidating, asking her intimate questions, and becoming hostile when she would not answer or agree to go out with him.

You ask to see Louis's GP notes. These reveal only that Louis also has several convictions for drunk driving, and that he was fined for an assault on his ex-wife.

Questions

1. What are the clinical, legal, clinico-legal, and ethical issues in the case?

> ### Clinical
> You and Dr Friedan have ruled out major mental illness, and any dementia or other organic disorder. Dr Friedan's report suggests it may not be safe to rely upon Louis's self-report, including in regard to symptoms of minor depression.
>
> Your assessments have also demonstrated that Louis presents differently with a younger female professional, and that, based on his suggested malingering, he may be more characterologically dishonest than he first appears. Repeated fraud convictions, drunk driving, and assault, combined with

misogyny and an attempt to charm the psychologist could indicate a mild degree of psychopathy. On the other hand, his behaviour is consistent with the values and attitudes of certain older 'macho' men, and might have been culturally acceptable when he was growing up.

You may need to ensure that your new suspiciousness of Louis does not lead you to overlook genuine depressive symptoms, if they emerge at a later stage: Louis' age, sex, social isolation, and impending prosecution put him at risk of adjustment disorder and depression.

Legal and clinico-legal

You can fulfil your instructions by writing a report that states that there is no evidence of mental illness or organic brain disorder, and that there is no reason to think Louis incapable of instructing solicitors.

Of course, Louis's lawyers have a duty to explore any possible line of defence. And it is not uncommon for lawyers to obtain psychiatric reports as part of case preparation, in order to work out a strategy. In this case, it appears that they are on a 'fishing expedition' to find any psychiatric condition that might help his case.

Your duty is to the court, to provide impartial, objective, and truthful expert testimony. You should never adjust or alter your opinion to suit the defence posture. If the lawyers do not like your opinion, they do not have to use your report.

In some situations, you may have an additional duty to warn potential victims,[1] but as Louis does not have any current partner, there is no identifiable victim to warn.

Ethical

In assessing Louis according to your instructions, you have unearthed possible additional evidence of dishonesty (which might be relevant to the trial) and of bad character (which might be relevant at sentencing, if he is convicted). You should put this in your report if it is relevant to your opinion on his condition and ability to give instructions, notwithstanding the uses to which it might be put by the court, but you should not include it if it is not relevant to your opinion.

If you do include it, Louis' solicitors are likely not to use your report. In this case, that would probably be the end of the matter, but if you believed that the trial would be unjust if the court were unaware of your evidence (e.g. if it were a trial for murder and you had uncovered evidence of a possible previous attempt by Louis on the victim's life), you might decide that the public interest in disclosure is sufficient to justify a breach of confidence on your part.[2]

---

[1] *Palmer v Tees Health Authority* [1999] All ER 722: see ethics case 14 for an exploration of this.

[2] In *R v Crozier* [1991] CrimLR 138, the judge found that Dr Crozier's breach of confidence was justified by the magnitude and severity of the risk of harm that he sought to prevent. You cannot assume that a court would think similarly in Louis's trial for fraud.

Right or duty to breach confidence in civil law context

Themes: *Huntington's Disease (p.116) [C]; duty of confidentiality (p.320) and negligence (p.548) [L]; demonstrating a reasoned decision (p.684) [CL]; and ethics of disclosure (p.320) [E]*

Case description

Arnold, a late-middle-aged man with no history previously of violence, is admitted to your MSU after conviction of GBH for seriously assaulting his wife. He suffers from depression, complicated apparently by narcissistic traits (not amounting to personality disorders (PD)). His wife has since died from an unrelated disease.

During the admission, he begins to show choreiform movements that worsen slowly but progressively. A neurological examination and MRI scan suggest Huntington's disease (HD), which is confirmed by genetic testing, to which he consents. In hindsight, you consider his depression to have been the initial presentation of Huntington's, which could well have predisposed him to violence.

The geneticist tells you that each of his two adult daughters has a 50% chance of having inherited the condition. They have participated in family therapy with their father at your unit, and you know they are both planning to start families.

Arnold refuses consent to disclosure of his condition to his children, and you are satisfied that he has the mental capacity to do so.

Questions

1. Can you—and if so, should you—breach his confidentiality and tell his children of his diagnosis?
2. What other clinical, legal, clinico-legal, and ethical issues arise in the case?

Clinical

All reasonable attempts must first be made to ensure Arnold fully understands, and has considered in detail, the ramifications of his decision, including the consequences for his children and potential grandchildren. This includes the impact on the family therapy currently underway, and on his relationship with his children if and when they discover for themselves that they have the disease. Also, his HD will now certainly be relevant to his discharge planning, which may thereby become known by the family.

If the decision is taken to breach Arnold's confidence then there is a significant risk of undermining the trust inherent in the doctor-patient relationship. But not breaching could undermine the trust between the family and the team.

Legal

The legal questions are whether there are *sufficient grounds* to breach Arnold's medical confidentiality, and even whether there is a *duty* to breach.

The precise grounds to be considered, and the threshold for the *right* to breach, may vary from one jurisdiction to another, but all centre firstly on whether there is 'a significant risk of serious harm to others'[3] if no disclosure were to be made. A related question is whether either disclosing *without* clear evidence of such a risk, or not disclosing *despite* such evidence, might give rise to negligence proceedings or a GMC/IMC investigation. A further question is whether you owe a *duty* to disclose to the children, either 'as third parties' or because they have been made 'patients' by way of the family therapy.

Whether your grounds are sufficient to justify your decision in either direction will turn on factual details, such as whether the loss of the chance to have genetic testing and to prepare oneself before the onset of HD can count in law as 'serious harm' from the perspective of one of the affected children, or perhaps whether the information would make the difference between that child choosing not to conceive and having a (grand)child with a 50% probability of developing a seriously harmful condition. And, probably crucially, upon whether you 'weighed' the factors reasonably.[4]

If you do not disclose, if and when his children later find out, they might seek to sue you in negligence, arguing that you owed them a duty of care because of their involvement in family therapy and in their father's CPA meetings. They might also sue you, and the genetics team, for failure to prevent a 'wrongful birth': the birth of a child you would not have conceived (or from a pregnancy you would have terminated) had the genetic test results been disclosed to you in time.[5] These questions raise broad policy considerations about the scope of duties to third parties (and how remote those third parties can be from the patient/proband undergoing genetic testing), and the impact of adopting them on the practice of medicine.

Clinico-legal

A defensible process for addressing this question is essential, ensuring that all perspectives are taken into consideration, and reasonably weighed, and that relevant professional guidance is applied.

Whatever decision is made, professional or legal challenge is a distinct possibility, and to minimise further anguish for Arnold and his family (and yourself), it will be important that you follow a process that is explicitly reasoned and seen to be fair. This may include, for example, you or other team members discussing the issue with Arnold in depth on multiple occasions; speaking to his children to get an understanding of their perspectives, beliefs, and wishes insofar as this is possible without at this stage disclosing Arnold's diagnosis of HD; and discussing the issues within your team to explore various perspectives.

Certainly, this is a case that falls into a category where advice should be taken from the legal department of your hospital. You may also properly seek advice from senior medical management, as well as from your Clinical Ethics Committee (if one is available).[6] You should also consult your medical defence body.

---

[3] See *W v Egdell* [1990] 1 ALL ER 835, and article 8 of the ECHR.

[4] Where the aversion of harm by the disclosure substantially outweighs the patient's claim to confidentiality, guidance (Medicine JCoGi 2019. *Consent and Confidentiality in Genomic Medicine*, Report of Royal College of Physicians and Royal College of Pathologists UK) makes clear that doctors have a professional, and since *ABC v St George's Healthcare NHS Trust and others* [2020] EWHC 455, probably a legal, duty 'to weigh'.

[5] The other category of 'wrongful birth' follows a negligently performed sterilisation or vasectomy, when the parents can claim for the pain, incapacity, and distress of an unwanted pregnancy, and for the loss of their right to control the size of their family, and, if the child is disabled, also for the costs of caring for them: *Rees v Darlington Memorial Hospital NHS Trust* [2003] UKHL 52.

[6] In *ABC v St George's Healthcare NHS Trust* it was evidentially crucial to the defence that such weighing was evident from the local Clinical Ethics Committee minutes (which were legally discoverable).

Ethical

Conventional bioethical approaches can provide a framework for discussing the legal questions, but even approaches that set out principles to follow[7] cannot offer a clear answer. However, so-called dialogical[8] approaches can help structure the process so as to maximise the chances of an answer emerging which is recognised as legitimate by all parties.

This case involves clear conflicts between Arnold's interests (in confidentiality, in having control over personal information, and in protecting himself from further anticipated opprobrium from his children) and his children's (in knowing that they may carry the Huntington's gene, and being able to make informed choices about whether to be tested and whether to have children themselves). There is also a conflict of interest between you and Arnold, in that you may wish to be relieved of the burden of knowledge that you are unable to share, and which you may one day be attacked for not having shared.

There is arguably an accelerating trend towards greater recognition of patient autonomy in Anglo-Saxon jurisdictions. But in this case the concept of autonomy helps little: the relevant ethical tension is between the autonomy of one party (Arnold) and that of others (his children).

Honesty is a core professional standard. Taken narrowly you can be honest to your patient if you respect their wishes, but this ignores your professional interactions with his family. Maintaining honesty with his family is impossible without disclosing the diagnosis. This may be justifiable but may be complicated if you are asked direct questions by his family about his health in professional meetings.

There is a possibility that, were one or more of his children to develop HD later in life, as with Arnold, their condition might present with depression or other abnormalities of mental state associated with an increased risk of violence towards others. From the perspective of your duty to protect the public, this could be a potential concern, and a further reason to seek disclosure of the genetic test results. However, it is a weak argument in that the probability of this scenario is very difficult to estimate, and likely to be low, as well as very distant in time.

---

[7] See for example Beauchamp T L and Childress T F (2013) *Principles of Biomedical Ethics*, Oxford University Press.

[8] Rudnick A (2002) The ground of dialogical bioethics, Health Care Analysis 10: 391–402.

3 Duty to supervise a patient in the community

Themes: *community forensic supervision (p.266)[C]; legal duty to treat (p.552), employment contract liability (p.557), and Bolam test (p.550) [L]; disagreement with tribunal decision (p.512) [CL]; and balancing duties to patient and public (p.296) [E]*

Case description

You are the consultant in a community forensic team. You have been referred Nick, who was admitted to a high-security hospital under a restricted hospital order four years ago, after conviction for manslaughter by 'diminished responsibility' of his female partner. He has schizophrenia, which has responded well to clozapine, and narcissistic PD, which has not responded to psychological treatment.

He was referred because a tribunal ordered 'conditional discharge' against the recommendations of the high secure team. It accepted the argument of an independent forensic psychiatrist that continued detention would not benefit him, and would worsen expression of his narcissistic traits. It deferred the discharge while a supervising psychiatrist was identified.

You assess him and, based upon his records, your interview and his behaviour in hospital, you come to the same conclusion as his treating team: that he remains at high risk of seriously assaulting or killing any woman with whom he forms a relationship. You also believe that he will not co-operate later with community supervision. You are unwilling to take on responsibility for his care.

His solicitor contacts you and asks about your reasons for refusal. She cites case law[9] in which it was found to be a breach of human rights not to facilitate the discharge of a patient whom a tribunal had decided should no longer be liable to detention. Your clinical director also contacts you, asking whether the hospital could be legally liable (given its duty to provide after-care[10]), and offering help and support with your decision.

Questions

1. Would it be legally and ethically defensible for you to refuse to take on Nick's care?
2. How should you respond to the solicitor's and clinical director's enquiries?
3. What else might you consider doing?
4. What other clinical, legal, clinico-legal, and ethical issues arise in the case?

---

[9] *Johnson v United Kingdom* (1997) 27 EHRR 296.
[10] Under s117 MHA in E&W, art112,113 MHNIO, and ss25–27 MHCTA in Scotland. There is no comparable duty to provide aftercare in RoI. This assumes that the hospital is a catchment area NHS service and not an independent hospital, which if it did not provide inpatient treatment might not be under any duty to take a patient on for treatment after discharge to the community.

> **Clinical**
> You have conducted a sound clinical assessment to reach your opinion, and your reasoning should be clearly set out.

> **Legal**
> You have individual legal and professional duties as a *doctor*, and separate legal duties that apply to you as an NHS/HSE *employee*. And there could be conflict between the two.
>
> The duty to provide after-care in the UK only applies to the NHS Trust, not to you as an individual clinician. However, were your employer to accept responsibility for treating Nick, and then to allocate you as the clinician responsible for delivering that treatment, your continued refusal could amount to a breach of your contract of employment, which might give rise to disciplinary proceedings and possibly also to professional proceedings at the GMC/IMC (although that is not (yet) the situation here).
>
> The legal test of whether a refusal to treat Nick would be negligent is the current version of the *Bolam* test[11]: is your professional practice in accordance with a practice accepted as proper by a body of responsible and skilled medical opinion?
>
> Case law makes clear that the Trust's duty is to make reasonable endeavours to comply with the proposed conditions.[12] If after doing so it cannot facilitate discharge subject to them, then the House of Lords has stated[13] that the tribunal will quite properly uphold continued detention.
>
> A related issue, which has been noted but not decided by the courts, is whether a psychiatrist is a 'hybrid public authority', and so must apply human rights law when exercising public functions, such as recommending the detention or release of patients.

> **Clinico-legal**
> The fact that the inpatient consultant is of the same view as you suggests that a refusal might meet the *Bolam* test. However, you might wish to consult official guidance, reports, and the research literature in order to ascertain whether your view conforms to a wider body of responsible, skilled medical opinion (e.g. in case others, while sharing your view about risk and the difficulties of supervision, might nevertheless agree to take Nick on).
>
> Your clinical director's anxiety is understandable. If necessary, you should politely remind them that the Trust only has to make reasonable efforts to facilitate discharge, provided it has, it would not be subject to legal criticism.
>
> In responding to the solicitor, you should make the same point, and perhaps also point out that the case law she cited is only authority for patients who no longer suffer from mental disorder; other cases have made clear that there is no breach of human rights if the patient continues to suffer from a mental disorder, such as Nick's personality disorder. You may wish to seek the support of your employer and/or its solicitors before writing.
>
> You should try to be helpful despite your refusal. For example, you and the inpatient consultant might make a joint statement of what you would want to see the patient achieve before you would support conditional discharge. Or, if you know of a colleague in another service who might hold a different opinion and agree to work with Nick (e.g. because they have access to alternative treatments), you could invite the inpatient team to refer to him.

> **Ethical**
> Emotion may play some part in your decision: for example, fear of the possible consequences for you if he were to reoffend or harm others while under your care. You should reflect on your feelings and pursue objectivity, for instance by imagining an alternative decision and your reasons for coming to it.

[11] As modified by *Bolitho* and (in relation to discussing treatment, as opposed to providing it) *Montgomery v Lanarkshire HB*. These are binding in the UK and of persuasive authority in RoI
[12] *R(K) v Camden and Islington Health Authority* [2001] EWCA Civ 240.
[13] *R v SSHD and another ex parte IH (FC)* [2003] UKHL 59.

Your duty to treat your patient is not absolute: you are under no professional or ethical obligation to provide treatment you think unjustified (e.g. because it would cause the patient harm or, as in Nick's case, it would place others at risk). You must balance the benefit to the patient against the harm to them or others.

Nick's autonomy and liberty will be compromised by continued detention if you refuse to treat him. You might argue that it will also protect him from the harm of reoffending, but this would be an extremely paternalistic position. The risk of harm to others is a much stronger argument.

4   What information to share with patients

Themes: *pharmacological treatments and side-effects (p.200) [C]; sharing and withholding information (p.320) [L]; obtaining informed consent (p.482) [CL]; and honesty in psychiatric practice (p.337) [E]*

Case description

Richard is a young man with severe paranoid schizophrenia. He has been in your low secure unit for six years, following conviction for GBH when psychotic. When free of symptoms, his risk of violence is low.

After an unsuccessful trial of haloperidol, he was given olanzapine: his passivity phenomena and hallucinations abated, and his delusions lessened. However, he developed priapism, severe enough to require emergency aspiration of blood by a urologist.

Olanzapine was stopped, and cautiously restarted a fortnight later, but he experienced priapism again, as did he on risperidone, quetiapine, and chlorpromazine. He stated he would refuse any drug that could cause priapism, as he found it unbearably painful, and waiting for it to happen was intolerable. He has since been treated with flupentixol, haloperidol, and zuclopenthixol, without priapism—but has severe residual psychotic symptoms that prevent him participating meaningfully in psychology, or using unescorted leave. Finally, last year, he was diagnosed with glucose intolerance. He accepted a low-sugar diet and blood glucose monitoring, and has achieved healthy readings.

You wish to consider clozapine. You know there have been reports of it, too, being associated with priapism.[14] However, you think he probably had elevated blood glucose when he experienced recurrent priapism, and you believe that now that his blood glucose is well-controlled the risk of priapism is acceptably low (you estimate it at roughly 5%–10%). You know that he will not entertain treatment with anything he thinks capable of causing priapism. However, you also believe that a more effective antipsychotic such as clozapine or olanzapine (to which he responded previously) offers the only realistic possibility of him living outside hospital. Richard retains the capacity to make treatment decisions.

Questions

1. Should you tell him there is a risk that clozapine could cause priapism despite his good blood glucose control, or withhold this fact?
2. Are there any justifiable alternative courses of action?
3. What other the clinical, legal, clinico-legal, and ethical issues arise in the case?

---

[14] For exampleSoon S, James W, and Bailon M-J (2008) Priapism associated with atypical antipsychotic medications: A review. *International Clinical Psychopharmacology* 23: 9–17.

Clinical

Your clinical opinion has balanced competing interests; your overall view is that a trial of clozapine is in Richard's best interest.

Legal

The law in the UK and Ireland used to focus exclusively on whether responsible clinicians could be in favour of the practice at issue[15] (in this case, withholding information on priapism). There has since been a steady shift towards recognising the patient as an active participant in treatment and not merely a passive recipient of medical expertise[16]; and, in 2015, the UK Supreme Court stated that in cases involving a decision to disclose or withhold relevant information the test is now 'whether, in the circumstances of the particular case, a reasonable person in the patient's position would be likely to attach significance to the risk; or the doctor is or should reasonably be aware that the particular patient would' do so. [17]

Clinico-legal

The process you follow matters: for a decision to withhold important information to be justifiable, all reasonable attempts must have been made to inform and educate Richard about the decision; to enable him to obtain information from other sources; to talk it through with others whom he trusts; and to take sufficient time for him (and you) to consider alternative perspectives.

It is not reasonable to assume that he will not reconsider on this occasion simply because he has not done so in the past. You can begin the discussion about 'another antipsychotic' without mentioning clozapine or revealing the risk of priapism, and encourage him to think not of drugs that do or do not cause priapism, but of switching from one with a low probability to another with a higher but still low probability.

If Richard will not consider another antipsychotic with a higher risk of priapism, you will need to consider your legal liability if he were to consent to clozapine without knowing of the risk, and then developed priapism again. Even if you believe a reasonable person in Richard's position would not attach sufficient significance to the risk to refuse the clozapine, it would be hard to argue that you were unaware that Richard himself does, whether reasonably or otherwise. It would therefore be unwise to withhold the information about clozapine's risk of causing priapism, despite the likely consequence.

Ethical

The underlying tension is between your clinical view of Richard's best interest (to receive successful treatment in order to recover and live more independently, despite the risk of priapism) and his view that running the risk of priapism is unacceptable, whatever the consequences. As a doctor, your ethical duty is to educate and if appropriate try to convince your patient to act on what you believe is the best medical advice, not merely to do whatever the patient wishes. The consequence of not attempting treatment with a more effective antipsychotic could well be lifelong residence in a hospital environment, which would not only limit Richard's liberty and quality of life, but also affect his family and friends, as well as both costing a great deal of public money and depriving him of potential income and lifestyle.

An alternative course of action would be to be open about the risks and benefits of clozapine treatment, and to try to focus the discussion not on a binary decision to take or not take it, but on what possible criteria would enable him to feel safe enough to try it (e.g. for him to have control over when

---

[15] Originally, A practice accepted as proper by a responsible body of medical men skilled in that particular art: *Bolam v Friern Hospital Management Committee* [1957] 1 WLR 582.

[16] *Sidaway v Bethlem Royal Hospital Governors* [1985] AC 871, per Scarman LJ; *Bolitho v City and Hackney Health Authority* [1997] 4 All ER 771.

[17] *Montgomery v Lanarkshire Health Board* [2015] UKSC 11.

a trial of treatment began; what the dose would be each day; whether and when it was increased; and to be able to terminate the trial and return to another drug at any time).

You could also offer a trial of another atypical antipsychotic that he has not yet tried with a slightly lower risk of priapism, such as aripiprazole, if he will not consider clozapine. Richard should be helped to understand that this offers a lesser chance of recovery and discharge, but still perhaps a greater one that he has without a change in treatment.

It is a core duty of a doctor to be honest. The discussion above suggests that you could—in certain circumstances and with certain conditions—lawfully be dishonest with your patient. But should you? There is a risk that you may fail to acknowledge your patient's remaining autonomy. You may be able to justify your conduct with respect to public trust but could your conduct, if you do deliberately deceive, be said you justify your patient trusting you?

5

Treating psychiatrist as expert witness at criminal trial

Themes: *personality disorder (p.78), disputed diagnosis (p.144), malingering (p.118), and homicide (p.46) [C]; contested diminished responsibility defence (p.624) [L]; and treating doctor as expert witness (p.652) [CL, E]*

Case description

You are a community forensic consultant supervising Kieran, a twenty-four-year-old man with antisocial and emotionally unstable personality disorder who has a history of psychosis when stressed. He was discharged from the MSU six months ago, after previous transfer from prison. Kieran has committed many offences since his early teens, and he abuses drugs and alcohol. Despite this he has no convictions for serious violence beyond an assault on a policeman when drunk.

He takes a low dose of an oral antipsychotic, prescribed by his GP, and lives in supported accommodation; his mental state has been good since discharge. He is single: his girlfriend left when he was imprisoned a year ago. However, staff in the accommodation now report that he has been sleeping poorly, and has spoken of feeling upset that his ex-girlfriend has a new partner.

The following week, you learn that Kieran has been remanded in custody, charged with the murder of his ex-girlfriend. You assess him in prison and agree with the team there that he is floridly psychotic, so you admit him to the MSU.

Six months later, Kieran's psychosis is much improved with antipsychotic medication, but he is now depressed because of the charge he is facing. He tells you that he had thought his ex-girlfriend was a demon who was going to kill his children, and that god wanted him to protect them.

Later, Professor Clarkson, who has assessed Kieran for the defence, contacts you. He says the established diagnosis of psychosis is wrong, and Kieran has psychopathy. He also thinks that Kieran is malingering illness, and could not plead diminished responsibility. Confidentially, he adds that his opinion is shared by Dr Hardman, who assessed Kieran for the prosecution.

Kieran's lawyers see from the medical records that your clinical view differs from Professor Clarkson's (whose report they are under no obligation to disclose). They instruct you to provide an expert opinion on diminished responsibility.

Questions

1. How could, or should you respond?
2. What other the clinical, legal, clinico-legal, and ethical issues arise in the case?

> **Clinical**
>
> Aside from your own records, you will have access to all of the clinical data contained in the report of Dr Hardman, but not in that of Professor Clarkson, since the defence will not disclose it and will assert that your communication with Professor Clarkson is legally privileged (meaning you cannot refer to it). Whether or not you accept the instructions, you should review your diagnosis in the light of both their views, to ensure Kieran receives the best treatment.
>
> If you accept the instructions, your report will need to take account of Dr Hardman's data and opinion, and respond to her claim that Kieran is malingering.

> **Legal**
>
> You are under no duty to accept the solicitor's instructions. If you do accept them, then if your opinion remains that he was psychotic at the time of the killing, you will need to address the criteria of diminished responsibility. These are set out and explored in criminal law cases 5–9.

Clinico-legal and ethical

You have ordinary clinical and ethical duties to make Kieran's care your first concern.

Beyond that, you have discretion over whether or not to accept the instructions. On the one hand, as a treating psychiatrist around the time of the alleged offence, you can give contemporaneous evidence on his likely mental state, and as the current treating psychiatrist, you are in a position to offer a bed should Kieran not be convicted of murder, and sentenced to treatment. On the other, you have an established therapeutic relationship that could bias your opinion, or at least give the appearance of bias—especially because a finding that Kieran's responsibility was not diminished could imply that your diagnosis and treatment of him had been inadequate. If you were to give evidence, it is likely that the cross-examining barrister would challenge your impartiality and objectivity because of this. Hence, guidelines often urge treating doctors not to accept instructions in respect of such serious legal proceedings relating to their patients.

Also, if you do not already have experience of psychiatric testimony in a murder trial, you are likely to find it highly complex—and, if you feel sympathetic towards your patient, distressing. You may also not be competent clinico-legally.[18]

In addition, you will need Kieran's consent to use his medical records for your report, and for any additional assessment you make, unless you have grounds for believing he lacks mental capacity to consent to this, and that providing a report would be in his best interest.

If you decline the instructions, either because of your ethical position, or because Kieran withholds consent, the defence might still consider subpoenaing you to provide a professional witness statement about your assessment *at the time* of Kieran's mental state. This would avoid the need for you to comment on malingering, or other issues, as you did not consider these at the time. For the defence to make use of such evidence, they would need a separate expert witness whose evidence was in favour of diminished responsibility.

---

[18] *Kumar v General Medical Council* [2012] EWHC 2688 (Admin).

6

Therapist as expert witness in civil litigation

Themes: *posttraumatic stress disorder (p.96) [C]; negligence, quantum (p.548) [L]; and clinical opinion on causation and psychological damage (p.700) [CL] acknowledging uncertainty (p.304) and treating doctor as expert witness (p.674) [E]*

Case description

You are a general psychiatrist with an interest in PTSD and mood disorders. You have a private practice in treating patients and medicolegal work.

Lola is referred to you by her insurers for assessment and possible treatment. She was travelling to work in a company car when it was involved in a serious accident in which two people were killed. Lola was uninjured but has not worked since the accident. At interview, she describes insomnia due to nightmares; hyperarousal related to traffic sounds and sirens, leading to her staying at home all day; and suicidal thoughts. She has lost weight and started smoking. Prior to the accident, she enjoyed good mental health, although she had previously experienced postnatal depression, which responded well to medication. Her parents divorced when she was five, but her mother remarried, and she describes herself as close to her family.

Lola engages well with treatment, attending all sessions, keeping a diary, and understanding the rationale for psychological treatment. You propose EMDR and CBT. Lola seems keen, but then misses some appointments. She says that her symptoms are worsening again, and disengages completely from therapy.

Soon after this, you receive a letter from solicitors representing Lola in a personal injury legal action against her employers (a prestigious investment bank). They ask your opinion about diagnosis, treatment, and prognosis, and they also ask specifically about work performance. They want to know how much of Lola's difficulty attending work is due to the accident, and how likely it is that she will recover with treatment.

You think that Lola's case is clinically mild, and that, with psychological treatment, she has a good chance of full recovery. However, if she does not engage, she will not recover, which might increase any compensation. Lola's lawyers send you a report prepared by the defendants' psychiatrist saying that Lola already had psychiatric problems before the accident, and her inability to work is not due to the PTSD for which you are treating her.

Questions

1. What clinical, legal, clinico-legal, and ethical issues are raised by this case?

Clinical

The clinical questions here relate to stress resilience and vulnerability, in the context of lack of good empirical evidence concerning how PTSD affects work performance. Occupational mental health evidence is sparse. Occupational resilience is idiosyncratic: some people with mental disorders find that work helps them recover from mental distress, whereas some find that they cannot work because of their distress.

It is well established, however, that PTSD and other mental disorders are more likely to occur in people who are vulnerable because of previous psychiatric disorders or previous trauma.

Some psychological treatment services do not recommend commencing psychological therapies until after any legal proceedings have concluded because of the perverse incentive not to recover lest it undermine a compensation claim.

Legal

Through her solicitors, Lola will seek to prove that others are liable to compensate her for her loss (psychological damage and loss of earnings). This could include claiming that another party involved in the traffic accident was negligent, or, if the driver of the car in which she was a passenger was negligent, then, because she was 'at work' at the time and in a company car, that her employer is vicariously liable. To receive compensation for such negligence she would also need to prove that the accident caused her mental disorder and loss of earnings, and to quantify the severity of that disorder and its effects.

Clinico-legal

These questions can be problematic even in nonpsychiatric personal injury cases. For example, if Lola had broken her leg in the accident, she could argue that the broken leg led to loss of earnings while her leg was healing. But if there were complications in the healing of the fractured limb, there would then be argument about the extent to which the accident had caused the recovery problems that would impact return to work and earning capacity.

The other empirical problem is the lack of an evidence base from which to comment. This enables defendants' lawyers to claim that vulnerability from pre-existing mental disorder or trauma was the true cause of the subsequent disorder rather than the accident. If they are unsuccessful in this, the 'eggshell skull' rule means that if the accident did cause the subsequent mental disorder, it is irrelevant if such an accident would not have caused disorder in a person without that vulnerability.

Ethical

The lack of empirical evidence required to address the clinical questions infers that experts must be honest about the degree of uncertainty attending their opinions; albeit each side will use such uncertainty to try to undermine their opponents' case.

The other main ethical issue relates to the duty to be impartial and avoid bias. Although treating therapists may hold the best-quality information about a person's likely clinical progress, they are at risk of being less objective than an external expert. So, if you provide an expert opinion on Lola, your impartiality is likely to be questioned in cross-examination.

Rather, in order to best help Lola, you need to protect your clinical relationship with her so that she can get better. If she is avoiding treatment to gain more compensation, she needs to be able to talk about that honestly in therapy, if she will, and she is unlikely to, if you are giving evidence in her case (although your clinical notes will be legally discoverable in any event). You will also need to help her discuss her ambivalence about recovery, which may reflect unresolved anger about the accident. So, in summary, if you act as her expert, Lola will lose you as her therapist, and this is not likely to be in her interest.

Personal injury work can be ethically problematic for experts. It can be very lucrative, as defendants are often wealthy corporations willing to pay highly for an opinion that will save them money in compensation. The strong financial incentive can be tempting for an expert acting for the defendant, as can the sense of fighting for a righteous underdog to the expert acting for the claimant.

7 Professional versus expert witness

Themes: *alcohol intoxication, withdrawal and dependence (p.76), and brain damage (p.112) [C]; professional versus expert witness (p.652) and fitness to have been interviewed (p.573) [L]; assessment for fitness to plead and stand trial (p.602) [CL]; and refusal to provide an expert report (p.680) [E]*

Case description

The police bring Nigel to A&E. He had been arrested thirty-six hours earlier, after being found in an alley next to the body of a man thought to be an acquaintance. The victim had died from head injuries. Several bottles of alcohol were close by, and Nigel smelt strongly of alcohol when arrested. Nigel replied, 'No comment' to all the questions put to him by the police, and claimed to have no memory of what had happened.

The A&E staff call you for advice. Nigel's medical records from previous contact with your hospital show that he is fifty years old and has a long history of very heavy alcohol use: two litres of spirits a day for fifteen years. He has suffered minor injuries after falling or getting into fights. He lives in a hostel.

Nigel received no medical treatment in police custody. However, the police officers accompanying him say he seemed confused, and that the hostel manager had said Nigel had been this way for weeks, and had then gone missing for a few days. In A&E, he is sweating, shaking, agitated, hypertensive, and tachycardic, and blood tests show poor liver function.

After assessing and treating Nigel, the police ask you for a statement, and his solicitor later instructs you to compete an expert psychiatric report.

Questions

1. Are there any limits on what you should include in your statement to police?
2. Can and should you refuse to provide an expert report?
3. Do you think Nigel was previously fit to be interviewed?
4. Is he likely later to be fit to plead and stand trial?
5. What other clinical, legal, clinico-legal, and ethical issues arise in the case?

Clinical

Chronic alcohol use is associated with brain changes involving the prefrontal cortex, limbic system, cerebellum, and hippocampus. Individuals with a history of alcohol misuse may present with impairments in memory, executive functioning (abstract reasoning, impulse control, and problem-solving), visuospatial functioning, speed of processing, and verbal fluency, whilst their general intellectual functioning tends to be intact.

Legal

Ordinary factual witnesses give evidence concerning what they saw or heard. Similarly, professional witnesses give factual evidence: a patient's presentation or the diagnosis recorded in their notes or the typical symptoms of a certain illness.

A professional witness can report an opinion they formed at the time of treating the patient, if that is relevant, but strictly speaking cannot give an opinion during the hearing on evidence from that hearing (though courts commonly blur this boundary). To do so, one must be an expert witness qualified by virtue of one's knowledge, expertise, or experience, to assist the court in matters outside its knowledge and experience.[19] Hence, an expert witness:

- is independently instructed by one or more parties, or by the court;
- provides an opinion on an issue within their professional expertise; and
- is a 'secondary' witness, giving an opinion on established facts (or if necessary, on each party's version of the facts).

All types of witness can be required to attend court and be both examined and cross examined.

Clinico-legal

By giving a statement to police about Nigel, you will be acting as a professional witness. You may describe Nigel's presentation in A&E, describing symptoms and diagnosis, and upon what you learned about his medical history, and you may comment upon cause, prognosis, and treatment. However, only if you accept the defence's instructions to act as an expert witness should you give an opinion on issues such as his likely mental state at the time of the alleged offence, his fitness to have been interviewed by the police, or his fitness to plead. The police themselves cannot instruct you as an expert.

If you accept the defence's instructions, you will need to make a further assessment of the defendant, in order to address questions they have asked that go beyond professional evidence (above). In particular, you will need to evaluate his memory problems and determine their aetiology. For example, if he has dementia or Korsakoff psychosis you should establish its severity, and the scope for improved cognitive function with treatment.

Ethical

Treating clinicians *can* act as expert witnesses in relation to their own patients. However, there is the potential for ethical and clinical conflict in doing so. It is therefore usually wise for a treating clinician to avoid acting as an expert, especially when the stakes are high.

Whether you can refuse will depend upon the jurisdiction in which the case is located. However, if you do not believe yourself to be competent to act as an expert, or believe that there are factors that would compromise your ability to be unbiased and independent, then you must refuse instruction, even if it comes from the court, albeit with an accompanying detailed explanation. You can also refuse if you consider it would seriously damage the therapeutic relationship with the patient, or if you lack the relevant expertise.

---

[19] *R v Turner* [1975] QB 834.

Professional versus contractual duty

Case description

You are employed part-time as a psychiatrist at an Immigration Removal Centre, which houses people awaiting deportation. One of the duties in your employment contract is to treat detainees suffering from mental disorder 'insofar as treatment is available, so as to facilitate deportation'.

You assess a twenty-one-year-old woman who, upon criminal conviction, was sentenced to deportation. Her destination is known to have a relatively good mental health care system. She is due to fly next week.

You assess her. She is suffering from an acute psychotic episode. Her medical records show that she has previously responded to haloperidol, in hospital. Despite her active persecutory delusions and auditory hallucinations, she is willing to accept haloperidol again (indeed, she asks you for it), and in your view she has the mental capacity to consent to this treatment.

The centre manager states that you must treat her in the expectation that she will be fit to fly next week.

You begin treatment. However, since in your view she warrants treatment in a psychiatric hospital, you also refer her to the local NHS service. You believe that continued detention in the IRC during treatment would at least slow her recovery—in other words, her health would be worsened currently by continued detention. The next day, the manager finds out about your referral. She angrily states that this will impede deportation and risk the company missing its removal target for the month, resulting in a financial penalty under its government contract. She notes that the woman slept well last night and suggests her condition is already improving; she tells you to withdraw your referral.

Questions

1. What are your contractual and professional duties?
2. Can you resolve the tension between them?
3. If not, how should you act?
4. What other clinical, legal, clinico-legal, and ethical issues in the case?

Clinical

Your assessment led to your clinical opinion about treatment needs, including admission. Nothing the manager has said (e.g. about good sleep) provides sufficient evidence to change this.

Legal

Mental health law can authorise transfer to hospital; it does not apply in the IRC, where any treatment not valid under common law as in an emergency must be based upon informed consent.

Detention in the detention centre while psychotic might amount to a breach of ECHR Article 3 right to freedom from torture and inhuman or degrading treatment.

Your contract of employment cannot override your professional obligations, though you could in principle face penalties for breach of contract.

Clinico-legal

The decision about recommending transfer to hospital involves considering both the patient's clinical needs and the legislation which provides the mechanism for transfer to hospital. You have reached the decision that transfer is necessary.

Ethical

Your professional duty is stated in the GMC/IMC documents on good medical practice,[20] which require you 'to make the care of the patient your first concern' (or in the wording of the IMC, 'your paramount professional responsibility is to act in the best interests of your patients'). Both bodies explicitly state that this overrides any duties to your employer. The Royal College of Psychiatrists gives more specific guidance on patients in immigration detention,[21] which includes that doctors in IRCs must report to the management any patients whose detention 'injuriously affects' their health.

Your contractual duty to treat the patient is clear, and there is no conflict in this with your professional duty to make the care of the patient your first concern, as you wish to treat her, and she consents to treatment. The conflict arises in the setting and purpose of treatment: you are recommending transfer to a psychiatric hospital for inpatient treatment for the purpose of recovery, whereas your employer (as represented by the unit manager) wants her treated in the detention centre.

It may be that the manager has, in effect, misinterpreted your contractual duty, which is that you have no duty to treat the patient other than in the manner you consider fit. In this case, the conflict would be between her interpretation and your interpretation of what the company can ask or instruct you to do. Alternatively, if her interpretation is correct, then your contract conflicts with the Detention Centre Rules 2001 under which the company is required to operate.

You should try to discuss this calmly with the manager, and if necessary, state in writing that, in your opinion, the detainee's health is being 'injuriously affected' by her detention and that she should be transferred, explaining tactfully that, in these circumstances, transfer is supported by the Detention Centre Rules.

If she does not change her position, you should prioritise your professional duty and proceed with the transfer, and, during this process, you should both consider discussing the situation with your medical defence body and should escalate the disagreement within your employer's management hierarchy.

[20] General Medical Council (2013) *Good Medical Practice: Duties of a Doctor*, GMC; IMC (2014) *Guide to Professional Conduct and Ethics for Registered Medical Practitioners*. Medical Council, Dublin.

[21] Council Report CR199. *Psychiatric Reports: Preparation and Use in Cases Involving Asylum, Removal from the UK or Immigration Detention*. Available at: https://www.rcpsych.ac.uk/docs/default-source/improving-care/better-mh-policy/college-reports/college-report-cr199.pdf.

9 Medically relevant but legally inadmissible information

> **Themes:** *personality disorder (p.78), paraphilia (pp.56, 102), and homicide (p.46) [C]; diminished responsibility (p.624), admissibility (p.382), and conflict of legal and medical paradigms (p.354) [L]; change of expert opinion (p.690) and duty to the court (p.678) [CL]; and data, evidence, and 'truth' (p.290) [E]*

Case description

You are instructed by the defence to prepare a report addressing 'diminished responsibility' for Kai, a twenty-three-year-old man charged with murder. Kai admits killing Rafe; he has claimed throughout that Rafe had just sexually assaulted him.

Kai has no past history of aggression or of violent behaviour, other than once, aged fourteen, using a table knife at school to threaten a boy who had teased him.

Based upon your own assessment and psychometric testing by an experienced psychologist colleague, you diagnose him with personality disorder, with prominent schizoid and avoidant traits. You find no evidence (including in the police report of their search of his computer's hard drive, which contains many homosexual images) to suggest potentially paraphilic sexual interests or behaviour; although you note his uncertain sexual orientation, in that he has occasionally tried unsuccessfully to have sex with women. The psychologist agrees. You both support a plea of diminished responsibility.

The psychologist gives oral evidence that Kai is a shy, withdrawn, and private young man in conflict about his possible homosexuality, who could have lost control after being sexually assaulted. He asserts there is no evidence of 'sexual deviance'.

While you are giving your own evidence under cross-examination, the jury is unexpectedly asked to leave. The prosecution explains that they have new evidence: the police have just found six highly sadomasochistic homosexual pornographic images amongst those on Kai's computer. The defence counter that the police have had six months to find such images, and that it would be unfair to admit them now. Both sides agree that you and the psychologist can see the images concerned. The judge adjourns the trial, and indicates that she will rule on the admissibility of the new material tomorrow.

Overnight, you ponder how this might change the evidence you will give in the morning. You recognise the uncertainty over whether Kai deliberately downloaded the images, or viewed them (just six amongst thousands of innocuous images). However, if he did, and they reflect sadomasochistic interests, this could be a factor contributory to the offence; you decide that would significantly weaken, but not abolish, your support for diminished responsibility.

In the morning the evidence is ruled inadmissible. You return to the witness box to continue giving evidence under cross-examination.

Questions

1. Do you continue to give evidence after the jury returns as if nothing has happened or do you ask to ask to stop, and amend your opinion?
2. If you continue, will you take account of the new evidence or act as if unaware of it?
3. What would be the implications for the trial of you deciding that you cannot continue without taking account of the inadmissible evidence? And are these implications relevant to your decision?
4. What other clinical, legal, clinico-legal, and ethical issues in the case?

Clinical

You have already come to an opinion; although have now somewhat revised it in the light of new information that you consider significant. Given that you are in the midst of giving evidence, you cannot reinterview the defendant.

Legal

The case represents starkly the clash of medical and legal paradigms that lurks within all medicolegal practice. The medical method is investigative: so that it properly takes account of any 'data' that could be relevant to the clinical questions, weighted by your degree of confidence in it. By contrast, legal process addresses 'evidence'; which can only be such if it is deemed 'admissible'; as being 'relevant' and also 'fairly' considered[22]). Hence there can be clinically relevant data that is legally inadmissible.

Clinico-legal

Kai's personality disorder is a 'recognised medical condition';, and it is reasonable for you to form the opinion that, in the context of his unresolved sexual orientation and the presumed sexual assault by Rafe, it could have caused him to experience an 'abnormality of mental functioning' that 'substantially impaired his ability to exercise self-control',[23] something which would have been 'a significant contributory factor' to the killing.

Here the paradigm clash confronts you with a profound dilemma. You should consider, within a psychiatric paradigm, the possibility that Kai has paraphilic interests (based upon your weighting of the likelihood that he intended to download the six images). Ideally you would have been able to explore any such possible interest with him in detail during your interview, as well as its causal relevance the killing. As that is not possible, considering the possibility of paraphilia requires taking a view on a factual matter (his intent to download the images) that the court will now not determine, because their existence is inadmissible.

If you continue your evidence under cross-examination based upon the admissible evidence alone, you will not reflect what is now your true clinical opinion, which is a breach of your duty to inform the court of a change of opinion.[24] Conversely, if you take account of the new information you will have to contradict the opinion you expressed in your evidence-in-chief,[25] at least in terms of the strength of your opinion. Moreover, you would need to express your new opinion conditionally ('if he intended to download the six images, then I now think …') but this would mean revealing inadmissible evidence to

---

[22] For example, relevant evidence might be inadmissible because it was collected unfairly (e.g. through unauthorised surveillance), because it is unreliable (e.g. testimony from a witness shown to have lied) or because it is presented in a way that gives a false impression, or because it may prejudice the jury's view of one party without adding significantly to what can be proved.

[23] Or to have amounted to an abnormality of mind that substantially impaired his ability to control his actions in Scotland, or that substantially diminished his responsibility for his actions in RoI.

[24] For example under s19.2(3)(c) of the 2015 version of the E&W *Criminal Procedure Rules*.

[25] Unless you decide that he could not have intended to download those images—but you do not have sufficient evidence to infer this, and in any case it is a matter for the court, not you.

the jury, which would breach your duty to the court and would probably result in a mistrial,[26] and perhaps your referral to the GMC/IMC. Even saying that you are aware of new evidence that has changed your opinion, without saying what that evidence is, would contradict the judge's ruling.

You could consider withdrawing from the case in order to avoid the dilemma, but this would cause the case to collapse and again *could* result in a formal complaint against you from the judge for breach of your duty as an expert witness.[27]

You might reasonably ask to speak to the judge in the absence of the jury (you should have prepared your instructing solicitor for this request in the event that the judge ruled the new evidence inadmissible). And you should then explain your dilemma to the judge, the conditional change in your opinion, and the effect of his ruling on your evidence. The judge might then consent (albeit reluctantly) to your withdrawal, with the trial continuing, although the defence will be very unhappy, or order a retrial or if both prosecution and defence agree, order an adjournment of several weeks to allow the new evidence to be considered by the defence and for new or updated expert evidence to be produced, allowing the evidence to be ruled admissible after all when the trial resumes.

Ethical

Many experts faced with this situation will find it ethically unacceptable to continue giving any evidence; that is, they will wholly privilege the medical paradigm. Others will accept that a clinician who gives evidence in a legal context is constrained by that context.

A similar ethical dilemma can arise in other circumstances, such as if the expert received a bundle of evidence, but after reading it, learns that some has been agreed inadmissible by both parties; if the inadmissible evidence is relevant to the expert's opinion, what should they do? It may be easier to withdraw at this stage than during the trial, as there may be time to instruct a new expert (from whom the inadmissible evidence can be withheld—though of course this leaves the dilemma of knowing that expert's opinion might be incomplete and even wrong in some important respect).

A weaker form of the same dilemma would be knowing from the outset that there is additional evidence that has not been shared with you because it is legally privileged: in that you will not know whether your opinion is valid and complete without knowing what is the additional evidence that exists (unless, for instance, the solicitor is able to tell you what category of information it is, and this is enough to make clear that it would not be relevant to your clinical opinion).

A further, but different, form of the dilemma occurs where the doctor is inhibited from carrying out a full clinical assessment by legal procedure. Hence, for example, where it would be proper, indeed required, in ordinary clinical practice to ask informants about a patient, in a legal context this may be ruled out (e.g. if the informant is also a witness).

[26] A trial that has to be abandoned because the court lacks jurisdiction, because the jury cannot reach a verdict, or because of a procedural error that is so prejudicial it cannot be remedied (e.g. the jury hearing prejudicial information that they would be unable to disregard despite instructions from the judge to do so).

[27] For example your duty to 'help the court with the overriding objective' of obtaining justice in the case.

10

Role of personal values in expert decision-making

Case description

Celine set a fire in her mental health hostel. Another resident died in the fire. She is now charged with murder.

The defence expert's opinion is that Celine was in an abnormal mental state at the time of the killing, and that her personality disorder is a 'recognised medical condition' that would explain her actions. He supports the defence of diminished responsibility.

The prosecution expert disagrees that personality disorder can amount to a 'recognised medical condition' for this purpose. She also places great weight on the view of some staff at the hospital to which Celine was admitted after the fire, that she 'had mental capacity' and was 'not unwell' at the time, whilst dismissing the contrary view of hostel staff as biased by being 'too therapeutically close' to her.

You have been asked by the defence solicitor to review both expert reports and to give advice.

Questions

1. What will be your analysis of the two reports?
2. Do you think either of the experts should have done or said anything different? If so, what?
3. What ethical considerations are there for the experts?
4. What ethical considerations are there for you in your role?
5. What other clinical, legal, clinico-legal, and ethical issues arise in the case?

Clinical

Despite their recognition as diagnoses in ICD11 and DSM5, and despite research evidence that treatments already exist that can significantly improve the experience of living with most forms of the disorder, some psychiatrists claim that PD are not 'true' mental disorders like psychosis. Patients with PD therefore face stigma and prejudice.

Legal

Diminished responsibility is considered in detail in criminal law cases 5–9. Personality disorder is not excluded as a 'recognised medical condition' in E&W or NI, nor as a cause of 'abnormality of mind' in Scotland, nor as a 'qualifying mental disorder' in RoI. This being in contrast to intoxication, which is excluded despite being recognised as a medical condition in both ICD11 and DSM5.[28]

The prosecution's psychiatrist is therefore mistaken about the law, and this should be raised in cross-examination by the defence barrister.

Clinico-legal

If you decide to offer advice you will be advising counsel within the adversarial envelope, not being 'an expert to the court'. And you should limit yourself to assessing the merits and flaws of the two psychiatrists' expert opinions.

There is an important ethical and legal question concerning how unconventional views about diagnoses (such as that PD is not a 'true' mental disorder) should be managed within the legal process. And the practice guidelines for experts require that experts make clear where there are important alternative views to their own, and the evidence they have used to come to their views.[29]

Lying behind this example of dubious expert opinion is the possibility that the psychiatrist has decided what she thinks the right outcome should be, and has 'made a psychiatric case' to achieve that outcome. Sometimes this can be quite subtle: overemphasising one clinical aspect and underplaying another, say, so as to lean more or less in favour of a condition amounting to 'substantial impairment' or an 'explanation'. Indeed, the prosecution expert might, under cross-examination, concede that PD could be a recognised medical condition, and then fall back to the (more tenable) position that nevertheless there is no valid way of distinguishing between PD impairing the ability to exercise self-control, and mere failure to do so.

Ethical

In this case, the prosecution expert is putting forward a view that may be shared by some other psychiatrists—even if not a 'responsible body' of psychiatrists. And anyone adopting such a minority position should question whether it is ethical to do so, especially when the consequences are severe (e.g. denying treatment or life imprisonment for murder).

Moreover, picking facts that bolster your argument while dismissing those that do not is also unethical (it conflicts with the general duty to be honest, objective and to act with integrity, as well as specific duties relating to report-writing). If the expert is influenced by a personal dislike of patients with PD (something many mental health professionals feel, because of their past experience of the behaviour of some such patients), then it is also unethical to have allowed these personal views to influence her professional judgment.

Accusations of bias and prejudice within the adversarial process are often nuanced. For example, a defence expert in a trial of a woman charged with murder was accused of giving biased testimony in favour of the defendant because she was a 'well-known feminist'. This attack implies that the expert has allowed their presumed personal views to influence their professional opinion; and the attacker should be challenged to show evidence of the implicitly alleged bias. (Such *ad hominem* attacks are usually a sign that the opposing case is weak.)

If you come to the view that the prosecution expert has made a flawed assessment and given a biased opinion, and she does not address this after it has been raised with her within the legal process, you may need to consider referring her to the GMC (similar cases of experts being blind to well-meaning but biased practice, such as *GMC v Meadows* and *R (Squire) v GMC*, have resulted in professional sanctions).

Lastly, be alert to the nature of your own position, giving advice to counsel. You have not assessed the defendant and cannot ethically offer an opinion on her diagnosis, treatment, or prognosis. Although you could perhaps be asked to give expert evidence as to the status of personality disorder within psychiatry.

[28] *R v Dowds* [2012] EWCA Crim 281.
[29] For example, in a criminal case in E&W, the *Criminal Procedure Rules*, Chapter 19.

11

Uncertainty about your opinion and resisting legal pressure

Themes: *diagnostic uncertainty (p.144) [C]; capacity to form intent (p.402), standard of proof (p.380), and expert witness rules (p.656) [L]; expressing uncertainty (p.304) [CL]; and conflict between good clinical practice and legal demands (p.306) [E]*

Case description

Finlay is a seventeen-year-old adolescent with no previous contact with psychiatric services. He is charged with arson with intent to endanger life. You accept defence instructions to report on his diagnosis, likely concurrent mental state, and capacity to form intent.

His GP records list nothing of note other than a consultation two years ago for mild depression, when he was offered six sessions with the practice counsellor, but attended only one. School records show that he was briefly excluded at age fifteen years after a playground fight, but had no history of serious behavioural problems, and he left school aged sixteen years with average exam results.

The offence summary states that he smashed a bottle of spirits through the letterbox of a fifteen-year-old girl from his old school, and ignited them with a match. Much of the house was consumed by fire, but the girl was sleeping over at a friend's home at the time, and her parents escaped without injury. Moments after the fire was set, the girl's phone received the text message 'Die, bitch', which was traced to a phone Finlay had bought a week earlier.

The girl told police she had been dimly aware of the defendant from school, and that a couple of weeks ago he had clumsily asked her out in front of her friends, and that she had snubbed him. None of the witness statements report anything he was seen doing, or heard saying, at the time of the alleged offence, and the custody records reveal no sign of mental disorder, beyond seeming unconcerned at the seriousness of the charge.

You assess him on remand. After two hours, you can detect no symptom of mental illness, but he does seem 'odd'. Prison officers report that he isolates himself from other inmates, and is sometimes teased, but mostly ignored. He has committed no breaches of prison discipline, and has not been seen by the in-reach psychiatric team, showing no sign of mental illness.

A week before your report is due, you are unsure of your opinion. Your differential diagnosis includes an autistic spectrum disorder, personality disorder, a depressive or mixed affective disorder, and no mental disorder.

Questions

1. What pressures might you be placed under?
2. How should you respond?
3. How will you explain your decision to the instructing solicitor and the court?
4. What other clinical, legal, clinico-legal, and ethical issues in the case?

Clinical

The diagnosis is uncertain, and making a diagnosis now will have significant consequences. Correctly diagnosing him with depression, for example, could lead to rapidly effective treatment, perhaps provided following a medical disposal—but conversely, incorrectly diagnosing him with depression could lead to an ineffective treatment that leaves unchanged his risk of further harming others in the future, while denying the victim and her family a sense of justice. Your uncertainty means that further assessment is indicated, and perhaps a second opinion.

Legal

The maximum length of time that can be spent in custody between the first appearance in court and service of the prosecution case is usually fifty days in E&W, with courts under pressure to minimise all delays.

Although your professional duties as a medical practitioner apply, your legal duty is to the court. This includes a specific duty to state any 'qualification' of your opinion, such as that you are uncertain of it or that it could change in certain circumstances.

Clinico-legal

How you should proceed will depend initially on how quickly you could obtain further information that would allow you to make a confident diagnosis (e.g. a specialist diagnostic interview for autistic spectrum disorders, or a period of inpatient observation). If you think this can be achieved swiftly, you should suggest requesting an adjournment. If not, you should recommend an alternative expert be involved at the earliest opportunity.

Despite additional information, you may remain uncertain diagnostically. If so, you could set out your differential diagnosis, and the evidence for and against each condition. The court will then wish to know whether, on the balance of probabilities, Finlay has a given diagnosis, and you should word your opinion so as to make it clear whether you think any of the diagnoses more likely than not to be present.

You should consider the possibility that a mental disorder may reveal itself clearly at a later stage, and allow for assessment and treatment at that stage (e.g. by recommending that the prison in-reach psychiatric team or a community team monitor him, depending on the trial outcome).

Ethical

There may be tension between your duty to adhere to good standards of medical practice and your duty to assist the court in determining legal issues in a timely fashion. Many mental disorders can only be diagnosed reliably after a period of assessment too long to be accepted by a criminal court. In the meantime, good medical practice is to make a provisional diagnosis and change it as necessary, but again, this is problematic for the court, which wants to rely on a definite rather than a shifting opinion. It may be possible to use expensive investigations to speed the process up, but again this may be resisted if the cost will come from the legal aid budget.

Be honest. Any external pressure from lawyers or the court to go beyond the degree of certainty you currently have should be resisted, so as not to fall below the standards of good clinical practice.

12

Dispute within forensic mental health team and evidence to tribunal

Themes: *personality disorder (p.78) and risk management (p.237) [C]; criteria for continued detention (p.461) and 'treatability' test (p.471) [L]; recommendation to tribunal (p.692) [CL]; and managing conflicting perspectives (p.312) and values-based practice (p.288) [E]*

Case description

You are the consultant forensic psychiatrist in a low secure unit, treating Chelsea, who was severely physically abused as a child, and by various male partners. You have diagnosed her with mixed cluster B&C personality disorder, but recognise her condition could also be formulated as complex PTSD. She has also had several depressive episodes. She was convicted of the attempted murder of a teenage girl during an episode of psychotic depression; having been unable to bring herself to complete the homicide, she tried to kill herself before the police arrived. She received a restricted hospital order.

After three years in an MSU she was transferred to you a year ago. Her depression had resolved slowly with antidepressant treatment. Her skills for independent living have improved slightly through occupational therapy, although she remains very socially isolated, with no children, no current partner, no family contact, and no friends outside hospital. However, despite numerous attempts to engage her in several modalities of group and individual psychotherapy, her personality traits (or persistent symptoms of PTSD) remain largely unchanged, and the psychology service does not recommend any further attempt at treatment.

She has applied to a tribunal for discharge from hospital; you and the social worker are considering whether to support her application. In team discussions, it becomes clear that the psychologist and most of the nurses believe she should be discharged because no further effective treatment is possible in hospital, whereas the social worker, OT, and junior doctor believe that her risk of becoming depressed again is significant, and that were she to do so, she would again pose a high risk of harm to herself and to others.

Questions

1. Should you act to resolve the disagreement?
2. If so, what approaches might help you to do so?
3. How should varying views be represented in evidence to the tribunal?
4. What other clinical, legal, clinico-legal, and ethical issues in the case?

Clinical

This scenario involves a tension between a 'clinical treatment' perspective (all that can be done has been done, so the opportunity for inpatient treatment should now be given to another patient) and a 'risk management' one (the risk of harm to others has not yet declined to an acceptably low level, so further action is required).

In this scenario, you have two relevant roles: you will have to give your own independent opinion and recommendation to the tribunal, but you are also the clinical leader of the team and should consider facilitating further discussion within (and perhaps outside) the team that might lead to consensus.

You should enable team members to go beyond disputes over facts and opinions, so as to identify and address the values and related perspectives that may be in play.

Legal

In E&W, the test for continued detention includes that 'appropriate treatment is *available*' for Chelsea, not that it is likely to be effective[30]; in Scotland, that available treatment would be likely to prevent her disorder worsening or alleviate its symptoms or effects; and in RoI, that treatment is likely to benefit or alleviate her condition to a material extent. No explicit treatability test applies in NI, though in practice the tribunal would implicitly consider it in Chelsea's case.

Clinico-legal

Given the lack of disagreement over the continued presence of severe mental disorder or the continued risk of harm to herself and others if she relapses, the key criterion will be whether detention is necessary to achieve the aims of treatment (including habilitation, rehabilitation, nursing care, and treatment for the consequences of mental disorder[31] and its manifestations: anything more than 'mere containment'[32]).

Whether a possible treatment is clinically appropriate, or the power of recall after discharge clinically necessary, depends upon the purpose of that treatment or recall, and therefore on the perspective of the clinician. If a significant risk of harm to others persists, how do you balance the need to keep others safe from Chelsea, with her right to liberty (given that continued detention for treatment might be indefinite)? The loosely drawn law allows for either to have priority.

You will be required by the tribunal to give evidence that represents your own opinion on the grounds for continued detention (or for discharge) under the MHA, but also to summarise and represent the views of the clinical team as a whole. If no consensus has been achieved, this means reflecting opposing points of view appropriately in your report.

Ethical

The values-based practice approach may assist. Everyone, including Chelsea, has a valid perspective, which must be heard and respected; even if Chelsea has no empathy for the girl she tried to kill, her view that she should be released should not simply be dismissed. Discussions should take place in a calm, reflective atmosphere, which may mean a special session outside ordinary team meetings or ward rounds, and this is particularly important where the stakes are high (e.g. where there is a risk of homicide). Minutes of the meeting should be available for the tribunal.

During the discussion, the facts on which a decision will be based should be agreed, as far as possible, before there is any (values-driven) interpretation of the facts or inferences drawn from them. This might mean, for example, beginning with a multidisciplinary presentation of Chelsea's case to date, and a summary of the risk history as a basis for a joint risk-assessment.

Disagreements of interpretation should then be brought out in a nonjudgmental fashion, trying to tease out the values each contributor thinks most important. If consensus cannot be reached, the remaining areas of disagreement and different perspectives should be described.

---

[30] *Nottinghamshire Healthcare NHS Trust v RC* [2014] EWHC 1136.
[31] *B v Croydon Health Authority* [1995] Fam 133.
[32] *R (on the application of W) v Rampton Hospital Authority* [2001] EWHC Admin 134.

13

Clash between clinician and organisational values

Case description

Since 2015, NHS Trusts have been required by counter-terrorism legislation to train staff 'to prevent people from being drawn into terrorism'. 'Prevent' training has been developed to help health care professionals identify people at risk of being drawn into terrorist activities. It is mandatory and must be repeated every two to three years.

You undertake the training and now have ethical concerns about it. You are suspicious of claims that it is possible to identify in advance people who pose a risk of terrorist violence, based on mental ill-health, and you fear staff will be encouraged to breach patient confidentiality on dubious grounds. You think that the programme focuses unduly on terrorism related to Islam, and overlooks other forms (e.g. related to white supremacism, or far-right views). You believe it may lead to discrimination and prejudice against young Muslim males with mental health problems, which contradicts your Trust's value of respect for cultural diversity. You have a significant number of young Muslim men under your care.

You approach your line manager to express your concerns; he disagrees, and points out that this is a nationally mandated programme for all NHS staff.

Questions

1. What should you do?
2. What other clinical, legal, clinico-legal, and ethical issues in the case?

Clinical

Your responsibilities as a mental health professional include considering the risks of harm to self or others that might arise from a range of mental health problems. Although terrorist allegiance and supportive beliefs are of course not evidence of mental disorder per se, it is possible that exposure to pro-terrorist images and online materials may destabilise those who are already in a vulnerable mental state due to depression, drug abuse, or psychotic illness.

In general, anyone voicing concerns about politically violent thoughts and preoccupations wants help with them. Such individuals may feel great shame and fear about such thoughts, and suicide risk may be greater than the risk of terrorist action. It is entirely reasonable to calmly explore with the patient whether they have made any plans to carry out terrorist actions, whether they have enacted them in any way, and whether they feel under pressure from anyone to do this.

Legal

Mandatory training, which has grown enormously over the last fifteen years, is a key indicator on which NHS bodies' performance is judged, and some funding can be withheld if staff do not complete agreed training relevant to improving health.

Prevent training is unusual in that it attempts to link public health with the risk of politically motivated violence. It was formally made mandatory in 2016. In theory at least, if a staff member failed to share reasonable and well-founded concerns about a patient's risk of violence to others, this might lead to an allegation of breach of a contractual duty, or even negligence.

However, the Equality Act 2010 places a responsibility on employers to take steps to prevent discrimination. If any training was found to discriminate against people with a protected characteristic (including religious beliefs) then this might breach the Act.

Clinico-legal

Whilst there may be very complex clinico-legal decisions to take in relation to individual patients and the Prevent programme, in this scenario there is no individual clinical aspect to your decision beyond consideration of your general duty of confidentiality.

Ethical

There is a conundrum here in balancing your duty as an employee against your personal values. Your employer cannot ask you to do anything illegal, but, equally, you accept a duty to comply with required training when you sign a contract of employment. In this case, your employer is asking you to undertake training in relation to actions that are legal, but potentially unjust and in conflict with your personal values. The Royal College of Psychiatrists and other bodies have voiced similar concerns to yours.[33]

The GMC & IMC require that you contribute to and comply with systems to protect patients.[34] However, they also require medical staff to raise concerns openly and safely. By raising your concerns, you are fulfilling your professional ethical duty; although, personally, you may not deem this enough.

Only you can decide to refuse to comply with the Prevent programme, which might lead to disciplinary proceedings. You may wish to discuss this first with a senior colleague or peer group, and you may also want to consult your professional indemnity body, who are unlikely to support you because the training is a national requirement.

Practically you may do more good, and prevent more discrimination, by offering training about risk assessment to staff in your Trust. You can then give good-quality information about the connection between mental disorder and violence (including terrorist violence), including in the context of also advising about the duty of confidentiality on all staff even in regard to risk assessment and management.

[33] Royal College of Psychiatrists (2016) *Counter-terrorism and Psychiatry.*
[34] *Good Medical Practice* (2013) General Medical Council.

14

Role of personal values in risk-formulation

Themes: *schizophrenia (p.73), ASPD (p.82), and depot medication (p.201) [C]; duties of care to patient and potential victim (p.544) and confidentiality (p.320) [L]; risk-formulation (p.146) [CL]; and duties to patient and potential victim (p.296) and values-based practice (p.288) [E]*

Case description

You are a CMHT consultant. Henry (from clinical case 2) has been on your caseload for a year, since conditional discharge from the MSU. When psychotic, he committed a serious assault on a woman unknown to him. He made a good recovery and was conditionally discharged[35] to a community placement, with conditions including accepting his depot medication. He engages well with one CPN, but has a poor relationship with his new social supervisor.

Henry suffers from paranoid schizophrenia, with features of antisocial personality disorder (ASPD). In the past he held down jobs and made relationships, but these often broke down because of his violence. Characteristically, he becomes intensely attached to a woman, usually younger than him; he first idealises her and then becomes jealous, believes she is unfaithful, argues, and becomes violent.

The MSU's risk assessment of him included unproven information about a sexual element to his index offence, and police suspicion that he was responsible for a number of rapes. The tribunal accepted the view that his illness was the major cause of his index offence, while acknowledging his ASPD.

You now face two dilemmas. First, Henry asks to switch from depot to oral medication. He says he finds it humiliating to be injected in the buttocks; he also asserts plausibly that his sexual function is worse on the depot. Half your team predict he will not take oral medication consistently; the others think that agreeing would maintain the therapeutic alliance, so reducing the risk of relapse.

Second, the social worker notes Henry's risk of violence to his newly pregnant girlfriend. He says she should be informed of Henry's past offending. He also disputes that mental illness plays any part in Henry's risk to women, attributing it instead to his misogynistic views. However, Henry refuses to consent to the team talking to his girlfriend; he claims he has told her about his history.

Questions

1. What courses of action are there and how might each be justifiable?
2. What other clinical, legal, clinico-legal, and ethical issues in the case?

---

[35] In E&W, NI, or RoI. In Scotland, the terms of his s53 compulsion order would be varied by the tribunal to authorise compulsory community treatment instead of detention in hospital.

Clinical

Choosing between depot and oral medication represents a common dilemma for clinical teams. You have a duty to minimise the risk of relapse, and of harm to others. However, Henry's sexual function is important, and may contribute to a successful and supportive intimate relationship. Feelings of shame and distress may hinder recovery as much as medication side-effects.

A detailed formulation, using structured measures such as the HCR20v3 or the RSVP may help unpick the factors underlying his risk of harm to women. His risk is likely to arise from a combination of misogyny, ASPD, and disinhibition due to psychosis; of these, reducing risk of psychotic relapse may be the easiest to achieve in the short-term. If you see the risk as predominantly due to ASPD and misogyny, Henry should be offered therapies to address them, and disclosure of risk to others will be essential to the treatment plan. If you see mental illness as the key factor (such that the risk is tolerably low when he is mentally well), you may be willing to refrain from disclosure in return for Henry's assurances about treatment compliance.

You might choose to put to Henry the link between his mental health and the perceived risk to his girlfriend: the less concerned you are about the risk of relapse (because he is on depot medication), the less you will need frequent and possibly intrusive contact with his girlfriend in order to safeguard her. Or you could try to move the discussion from a binary choice between depot and oral, to one involving multiple factors such as the dose, the timing, the specific drug, the criteria for switching, for example, within which he could exercise choice over some aspects, provided that you are content with the overall plan.

Legal

You have a duty of care to Henry, coupled with expecting him to take medication you prescribe, backed up by the power of recall to hospital[36] if he refuses. However, having a legal power does not mean you have a duty to use it, and the law will only defend you doing so if a responsible body of medical opinion would support your decision.

You may[37] also have a duty of care to Henry's girlfriend, as an identifiable individual[38] who may be at risk from him, especially if his mental state deteriorates. You can lawfully breach confidence in regard to the risk that Henry may pose to her if failure to do so would result in a significant risk of serious harm.[39]

The law also allows police to make similar disclosures, either at the suggestion of partner agencies such as the NHS, or on the application of the girlfriend or concerned friends or relatives. In E&W this is covered by the Domestic Violence Disclosure Scheme (commonly known as 'Claire's Law').

Clinico-legal

If you try but fail to persuade Henry to consent to disclosure of his history to his girlfriend, you should consider whether to disclose without his consent. The NHS Code of Confidentiality and the GMC state that health care professionals can breach confidentiality to prevent of serious crime if the risk is sufficiently great.

Whether that threshold is passed will be influenced by your clinical assessment of the current risk of violence to his girlfriend in the absence of psychotic symptoms, and how likely (based upon the agreed treatment plan) you are to be able to prevent relapse of his psychosis.

[36] In E&W, NI, or RoI. In Scotland there is also a power to force treatment in the community if a patient fails to attend an appointment for treatment (s112 MHCTA).
[37] Other jurisdictions, most famously California in *Tarasoff v Regents of the University of California* 17 Cal 3d 425, have subjected professionals to a duty to warn identifiable potential victims. Case law in the UK and RoI has not found such a duty to date (e.g. *Palmer v Tees Health Authority* [1999] All ER 722; *Surrey CC v McManus* [2001] EWCA 691; *K v SSHD* [2002] EWCA Civ 775). However, the issue keeps resurfacing, and a case returning to the High Court at the time of writing may result in such a duty, at least concerning warnings related to genetic conditions (*ABC v St George's Healthcare Trust and others* [2017] EWCA Civ 336, issues from which are discussed in ethics case 2).
[38] There is almost certainly no legal duty in the UK and RoI when no specific victim is identifiable.
[39] *W v Egdell* [1990] 1 AllER 835. See ethics case 2 and civil case 2 for a fuller discussion.

Ethical

An ethical tension arises from the team's responsibility not only to improve Henry's mental health but also to reduce his risk of violence towards women from any cause, not just his psychosis.

It is common in such cases for teams to split, with one view perceiving the risk as arising from attitudes unrelated to mental disorder, and another from mental disorder. There may be strongly differing opinions about coercion and disclosure, reflecting team members' different values and technical approaches. This may be best addressed by adopting a values-based approach: emphasising resolution by reflection on the personal, professional, social, and legal values that are in tension, and not seeking simplistic answers in terms of law, local policy, or clinical facts. It is as well to remember that in forensic practice there are rarely single formulations of violence, and it is wise to try to keep all risk factors in mind as relevant.

15 Continued detention after changed diagnosis and risk assessment

Themes: *substance misuse (p.76), psychosis (p.72), and risk assessment (p.237) [C]; diagnosis as a basis for detention (p.144) [L]; detention despite nonengagement in treatment (p.510) [CL]; and unjust detention (p.338) [E]*

Case description

You are asked to provide an opinion on Markus, a twenty-three-year-old man detained in the MSU. Markus was well known to CAMHS from age twelve years, when he presented with suicidal thoughts and substance misuse due to attachment problems and depression. His father was violent to his mother, and possibly also to the children. He and his family did not engage in family therapy. He later became a regular user of cocaine, amphetamines, and spice, and then presented to mental health services with paranoia.

He served several short sentences for theft, burglary, assaults, and drunk & disorderly behaviour. His index offence was robbery (threatening a man with a knife, demanding his headphones). Since he was on licence after release from prison three weeks earlier, he was also charged with breach of licence. He was transferred to hospital for treatment of psychosis, engaged well with all treatment, recovered swiftly, and became insightful, pleasant, and helpful on the ward. At this point he pleaded guilty and received a restricted hospital order.

Two years on, the clinical picture is very different. There are periods when Markus is still pleasant and co-operative, and this has led to him gaining community leave to his family, which he uses well. But he is often rude and verbally aggressive to staff, and he denies that he ever had any mental disorder. He refuses medication, and an extended drug-free trial has not resulted in relapse. He complies with ward rules, but only minimally, and often challenges boundaries with staff. He is secretive about what he does when on leave, and there are concerns that he is dishonest with the team.

Markus has applied to the tribunal for absolute discharge on the ground that he does not have mental disorder. He has an expert report supporting this position. The week before the tribunal, he smashes up his room and hits a member of staff, with no apparent trigger.

Questions

1. What clinical, legal, clinico-legal, and ethical issues arise in the case?

Clinical

Clinically, one could make a good case that Markus has an ASPD, with some borderline traits. Formal psychological testing might confirm this.

Markus' violence shortly before the hearing may represent self-sabotage, and if so, would fit with the formulation that he has personality disorder: this would have made him vulnerable to psychosis when in prison, and could now mean he has formed an ambivalent attachment to the MSU and its staff, which is threatened by the prospect of discharge.

Legal

Mental health law requires mental disorder as a basis for detention; it does not matter if the disorder changes during the period of detention. Provided you have sufficient evidence of personality disorder, this could provide a ground for continued detention, if coupled with evidence of risk of harm to others, and the availability of appropriate inpatient treatment.

Clinico-legal

Although most people with psychotic disorders are not violent, and most perpetrators of violence are not mentally unwell, when a young man presents with psychotic symptoms on remand for a violent offence it is often assumed that they must be linked, and that a hospital disposal is therefore appropriate. Markus's case shows the wisdom of assessing this carefully at the sentencing stage, and only recommending a direct hospital disposal if confident of the link.[40] Prisons are stressful places, especially for people with personality dysfunction, and so it is common for inmates to experience brief psychotic episodes.

If on reviewing the expert report you agree that Markus no longer suffers from any mental disorder, then you must support 'absolute discharge', despite the risk of harm to others, and despite the likelihood that he could become mentally ill again in the future.

However, if you are satisfied that he suffers from PD, and believe it can successfully be treated in hospital, you should recommend continued detention. If you do not think this, you might nevertheless seek to oppose absolute discharge, and recommend conditional discharge instead, on the ground that his mental disorder makes the power of recall necessary; conditions could include identified accommodation, compliance with CPN support, and continued work on substance misuse. The MoJ would be likely to oppose both absolute and conditional discharge, given his risk of harm to others.

Ethical

Ethically, there are two issues to consider. First, if Markus cannot, or will not, engage in treatment, then it may not be just to continue detaining him, even if treatment is available, and even though detention would be lawful. Further, the treatment available in the MSU may not be of the right sort for Markus; many MSUs have therapy regimes that are geared towards people with psychotic disorders, and may not be as effective for people with ASPD. It is for this reason that personality disorder pathways exist in prison and some specialist secure services, aimed at people like Markus.

Second, it is worth noting that Markus has now spent more time in hospital for this offence than he would if imprisoned. This militates against any argument that it would be just to detain him potentially indefinitely in order to protect the public.

---

[40] In E&W, courts are now likely to imprison people like Markus, or impose a hybrid order, following the *Vowles* judgment, so the team might not face this dilemma. See ethics case 18.

16

Monitoring as 'treatment' justifying continued legal restrictions

Themes: *ASPD (p.82), substance misuse (p.76), and community risk management (p.240) [C]; conditions of discharge (p.511) and definition of treatment (p.482) [L]; benefits and harms of coercion (p.186) [CL]; and conflict with role as a doctor (p.298) [E]*

Case description

Brian, a forty-five-year-old man, was convicted of attempted murder seven years ago. He has sixty previous convictions for acquisitive, drug-related, and violent offences. He has a diagnosis of ASPD, and on the basis of this, was sentenced to a restricted hospital order[41] and admitted to your MSU.

He had used crack cocaine and cannabis heavily in the past; the cocaine disinhibited him but did not cause mental illness. His PCL-R score was 16, and you regard him as belonging to the 'anxious antisocial' group. He completed a basic group on coping with emotions, but refused to attend any subsequent psychological treatment. He was never seriously aggressive or violent as an inpatient, although he made occasional threats when staff displeased him. He was therefore conditionally discharged to your community forensic team two years ago.

Since discharge, he has not been involved in any offending behaviour or other incidents of aggression or violence, to your knowledge or that of the local police (with whom you used to discussed him every six months, until he was dropped from the multiagency agenda three months ago[42]). He has now resumed using cannabis, and occasionally crack, although this has had no apparent impact upon his mental state or behaviour. He has consistently declined offers of psychological treatment, and has become increasingly reluctant to attend appointments.

He has now applied to a tribunal for absolute discharge, or failing that, removal of the condition requiring him to attend appointments and home visits. His solicitor's skeleton argument[43] is that simply monitoring Brian's risk of harm to others does not amount to 'treatment', and so is not a legally valid condition.

---

[41] This was a relatively common occurrence in E&W before the *Vowles* and *Edwards* judgments: see ethics case 18. The scenario is not possible in RoI, where ASPD is insufficient for an order under s4 or s5 CLIA.

[42] In the UK, this would be the Multi-Agency Public Protection Arrangements (MAPPA, or PPANI), at which he would have been discussed at 'level 2' meetings until he no longer met the level 2 threshold. There are no equivalent arrangements in RoI, though the Probation Service has links with many community-based organisations which can allow information-sharing.

[43] An advance summary of the arguments to be advanced at a hearing. In E&W, this is compulsory at immigration tribunals, for instance, but optional for mental health tribunals.

Questions

1. What are the clinical, legal, clinico-legal, and ethical issues in the case?
2. What will you recommend to the tribunal?

Clinical

Cases of 'stuck' patients with ASPD such as Brian are common, and can lead to a sense of hopelessness. However, ASPD can respond to treatment, which should always be offered (including by referral to other specialist teams if necessary).

Since Brian appears unlikely to co-operate for the foreseeable future, this could entail waiting for several years or more before he moves from being 'precontemplative' to contemplating treatment.

If and when he does accept psychosocial treatment, you and his care co-ordinator would use your regular appointments and visits to monitor the impact of treatment, to enable him to reflect and discuss what comes up, and to support his continued engagement. Until that point, however, your sessions can only offer basic counselling, plus monitoring of his mental state, drug use, and reported behaviour.

Legal

Mental health law makes clear that, to count as legally enforceable treatment, proposed interventions must be for mental disorder, its symptoms or manifestations, and/or its consequences.[44] E&W has the widest legal definition of *medical treatment*: 'treatment including nursing care, psychological intervention and specialist mental health habilitation, rehabilitation and care, the purpose of which is to alleviate, or prevent a worsening of, the disorder or one or more of its symptoms or manifestations'; other jurisdictions have very similar but slightly narrower definitions.[45]

There is no case law on the specific point of whether monitoring alone can amount to treatment. However, the E&W Code of Practice explicitly envisages monitoring as *part* of community treatment for patients with personality disorder[46]; and the Code has been approved as authoritative for similar purposes by the Upper Tribunal.[47] It is therefore possible that a tribunal would find that monitoring *alone* amounted to community treatment for PD; although, it would retain a discretion to discharge Brian or to remove the condition, nevertheless.

Clinico-legal

Just because it might be lawful to recommend the conditions continue, you do not have to recommend this; and you should only do so if you believe it is beneficial for Brian to be required to attend appointments and accept visits. So ask yourself 'how are the aims of medical treatment advanced by it, given the likely harm to the potential therapeutic alliance caused by the coercion?'

For instance, if your assessment is that you should use occasional visits to assess whether he is contemplative about change, and to take any opportunities offered by life events to prompt him to undertake such contemplation, and that there is no prospect of any improved therapeutic alliance if

---

[44] For instance, severe weight loss in anorexia can be treated by refeeding, as a consequence of the illness (and a prerequisite to psychological treatment, because very low weight causes cognitive rigidity): (1994) *Re KB (adult) (mental patient: medical treatment)*, BMLR 9: 144. A court even held that in certain circumstances self-starvation was a consequence of severe borderline PD for which refeeding was a treatment: *B v Croydon Health Authority* [1995] Fam 133.

[45] In Scotland, 'nursing, care, psychological intervention, habilitation or rehabilitation'; in NI, 'treatment, care habilitation or rehabilitation'; in RoI, treatment includes (but is therefore not limited to) 'the administration of physical, psychological and other remedies … intended for the purposes of ameliorating a mental disorder'.

[46] Section 21.14, referring to 'day-to-day support and monitoring for the patient's social as well as psychological needs'. Department of Health (2015) *Mental Health Act 1983: Code of Practice*. The Stationery Office.

[47] *DL-H v Devon Partnership NHS Trust and another* [2010] UKUT 102 (AAC).

coercion were removed (after this length of time), then you might recommend maintaining the condition, on the understanding that appointments might be relatively infrequent (perhaps only monthly).

Conversely, if the only value you can see in the appointments is picking up signs of increased risk of reoffending, and risk of harm to others, and you think he is more likely to develop a better relationship if free to choose not to see you, then you might recommend absolute discharge.

Ethical

This kind of stalemate can persist for a number of years with patients with personality disorder. Arguably, prolonged refusal to engage in treatment makes continued coercive attempts at treatment ethically dubious, even if lawful.

You should consider what the reasons for refusal of therapy are, what steps might be taken to try to change Brian's views, and their likelihood of success. A helpful way to think about this might be values-based practice: even if the patient will not take part in the discussion with you, try to consider matters from his perspective and think about what values might be in play for him, and how a compromise might be feasible, and ethical.

Finally, you might consider whether in recommending monitoring alone you would still be operating as a doctor, and if not, whether that should impact your recommendation to the tribunal.

17

Assisting police and prosecution of a patient

Themes: *learning disability (p.110), schizophrenia (p.73), and violence (p.26) [C]; actual bodily harm (p.416) and criteria for prosecution (pp.398, 380) [L]; criminal 'capacity' (p.610) and police access to medical records (p.596) [CL]; and ethics of assisting police (p.314) and role of personal values (p.330) [E]*

Case description

Colin has diagnoses of paranoid schizophrenia and mild intellectual disability. He was previously convicted of five offences; most seriously assault occasioning actual bodily harm, for which he received a hospital order. His psychosis improved after fifteen months, and he was discharged to a care home having six other residents. He needed help with bills but was otherwise independent, attended college, and used a day centre for people with intellectual disability.

Unexpectedly, Colin became disturbed and aggressive, and hit a staff member with a chair. He was assessed in the police station and admitted to your low secure ward.

It transpired that his father had died three weeks earlier, and he had not found out until after the funeral. He wanted to see his father's grave but did not know where it was. He continued to take his antipsychotic medication, and there is no evidence of any recurrence of psychotic symptoms.

He was initially very disturbed on the ward; he smashed windows, and punched two members of staff when they told him he could not have leave to search for his father's grave. This was reported to the police.

The police ask you for a report to help to decide whether Colin should be prosecuted. They have also requested copies of his medical records. They ask:

- Did Colin have capacity to commit the crime?
- Did Colin know what he was doing when he assaulted staff?
- Did Colin know the difference between right and wrong?

Questions

1. How should you respond?
2. Should you give an expert opinion if you are the responsible clinician?
3. What other clinical, legal, clinico-legal, and ethical issues arise in the case?

Clinical

Some of the questions posed are clinical, and you already have the clinical data necessary to answer these. For example, his mental disorder has already been determined.

Legal

The police conduct enquiries into any alleged crime, and submit evidence to the prosecution authority.[48] To proceed, there must be sufficient evidence, and prosecution must be in the public interest.

The 'evidential test' is whether there is a realistic prospect (greater than 50% chance) of conviction. This includes the probable impact of any possible defence, including any mental condition defence. The 'public interest test' considers the seriousness of the offence, the culpability of the defendant, the circumstances of any the harm caused to the victim, the age of the suspect, the impact of the offence on the community, and whether prosecution is a proportionate response.

The questions the police have asked you go beyond information you will have collected for Colin's clinical care; so, if you answer, you will be acting as an expert witness, and have corresponding duties to the court.

Clinico-legal

You should be clear about the clinical data upon which you would base any medicolegal opinions you may express.

Your response to the police request for copies of Colin's medical records should be limited to the minimum necessary for their investigation. Your employer should have a department that will check this, seek Colin's consent, and respond on your behalf; if Colin refuses consent, you may be asked to assist in determining whether there are grounds for disclosing some information nevertheless (e.g. if it is necessary for the prosecution of serious crime).

If only submitting factual information to the police as a professional witness (again, with consent or because there are lawful grounds to disclose without consent), this can be in the form of a witness statement. However, any answers to questions posed to you as an expert witness should be within a report.

The police question about capacity is ill-defined. A general statement about mental capacity as commonly understood in psychiatric services is not directly relevant; rather, the question implies that Colin may have lacked the legal capacity to form intent, or some other relevant state of mind (e.g. recklessness). Ask for instructions that set out the relevant legal test.

Likewise, the questions about 'knowing what he was doing' and 'knowing the difference between right and wrong' need context to explain what the relevant legal issues may be. The language may hint that the police think that the legal defence of insanity could be relevant, but, again, this needs to be set out clearly, so that you are in a position to properly help the court.

Ethical

Having mental disorder, even if detained under the MHA, does not mean that a person cannot be held responsible for criminal acts. Provided that he was capable of not committing the crime (a functional test, incorporating tests e.g. 'capacity to form intent' as above), then fairness and nondiscrimination argue that Colin should be eligible for prosecution like anyone else.

You must balance your role as Colin's doctor *and* any responsibility to assist the police and protect others, including hospital staff. The difficulty in this case is not whether you should offer any assistance to the police, but, rather, what evidence you can offer consistent with your responsibilities.

You should think very carefully about what information might be needed by the police, and ensure you follow your organisation's procedure for this. Especially if Colin has not given (or is unable to give) consent, you should not simply hand over reports prepared for other purposes, and should not allow the police to read or access notes in the hospital.

There is no consensus on whether you should give expert opinion on patients under your care, though it is broadly acceptable for minor offences and widely cautioned against in the most serious cases (wherein the risk and consequences of unintended bias are greater). There may be pressure from police and prosecutors who might feel 'entitled' to your opinion, and understandably are not aware of the ethical concerns you may have. It is important that you establish your own professional position. If there is Trust policy or guidance suggesting you take an approach that you are ethically uncomfortable with, then you should seek advice from a colleague or your defence organisation. Ultimately you can be forced to give factual information, but you cannot be forced to give an expert opinion.

---

[48] For example the Procurator Fiscal in Scotland, or the Crown Prosecution Service in E&W.

18 Risk assessment informing sentencing after GBH conviction

Themes: *abuse and trauma (p.32) and posttraumatic stress disorder (p.96)[C]; hybrid orders, Vowles and Edwards (pp.504, 754, 770), and mitigation (p.638) [L]; risk assessment for penal purposes (p.670) [CL]; and giving an opinion on subthreshold symptoms (p.668) and resisting commenting on culpability (p.664) [E]*

Case description

Savannah has been convicted of GBH following an incident in a nightclub.

When Savannah was three years old, she was raped by her father's adolescent nephew. Her mother told her father, but her father disbelieved her and continued to allow his nephew to have regular contact with Savannah. She confronted her father about what had happened much later, and he apologised. She has worked for an airline for some years without problems.

She drank socially as a teenager, but when she met her former partner, her use of alcohol increased. For several years she drank three bottles of wine a day, and frequently suffered withdrawal symptoms.

Savannah's relationship with her former partner was very abusive of her: he caused her to miscarry through assaulting her, and his demeanour could change in an instant. She lost confidence in herself and became depressed, and was prescribed antidepressant medication for several years. She sleeps poorly and often has nightmares about him. She is 'scared of everything' and avoids others.

On the night of the alleged offence, Savannah visited a nightclub with a female friend, and they had some drinks. At the end of the evening, Savannah and her friend were approached by a male security guard, who Savannah said, 'was seven-foot tall and very threatening ... he was in my face'. Savannah believed that he unfairly targeted her, telling her to leave although other people were still dancing. This led her to challenge him. She said, 'I wasn't angry ... I just wanted to know why ... then he got in my face ... he started to take things out of his coat ... I felt he was preparing for something ... to hit me ... like my ex.... I felt threatened ... petrified ... I thought I was going to be attacked.' She could feel her heart in her chest, and started to sweat profusely. He grabbed her arm; she tried to throw her drink to make him 'back off'. The glass smashed and cut his face badly.

You are asked by her solicitor to provide a report addressing whether Savannah might have PTSD, and to give opinions on her risk to others and on disposal.

Questions

1. What are the clinical, legal, clinico-legal, and ethical issues in the case?

Clinical

Posttraumatic stress disorder (PTSD) develops following direct or indirect exposure to actual or threatened death, serious injury, or sexual violence, of a nature that would cause distress in anyone. It comprises re-experiencing, hyperarousal, and avoidance symptoms, and can include episodes of dissociation. It is associated with abuse of substances, particularly alcohol, to reduce anxiety and arousal, and irritability.

Resilience to trauma varies; around 25%–30% of people experiencing something like Savannah will develop PTSD. If the trauma occurs chronically in childhood, then personality development can be distorted, resulting in personality disorder. PTSD arising from a large number of persistent but individually less severe traumas is termed 'complex PTSD'.

PTSD causes people to be anxious and fearful, and often reluctant to discuss the trauma. The clinical interview should therefore be conducted in a calm and quiet manner. Some people, especially those who have experienced sexual violence, might be troubled by the presence of anyone who resembles their abuser(s), for example a male interviewer in the case of a woman raped by a man.

Based on Savannah's history and informant accounts, analyse:

- the frequency and duration of different types of trauma;
- when the events took place;
- Savannah's perception of the trauma and injury;
- how any symptoms experienced since relate to trauma;
- personal and family relationships, since sufferers often 'withdraw';
- how any dysfunction and disability relate to symptoms; and
- comorbidity, in particular depression or substance misuse.

Psychological tests such as the TSI or IES-R[49] can help collect these data. Some signs might be observable: for example, a hyper-startle response to noise, or apparent dissociation. Often, sufferers will experience a change in their mental state when discussing their trauma; so that they may be very anxious or appear dissociated.

Establishing a history of the offence is important, addressing how Savannah's behaviour might have related to her apparent PTSD, which can be done through clinical interview of her, and witness statements. Less commonly, it might be possible, with the defendant's or prosecution permission, to interview witnesses. You should particularly address her apparent level of arousal, and any suggestion of dissociation.

Do not consider your instructions a barrier to completing a full clinical assessment: for example, although your instructions only require an opinion on whether or not Savannah suffers from PTSD, if you consider that personality disorder (perhaps with transient psychosis) is a possible diagnosis, then you should assess her for this.

If she suffers from more severe PD with transient psychosis, a period of treatment in hospital might be appropriate, but, otherwise, treatment is likely to be psychological, and to be delivered in the community.

Legal

Evidence of mental disorder can found a recommendation for hospital treatment, contribute to an assessment of risk of future offending, or be offered in mitigation of sentence. Expert witnesses must keep strictly to proper boundaries of expert evidence (e.g. not directly suggesting mitigation).[50]

---

[49] *Trauma Symptom Inventory* and *Impact of Events Scale—Revised*.
[50] Thus it is unacceptable to give evidence <u>during trial</u> on possible future clinical decisions (e.g. on discharge from hospital if sentenced to treatment), because it can sway the jury in their verdict: *R v Edgington* [2013] EWCA Crim 2185. Such evidence should only be given before a judge who is deciding sentence.

Two landmark judgments, *Vowles*[51] and *Edwards*,[52] have greatly influenced how courts approach recommendations for medical disposal in E&W. Previously, most courts would only override medical recommendations if given strong reasons to do so. Now the judge must consider the extent to which the offender needs treatment; her degree of culpability; the extent to which the offence was attributable to mental disorder; punishment required; and the need for public protection (courts address 'dangerousness' not 'risk assessment'). Only if a hybrid order or imprisonment is inappropriate can the court make a hospital order.

Clinico-legal

Ensure your opinion does not read as a list of facts to be pleaded in mitigation, a sign of lack of expert objectivity. Likewise, your risk assessment must only relate to risk of harm arising from mental disorder; probation officers and forensic psychologists may comment upon risk arising from other sources.

It will be particularly helpful if you include 'scenarios' in which violence is a significant possibility; structured instruments such as the HCR20v3 can assist with this. For Savannah, this might include feeling hyper-aroused, being irritable, dissociating, misinterpreting potential victims' behaviour, and experiencing flashbacks triggered by such misinterpretations, especially if intoxicated. Particular interventions that may help in managing elements of these scenarios should also be included.

Although your report is for sentencing, it may include evidence that could[53] have supported an alternative finding at trial, such as insanity, or insane or sane[54] automatism (if she had been dissociating at the time of the attack). If this is your opinion, mention it to your instructing solicitor, even though it goes beyond your instructions. It will be up to them how to respond to this.

Ethical

It is acceptable to give an opinion even if you cannot diagnose PTSD, provided there are relevant aspects of the defendant's mental state, so long as you remain within a clinical paradigm.

Individuals who have experienced severe trauma more readily perceive threat, and can become irritable and aroused as a result. And this can occur even if other symptoms of PTSD are absent. However, it is important to be clear in your opinion whether you have made a diagnosis or whether you are describing lesser psychological consequences of trauma.

Where you recommend disposal, you should be careful only to recommend treatment options and never punishments; although you may choose to note that, if the court passes a punitive sentence, elements of treatment may be available, and you may conditionally recommend them (e.g. 'should the court be minded to pass a community order, I recommend consideration of a mental health treatment requirement … '). You should resist pressure to comment upon 'culpability' (see above), which is not a clinical construct, though you might reasonably comment upon causation of the offence arising from mental disorder.

---

[51] *R v Vowles and others* [2015] EWCA Crim 45.

[52] *R v Edwards* [2018] EWCA Crim 595.

[53] *Could* is the operative word here—the law in all four jurisdictions on insanity and insane automatism with a nonpsychotic mental disorder and the presence of voluntary intoxication is highly complex, and such defences would be unlikely to succeed in Savannah's case.

[54] Dissociation can be a sane automatism if the defendant is 'predisposed' to such by a previous unusual external stressor, such as rape (*R v T* [1990] CrimLR 256).

19

Risk assessment for sentencing of patient currently in treatment

Themes: *clinical risk-assessment (p.163) and recovered mental disorder (p.264) [C]; dangerousness (p.672) [L]; report on sentencing (p.670) [CL]; and conflict between patient welfare and duty to court (p.298) and declining instructions (p.680) [E]*

Case description

A solicitor contacts you about one of your community patients, who has just been convicted of a serious assault. The court has ordered her to obtain a psychiatric opinion on your patient's diagnosis, prognosis, treatment plan, and risk of future violence towards others.

She explains that, because he had previously been convicted of a still more serious assault,[55] the court is very likely to impose a long custodial sentence, with the length influenced by the risk assessments in the presentence report and psychiatric report.[56]

You happened to have reviewed the patient concerned the day before the offence and you are sure that he was mentally well, and had been for some time. The prison also reports that he is well. Although you would agree to reassess him for the purpose of completing a psychiatric report, you are sure that you would have no grounds for recommending any form of psychiatric disposal, such as an order for admission to hospital.

Questions

1. Should you accept the instruction to prepare a psychiatric report?
2. If yes, how would you approach the report?
3. If no, how would you respond to the court?
4. What other clinical, legal, clinico-legal, and ethical issues arise in the case?

Clinical

You have an existing clinical relationship with this patient, but it is unlikely that either you or he will have anticipated you needing to prepare such a report. If you accept the instructions, you will need his consent, and your thorough reassessment of him and his risk of violence will amount to a change in your relationship with him.

---

[55] Wounding with intent (E&W and NI); assault to the danger of life (Scotland); assault causing serious harm (RoI).

[56] This combination of offences would allow the court to consider an extended sentence of imprisonment under s226A Criminal Justice Act 2003 in E&W, s210A Criminal Procedure (Scotland) Act 1995, or art14 Criminal Justice (Northern Ireland) Order 2008 (p.IV.79). There is no equivalent extended sentence in RoI, though the court could take into account similar information in deciding what length of determinate sentence to impose.

Legal

The court will use any relevant information in your report in deciding the length of sentence. At this stage you have no legal duty to provide such information, merely an invitation to compile a report. The court may also infer mitigating and/or aggravating factors from your report. Even more indirectly, the court might use your description of his mental health to determine his degree of 'culpability'.

Dangerousness is defined in law in E&W as a 'significant risk to the public of serious harm (i.e. death or serious physical or psychological injury)' from an offender, which courts tend to perceive as akin to a character trait of the individual, and so may need to be persuaded of the merits of instead analysing 'risk of harm', which is partly situational.

Clinico-legal

You might reasonably decide to decline the instructions because you do not wish to provide evidence that would result in punishment, without the likelihood of treatment or care, viewing this as falling outside ethical medical practice. In this case the court might take evidence from a psychiatrist who knows your patient less well and has a different ethical stance, or use the medical records without an expert to interpret them or use no psychiatric evidence at all, including evidence on the likely impact of long imprisonment on the defendant's mental health.

Another option would be to offer to compile a report, including giving an opinion on the likely effects of prolonged or even indeterminate imprisonment on your patient, but without adding a risk assessment. The court might or might not be willing to instruct you on this basis. If you do this, you would then be able to put before the court evidence demonstrating the patient's vulnerability to the psychological impact of a long period of imprisonment, and the need for support from a prison psychiatric team, without providing evidence of risk of harm to others.

Ethical

Ethically, it is accepted practice to present evidence to the court of risk of harm where this is required to explain a recommendation for treatment (e.g. where you are recommending treatment in hospital under a restriction order), as the likelihood of the information being used solely for punishment is lower. However, many psychiatrists would consider it unethical to give such evidence where there is no realistic prospect of treatment or care, especially when you have a pre-existing duty of care to your patient.

If you do compile a report, with or without a risk assessment, you must ensure the patient gives his consent, fully informed about the possible outcomes. If you decide to include a risk assessment, this must be detailed to a clinical standard, based upon longitudinal information from a wide variety of sources, which may need to go beyond what you have gathered in the routine course of clinical care of the patient; you should also consider a team approach, rather than doing it in isolation.

Your report must be completed with the requirements of expert evidence in mind. Your duty to the court means you must not be selective in the information you present, or unduly emphasise anything tending to benefit your patient's interests. Another expert without the pre-existing relationship with your patient might be at lower risk of such bias.

If you decide to refuse the instructions, you should explain your reasons for doing so in detail.

20

What is a 'good-enough' treatment outcome for patient progression?

Themes: *drug-induced psychosis (p.72), community leave (p.191), and risk assessment (p.163) [C]; conditional discharge (p.511) [L]; and respect for patient's values (p.288) and disputes within team (p.312) [E]*

Case description

Konrad is a forty-year-old white man convicted of GBH with intent. He attacked an Afro-Caribbean man with a hammer when paranoid and hearing voices. The prosecutor accepted a guilty plea to GBH, withdrawing the original charge of attempted murder. The judge made a restricted hospital order.

Konrad's diagnosis is paranoid schizophrenia, with symptoms exacerbated by alcohol, cannabis, and cocaine use. His father, who was violent to him as a child, also suffered from schizophrenia. Konrad has never accepted the diagnosis, although he does acknowledge drug-related psychotic episodes, and has accepted medication in the medium secure unit. Eighteen months after being sentenced, having had psychological treatment and escorted leave, he was then transferred to your low secure ward.

Konrad has applied for conditional discharge. You are worried about Konrad's management by you in the community because he will only take oral medication. He also holds racist attitudes and can be dismissive of nonwhite staff. He insists he will never abuse drugs again; he refuses to attend the substance misuse group, but does talk about his drug use in individual sessions with the psychologist.

Most of the clinical team, including the social worker and psychologist, believe he has made sufficient progress to be discharged soon, after a period of unescorted leave. The social worker has identified potential accommodation.

You are conscious that the therapeutic alliance with Konrad may be threatened if he sees as you as delaying discharge. However, are unsure his recovery is 'good enough', meaning that he is still at significant risk of stopping medication and using substances (and hence of further psychotic episodes and possibly assaults on non-white people).

Questions

1. What alternative courses of action are there, and how might each be justified?
2. What should you do?
3. What other clinical, legal, clinico-legal, and ethical issues in the case?

Clinical

The clinical issues are not complicated: Konrad has engaged in treatment and responded to it. He seems to accept the risk of drug-related psychotic episodes. However, you perceive the risk as higher than he does (and perhaps also than the rest of the team does).

Legal

The key legal issue at the forthcoming tribunal will be whether continued detention in hospital under the MHA is justified: does Konrad have a mental disorder that warrants continued detention?

Clinico-legal

Konrad's lawyer may well seek to argue that he does not have a mental disorder at all, having recovered from psychosis, or that, if he does have schizophrenia, it is of neither a nature nor degree sufficient to warrant continued detention. As he has recovered, it would be difficult to argue 'degree', but you may argue that the 'nature' of his illness (i.e. the likelihood of it relapsing, and the resultant risk of harm to others) warrants further inpatient treatment[57]—ideally to establish depot medication or alternatively to reduce the chances of drug use through further psychological treatment.

Ethical

Your view is essentially that Konrad must adopt a higher standard of behaviour for you to be sure he will represent a low risk in the community, not just show no behaviours similar to the index offence; he must also accept depot medication and convincingly eschew illicit drugs.

The disagreement within your team may also be an ethical issue: how just are the decision-making processes within the team, given the impact of the final recommendation on Konrad's liberty? Will your view predominate, or will others be given due weight? If you do not reach a consensus, this is likely to become an issue at the hearing, especially if Konrad's solicitor instructs an expert who reaches a different conclusion to your own.

You should, if possible, reflect on the reasons for your view, and explore them in a joint meeting with equal respect for the values of other team members. In particular, is your view influenced by a desire for Konrad to be safe not only for himself and others, but also to avoid any inquiry or damage to your professional reputation?

The case highlights the need on occasions for 'positive risk-taking' as part of the recovery process in forensic settings. That is, you have a duty to ensure that Konrad is not unfairly held back because of your anxieties. And supporting Konrad, and his good relationships with the team, may do more to reduce risk than insisting he accept depot medication.

---

[57] *R (Smith) v MHRT South Thames Region* [1998] EWHC Admin 832 determined that 'nature' and 'degree' are disjunctive. And 'nature' includes both the diagnosis and its previous impact upon behaviour.

21 Assisting the detection, prevention, or prosecution of serious crime

Themes: *violent thoughts (p.26), extremism (p.42), and mood disorder (pp.92–95) [C]; duty of confidentiality (p.660) [L]; disclosure of information (p.320) and professional or expert witness (p.652) [CL];and balancing justice and duty of care (pp.296, 298) [E]*

Case description

You are the consultant in a community mental health team. Giles's GP has referred him to you because of his 'violent thoughts'. Giles tells you these have worried him since the age of thirteen, when his parents divorced, and he lost contact with his father. He tells you of his fantasies of making a bomb and putting it on a crowded train, or in a shopping centre. He feels drawn to racist websites that advocate expelling immigrants, especially Muslims.

You take the view that Giles's views are ego-dystonic, driven by a mood disorder, and do not constitute a threat to others. Your hypothesis seems validated when Giles's mood improves on an antidepressant, and the violent thoughts recede. Giles engages well with his CPN (who is of Asian background) and meets with a support worker regularly who helps him attend a recovery college.

Nine months later you are about to refer him back to his GP when a local mosque suffers a fire, and the police suspect arson by a local racist group. The local news features CCTV footage of possible suspects; you think you recognise Giles, but can't be sure. The following week, the CPN calls to say that Giles seems unusually agitated and hostile, and did not attend his usual appointment with his support worker. You see Giles, who breaks down in tears, and says he played a part in what happened. He is intensely distressed.

Questions

1. What alternative courses of action are there, and how might each be justifiable?
2. What should you do?
3. What other clinical, legal, clinico-legal, and ethical issues arise in the case?

Clinical

Clinically, your first duty is to Giles and his mental health; so your initial concern must be the deterioration of his mood. If he has committed a crime he now regrets, he may be at risk of impulsive, perhaps lethal, self-harm. Make time to talk calmly to Giles, ideally with his support worker. If Giles is depressed, consider treatment, if necessary in hospital.

Law

NHS/HSE advice to staff about managing confidential information supports disclosure of confidential medical information in order to prevent, detect or prosecute crime involving the risk of death or serious injury.[58] You have reasons to think that Giles may have been involved in a serious crime, and the police would probably find this information relevant. You do not have a legal duty to disclose at this stage, however, only the right to disclose if you consider the criteria above to be met.

Whatever you decide, you still have a duty of care to Giles.

If Giles were arrested by the police, and they then asked you for his medical records or other information, you should seek Giles's consent to disclosure, but if refused, you would be justified in disclosure anyway for the purpose of detecting serious crime.

Clinico-legal

One approach would be to try to persuade Giles to go to the police himself, with your support. This would have the advantage of being transparent, honest, and clinically helpful to Giles. You could advise him on finding a criminal solicitor. If he declines, you should weigh up your suspicion and your clinical knowledge of Giles; if you decide to inform the police, you should tell Giles beforehand, if safe to do so (giving him a final chance to go to the police himself, but also risking him going into hiding, which could disrupt treatment and place his health at risk, as well as perhaps others). You may wish to have a witness to the conversation and to keep a note.

If Giles then wants to leave, you cannot detain him; unless you think he requires a MHA assessment because he is relapsing, or relapse is imminent.[59] If he is detained, then this might initially have to be on a general psychiatric ward, but you should discuss him urgently with forensic colleagues. Given the lack of forensic history or evidence of immediate risk of harm to others in hospital, secure services are unlikely to admit him until he has been charged.

You and the treatment team will almost certainly be called as professional witnesses of what Giles told you, and of his mental state at the time of the alleged offence. Further questions, such as about the availability of an insanity defence or a psychiatric disposal, would be better answered by a forensic psychiatrist lacking a prior relationship with him.

Ethical

The obvious ethical tension lies in your duty to justice and public protection being in conflict with your duty to Giles's confidentiality and welfare; he may feel you have betrayed him if you disclose all that you know of him without his knowledge or consent. However, he does not have to like your actions, and you can validate his fear and distress and reassure him that you will continue to support him as his psychiatrist.

The tradition that confidentiality involves keeping dangerous secrets has long been abandoned. GMC/IMC and RCPsych guidance makes it clear that doctors may disclose patient information in the public interest, but that there needs to be a reflective process before disclosure that balances the costs and benefits of doing so. Being honest and transparent with patients about risk management is crucial because it treats them with respect. What people most resent is professionals talking about them behind their back in a way that they experience as deceitful.

---

[58] Provided that only the minimum necessary is disclosed, and to an appropriate authority.

[59] Or if you exercise your power to make a 'citizen's arrest' pending the arrival of the police: this is lawful because an arrestable offence has been committed, and you reasonably suspect him of it.

22 Professional boundary violations and workplace discrimination

Themes: *strongly held beliefs (p.42) [C]; equality and discrimination law (p.556) [L]; boundary violations by staff (p.302) [CL]; and personal and professional values (p.330) [E]*

Case description

You are the consultant for a secure ward. A patient tells you that a nurse, Jim, has asked to pray with him a few times. The patient says that he does not mind because he also identifies as Christian, but thought it was 'a bit unusual'.

You raise this with Jim, who confirms that he does pray with patients, if they agree. He also describes discussing religious matters with colleagues, including the role of Christianity in recovery and treatment. He asks you whether you are a Christian.

Four weeks later, a junior doctor says Jim pressurised her to come to his church. She felt uncomfortable, but was able to say no. She also mentions she has heard patients on the ward refer to Jim as 'The Prophet'.

You bring this up with Jim, who insists he has done nothing wrong. He adds that you are distressing him by infringing his freedom to practise his religious beliefs. You make a formal complaint against Jim. During the ensuing disciplinary process, two junior nurses report that Jim asked them to pray during supervision. Jim subsequently raises a grievance against you, citing religious discrimination. You used to have a good working relationship with Jim, and he was previously seen as a competent colleague who was popular with patients.

Questions

1. What are the legal and professional issues in this case?
2. What are the alternative courses of action?

Clinical

Observing religious belief is complex in mental health services because mental disorders can impact belief and identity, and because some symptoms can have religious content or a religiose quality. Treatment involves careful consideration of the impact of patients' beliefs on how they understand their condition.

For some people, prayer or other religious rituals may be helpful. This is best supported by chaplains, imams, or others from the appropriate religious tradition, rather than by clinicians stepping out of their clinical role.

Legal

The Equality Act 2010[60] protects certain characteristics, including religious faith. The ECHR also contains rights to hold and manifest religious beliefs (Article 9), and to freedom of expression of those beliefs (Article 10). Any alleged infringement of those rights at work would be considered legally at an employment tribunal.[61]

The nurse claims discrimination based upon membership of a religious group. But neither Jim's distress nor a complaint about Jim's religious practice at work is evidence of discrimination in itself.

Also, the rights are not absolute, and may be 'qualified' depending upon context. In the context of mental healthcare, an employer may be justified in asking professional staff not to express their religious beliefs at work, for the clinical reasons in the previous section. Jim would have to show that he was being treated *differently* because of his beliefs; whereas the Trust might reasonably claim that, in the context of mental health care, where values and conflicts of values are so common, and where patients are often vulnerable, it is entitled to require *all* staff not to express personal beliefs at work. The key legal test is whether such restrictions are 'proportionate', 'appropriate', and 'necessary' in the circumstances.

Clinico-legal

Having not resolved the issue with Jim yourself, and now being the subject of a grievance, you should not discuss the issue further with him. However, his line manager should consider informal discussions as the first step in the disciplinary process, and attempt to reach agreement on keeping religious practices personal (e.g. done alone, and only during breaks during his shifts). Depending upon local policies, this might have to wait until after the grievance against you has been resolved.

If Jim's line manager cannot reach an informal resolution with him, then a formal investigation will be necessary, and this might result in instructions to Jim not to conduct religious practices during work time, or with others on hospital premises. If Jim does not accept this, he can appeal internally and then to an employment tribunal (e.g. for constructive unfair dismissal[62]).

Ethical

For many people, religious faith is part of their personal and cultural identity, which connects them to family and social groups. Religious groups have sometimes been vulnerable to persecution; so that the duty to respect religious faith and culture is an essential aspect of respect for diversity more generally.

Boundary crossings and misdemeanours may be especially problematic in secure services because offending and risky behaviour also involve boundary violations. Making and maintaining professional boundaries has particular importance in secure care, where staff and patients spend long periods of time with each other, and there is the potential for personal relationships to develop.

The religious beliefs of staff are clearly a personal matter for them, and disclosure of such personal material is the commonest kind of professional boundary violation. In itself, telling a patient about one's personal faith may not be harmful, but it does reframe the relationship with the patient in a different and unpredictable way. Jim could not be sure that his avowal of faith, or practice of his beliefs, at work would not be misunderstood by patients, or colleagues, and, indeed, there is evidence that it did have a negative impact upon both colleagues and patients. Further, the fact that a member of the clinical team shares a patient's faith does not mean that they are expert in linking faith and recovery.

Although sharing some aspects of personal circumstances can be good for therapeutic relationships by 'making a connection', if it promotes a personal rather than professional relationship, then it will be counter-therapeutic. Disclosing a shared interest or allegiance to a sports team may be on the acceptable side of the line, depending on the circumstances; sharing deeper aspects of personal identity such as religion, sexuality, or politics will seldom be.

---

[60] Employment Equality Acts in RoI.

[61] In E&W or Scotland; in NI at a Fair Employment Tribunal; in RoI, at the Workplace Relations Commission.

[62] That is, that he felt forced to resign because of the (to him) unreasonable disciplinary decision.

23

Obesity—weighing treatment benefits against side-effects

Case description

Lucas is a forty-two-year-old man who has been detained under a civil section in the MSU for over two years. He was admitted from the PICU because of frequent assaults on staff, and because he did not appear to respond to antipsychotic medication. He has no insight into his condition or need for treatment; he claims that staff are trying to poison him to prevent him inheriting a large estate in America bequeathed by his father, who he claims was Elvis Presley.

Lucas is the youngest of three adult children. He was diagnosed with schizophrenia aged twenty-one. He left school at age sixteen and has no qualifications, though he is intelligent and enjoys reading comics and watching films. Both his older siblings also have schizophrenia, although they both have part-time jobs and have not needed lengthy inpatient care. His mother committed suicide when he was twenty-five years old; and his mental health has been much worse since then, with long periods detained in hospital, plus assaults on his father and older brothers. Lucas has never been charged with these offences, despite once fracturing his father's jaw and slashing his brother's arm. His father remains supportive but is frightened of Lucas.

In the MSU, Lucas remains psychotic despite high doses of first- and second-generation antipsychotics. He continues to be verbally aggressive and unpredictably violent, though less so than when on lower doses within BNF limits. He drinks large volumes of carbonated drinks because of his fear of being poisoned by staff, and eats only bread and potatoes. As a result of this, and his medication, he now weighs nearly nineteen stone, with a BMI of 31. Many staff have good relationships with him but also experience intimidation by him.

Lucas has developed diabetes and hypertension, but will not comply with his diet or blood tests. He denies that he has these conditions, and says he is 'fighting fit'. The team is concerned that Lucas will experience more complications of obesity, or even die suddenly.

Questions

1. What are the clinical, legal, and ethical implications of this case?
2. What should you do?

Clinical

Patients in long-stay residential secure care are at increased risk of leading sedentary lives from restrictions on their movements because of security needs and the unavailability of staff to supervise exercise. Moreover, very many forensic patients are prescribed medication that may improve symptoms and risk of violence–but which increase appetite and the risk of metabolic syndrome. Anecdotal evidence suggests that patients may increase their body weight by a third within six months of regular use of second-generation antipsychotics, especially at high doses, but that such doses are often maintained because of the risk of violence.

Legal

Mental health law distinguishes between treatments for mental disorder and those for other conditions.[63] Such treatments can be forced on dissenting patients even if they have mental capacity,[64] unlike those for other conditions, which can only be compelled if the patient lacks capacity[65] and (in the UK) it is in their best interest.

Treatment for mental disorder can, in limited circumstances, also include treatment of the physical consequences of mental disorder[66]; although this does not extend to *the side-effects of treatment*, such as of diabetes and hypertension. Moreover, it can be given despite potentially harmful consequences (e.g. an undesired loss of sex drive, or diabetes), provided merely that the 'purpose … is to alleviate, or prevent a worsening of, the [mental] disorder or one or more of its symptoms or manifestations [such as behaviour]'.[67]

Treatment for the diabetes and hypertension must therefore be with Lucas's consent or, if he lacks capacity, in his best interests[68]. This could include restraining him to take blood or administer medication if that were necessary to prevent harm and was proportionate to the likelihood and seriousness of that harm.

Clinico-legal

A team responsible for a detained patient therefore holds a great deal of coercive power under mental health legislation. And you must balance the risk of harm to others against the risk to the patient's life and wellbeing, now and in the future.

In regard to treatment of his hypertension and diabetes, this is an anxiety-provoking situation without an obvious or good solution; managing everyone's anxiety will be important.

You should maintain a good therapeutic relationship with Lucas, bearing in mind that others may have better relationships because they are not identified with your coercive power (e.g. the support worker or physical skills trainer).

---

[63] This is explored further in mental health law case 2.

[64] Subject to safeguards such as an independent second opinion after three months and restrictions on treatments such as ECT and psychosurgery, plus additional rules for emergency treatments. In Scotland, there must be 'significantly impaired' decision-making ability, though this is probably a lower threshold than full mental capacity.

[65] Compulsory treatment and isolation for people with certain high-risk infectious diseases is an exception to this general rule: s37 Public Health (Control of Disease) Act 1984 in E&W; s39 Public Health etc (Scotland) Act 2008; s3B Public Health Act (Northern Ireland) 1967; and s38 Health Act 1947 in RoI.

[66] For example enforced refeeding has been held to be lawful under mental health law in a capacitous patient with borderline PD who used food refusal as a form or self-harm (as treatment for a consequence of mental disorder, and a precondition to successful psychological treatment): *B v Croydon Health Authority* [1995] Fam 133. However, with rather circular logic the courts have ruled that any medical treatment involving a deprivation of liberty 'beyond what is properly within the ambit of' the MHA requires a prior application to the High Court.

[67] This is the test for E&W. The wording in Scotland, NI, and RoI differs slightly but is still based upon the intention rather than the actual effect of the treatment.

[68] In the UK. In RoI, it would have to be in accordance with his prior expressed or likely wishes.

Ethical

This is arguably one of the most serious contemporary ethical dilemmas in inpatient psychiatry. Patients are forced to take high-dose medications where the risks include death or serious morbidity, and the principal benefits accrue to others (through a reduction in the patient's aggression and violence).

In prescribing for Lucas's schizophrenia you must weigh the benefits and risks to him and to society, including staff: an onerous responsibility, and one that goes beyond ordinary medical practice. By contrast, in prescribing for Lucas's diabetes and hypertension you must (assuming Lucas lacks capacity and refuses treatment) weigh up only the likelihood and seriousness of the harm to Lucas himself—taking into account the possibility that treatment would have to be imposed on a daily basis.

Ethically, you have a duty to make Lucas's care your first concern, and that means improving his physical health as best you can. A good starting point is a transparent process of consulting all the stakeholders, and ensuring that everyone's views are heard and represented. This includes an advocate for Lucas. It might also be appropriate to involve his family, and to consult the hospital safeguarding team. Discussions and advice should be well documented.

What the discussions and consultations need to establish is what risk is predictable, and what risk can be tolerated, and by whom, while promoting an effective therapeutic relationship with Lucas that keeps him as involved as possible.

24

When all options stink

Case description

Gordon is a thirty-seven-year-old man serving life sentences for two murders. The first victim was a stranger; the second offence occurred in prison. He has been held for the last six years in prison Care and Separation Units (CSUs) because of his high risk of serious violence. Nevertheless, he has assaulted numerous prison officers.

He has repeatedly been referred for psychiatric treatment because of a suspicion of psychosis. During a period of assessment in a high secure hospital, he became slightly less aggressive on antipsychotic medication, but he refused consent to all treatment, would not engage in psychological work, and seriously assaulted several nurses. He was diagnosed with ASPD and remitted to prison. All requests for further hospital treatment have since been rejected, even though it is generally accepted that the severity of his condition determines that he lacks the capacity to make treatment decisions.

He is rarely allowed to associate with any other prisoners and has no visitors, being estranged from his family. He says that he will not accept any treatment anywhere, although he has instructed his solicitor to pursue transfer to hospital; staff think this is because he felt more able to intimidate nurses than prison officers.

His solicitor has initiated judicial review of the decision not to transfer, on the ground of a breach of Gordon's Article 3 right to freedom from inhuman or degrading treatment.

You are a high secure consultant who has not previously been involved. The court has instructed you as a single joint expert to give an opinion on diagnosis, treatment, and hospital transfer.

Questions

1. What are the justifiable alternative courses of action?
2. What should you do?
3. What other clinical, legal, clinico-legal, and ethical implications of the case are there?

Clinical

Gordon poses persistent risks to others that make medical care extremely difficult. The clinical question is twofold: is there a clinical need for hospital treatment in principle, and if so, can this be provided safely? There may be no level of hospital security capable of managing the risk of harm he poses.

There has been a clear longstanding difference of clinical opinion on diagnosis and treatment need between prison and hospital staff. However, it might be that the apparent difference in the clinical formulation represents a difference in opinion relating solely to where the care should be provided (that is, formulation is driven by the 'wished for' placement).

Some services offer an 'appeal' forum where disputed decisions on admissions can be discussed, and that might be helpful in Gordon's case.

Legal

Mental health law provides for transfer from prison to hospital, which would then permit antipsychotic treatment to be enforced. 'Appropriate treatment' only needs to be 'available' (in E &W); his anticipated refusal is not relevant.

The decision not to detain him (and therefore implicitly to respect his refusal of treatment despite his lack of capacity) is a decision by a psychiatrist or hospital acting as a public authority, and is therefore subject to judicial review on human rights grounds: in this case, the possibility that repeatedly refusing to transfer him to hospital amounts to inhuman or degrading treatment in breach of Article 3.[69]

Mental health law does not allow for enforcement of treatment in prison in the UK or RoI. Treatment can be given under mental capacity law, but it could only be enforced if it was considered necessary to prevent harm *to Gordon* (not to others, except in RoI), and was a proportionate response to the likelihood and seriousness of that harm.[70,71]

Clinico-legal

There is a need for discussion between the different interested parties, and this might include the Ministry of Justice. It may also help to ask the opinion of a neutral third party—which is effectively what the court has asked of you.

You should conduct your own independent assessment of Gordon before forming your own opinion on diagnosis, treatment, and prognosis. It would assist the court, though, if having formed your own view you then took part in a discussion with the other interested parties, as this might lead to a resolution of the dispute over hospital treatment. Even if it did not, it should clarify and perhaps narrow the areas of disagreement, thus simplifying the task before the court.

Ethical

Gordon has few remaining rights, given his prison sentence. He should be offered care with dignity that is as effective as possible, both in treating him and reducing his risk to others. However, there is tension between his care needs (as seen by others) and the safety of potential caregivers (and the reputations and legal liability of their employers). A fair process is required to balance these competing interests.

When all options are poor and the stakes are high, as with Gordon, this can lead the people faced with the difficult decision to adopt inflexible positions (which can resemble the patient's own psychological conflict). The only way for a satisfactory outcome to be reached is for all parties to be open to alternative perspectives. There is no easy route to this, but values-based approaches offer an often-successful route.[72]

[69] European Convention for the Protection of Human Rights and Fundamental Freedoms (ECHR). Article 3 prohibits torture and inhuman or degrading treatment.

[70] In Scotland, the law omits the requirement of proportionality, instead stating force must be threatened or used 'for the minimum time'. The law in RoI only allows force to be used in 'exceptional emergency circumstances' to prevent an 'imminent risk of serious harm'.

[71] It is also *possible* (at least in the UK) that a residual common law power exists under the doctrine of necessity, to enforce such treatment on people with capacity in prison, if it is necessary to prevent serious harm and it is a proportionate response to harm's likelihood and seriousness.

[72] See part A.

B.3
Criminal law cases

1

Preparing an expert report on a vulnerable defendant

Themes: *assessing risk of sexual offending (p.172) and learning disability (p.110) [C]; fitness to plead (p.602) [L]; and hospital and other disposals in unfitness to plead (p.604) [CL] and stigma in capacity assessments (p.322) [E]*

Case description

Owen is a sixty-two-year-old retired man with mild intellectual disability. He lives alone in the family home; his mother died five years ago. He worked for many years in shops. He has had no contact with mental health or learning disability services for many years. He does not misuse substances. He enjoys attending a local church and day centre. He and his dog Fred are members of a walking group.

Owen's only known relative is his fifty-seven-year-old sister, Jean, whom he has not seen since 1990. Six months ago, Jean reported Owen to the police for sexual offences when he was thirteen and she was eight years old. Jean had sought therapy after their mother died, and during that she disclosed how, over a two-year period, Owen had sexually assaulted her by digital vaginal penetration and masturbating in front of her, including ejaculating on her. She had told her mother after the first episode but was smacked for 'making up stories'. The abuse stopped when they were both sent to boarding schools; although Owen sent her three cards during his first term saying he loved her and wanted to marry her.

You are approached by Owen's solicitor, who informs you that Owen attended a police station voluntarily, and was interviewed with an appropriate adult and solicitor present. Owen predominantly said 'no comment' in response to questions, but also said, 'I'm sorry' a few times. The police have a contemporaneous witness statement that supports Jean's allegation. Owen has no prior criminal record of any kind.

She instructs you to give your opinion on diagnosis, fitness to plead, and special provisions for the trial, and whether Owen was capable at the time of the alleged offences of understanding whether such abuse would be wrong.

Questions

1. What are the clinical, legal, clinico-legal, and ethical issues in this case?

Clinical

It is obviously difficult after so many years to gain the kind of contemporaneous medical evidence that would normally form part of your assessment (e.g. school, social service, and GP records); although this should still be attempted.

The history suggests that Owen's intellectual impairment has had only a limited impact upon his social functioning. Obviously, it would be useful to gain much more information about the family, if possible, including what happened to Owen's father, and why he and Jane were sent to separate boarding schools.

You should advise the solicitors to instruct a qualified clinical psychologist who can administer and interpret cognitive tests, as well as assess his level of daily functioning and his sexual knowledge, attitudes, and interests.

On the currently available information, this appears to be sexually inappropriate behaviour by a pubertal boy in a particular context, possibly after the departure or death of his father. The fact that the behaviour did not recur at other times or in other contexts suggests that Owen is not sexually deviant; although this does not diminish the impact on Jean of the experience.

Such inappropriate sexual behaviour is not unusual in teenage boys, with their victims usually being younger family members or girlfriends. It often reflects family tension or discord, teenage confusion, and mood dysregulation. Desistance from this kind of behaviour is the norm.

Legal

There is more than one type of charge that Owen could face for sexual assault. You should bear in mind that the law that applied at the time, around forty-seven years ago, will be the law under which Owen is prosecuted—with older legal tests (and generally lesser penalties for sexual offending[1]).

The test of fitness to plead[2] is essentially cognitive, and any lack of memory of the alleged offence is not directly relevant.[3]

If he is found unfit to plead, there would then be a trial of the facts, involving evidence from his sister. If the court is satisfied that he did the acts alleged, the possible disposals[4] are a hospital/compulsion order (with or without restrictions), a guardianship order (or in E&W the similar supervision & treatment order), or absolute discharge.

Clinico-legal

Unless the police (for example) unearth letters from the time containing evidence of Owen discussing his view of the sexual assault, it is likely to be impossible to say anything concerning what he understood about his behaviour at the time, and whether he knew that what he was doing then, if true, was wrong.[5]

The more meaningful questions are whether at age sixty-two years Owen now understands what he is accused of doing and can understand questions put to him by his lawyers, including the meaning of a guilty plea, and can give evidence on his own behalf.

On the face of it, you are likely to find Owen fit to plead, assuming that you find no other mental disorder and his cognitive impairment is mild (as might be suggested by the fact that he has worked in retail). However, even if his impairment is mild, it would seem sensible for him to have support at court such as a registered intermediary, given how traumatic the process is likely to be. You might also respectfully advise his solicitor against him giving evidence himself, especially if the psychologist finds evidence of suggestibility or compliance.

If he pleads guilty (as he is likely to be advised to do) you may wish to assist the court by liaising with probation and social services to facilitate a community order. You may need to help social services in particular to understand the low risk of future offending, and support his entitlement to continue receiving social care (e.g. to keep attending the day centre).

[1] For example, the current English offences of assault of a child under age thirteen by penetration and of inciting a child under thirteen to engage in sexual activity were not created until 2003. As Owen did not penetrate Jean with his penis, the only relevant offence at the time was indecent assault on a woman, which carried a maximum sentence of five-years' imprisonment if the victim was under thirteen, in contrast to the fourteen years available today (and life imprisonment for assault by penetration).

[2] Explored in detail in criminal law cases 3 and 4.

[3] *R v Podola* [1960] 1 QB 325.

[4] Except in RoI, where the only possible disposal is committal for treatment (though this can be outpatient treatment).

[5] This is relevant in E&W because under the law at the time children aged ten to fourteen could only be prosecuted if they knew what they were doing was wrong (a doctrine known as *doli incapax*).

If instead you had found evidence that Owen was unfit to plead, you would have liaised with social services about possible guardianship or supervision. A hospital order would be inappropriate unless his condition suddenly deteriorated.

Ethical

The main ethical issues relate to Owen's capacity to participate in a process which is likely to be stigmatising, risky, and distressing for him, and in which he should be supported. The case describes a man whose life is about to be dramatically changed, given that he is accused of a highly stigmatising offence. The fact that he was technically a child himself at the time of the alleged offence, was cognitively impaired, may then have been under some emotional stress, and has been pro-social ever since may be ignored. Instead, some people and agencies may assume Owen to be a predatory paedophile, despite the evidence.

Forensic psychiatrists have a duty to provide realistic evidence of risk, and to help avoid the emotive nature of the offences affecting risk assessments and management. He was a member of a vulnerable group before because of his cognitive impairment; he will also likely now be a member of an even more vulnerable group, namely convicted sex offenders. Sadly, people like Owen often lose all their social supports after legal conviction for historic offences, which increases the risk to their health and wellbeing.

2

Assessment for suggestibility and compliance

Themes: *intellectual disability (p.110); suggestibility and compliance (p.160); cultural differences in assessment (p.126) [C]; admissibility of confession (p.608) [L]; reliability of confessions (p.608) [CL]; and boundary of expert evidence (p.686) [E]*

Case description

Mustafa is a sixteen-year-old boy of Pakistani origin awaiting trial for the murder of his nineteen-year-old female cousin. During police interviews he confessed to involvement in the killing.

Mustafa came to the UK aged nine years, and has not seen his parents since. He lived with his maternal aunt and uncle. He attended mainstream school, but his reports suggest that he needed significant help (special classes and in-class support), and that he failed to achieve literacy. Educational psychology reports suggest he has learning difficulties. He has no previous forensic or substance misuse history.

Clinical psychology assessment has found a full-scale IQ in the 'extremely low' range, with a reading age of around seven. His immediate recall on the suggestibility test was below the first percentile; his yield and shift scores[6] were above the 95th percentile, and his total suggestibility score was between the 75th and 80th percentiles. He also scores above the 90th percentile on measures of compliance. There is no evidence of impulsivity, hyperactivity or of overt mental illness.

Mustafa said that he thought that the police had told him that he could go home if he gave a statement to them about what happened to his cousin. He said he felt under pressure to talk to them and did not understand a lot of their questions.

His solicitor has instructed you to assess Mustafa and prepare an expert report concerning the reliability of his confession.

Questions

1. What clinical, legal, clinico-legal, and ethical issues arise in the case?
2. How should you proceed?

Clinical

Interrogative suggestibility represents the extent to which an individual comes to accept or believe information communicated to them during formal questioning (e.g. a police interview or cross-examination).

---

[6] Measures of his tendency to incorporate into memory the suggestive information embedded in the question (yield), and his sensitivity to subsequent critical comments about his earlier performance (shift).

Suggestibility is more likely in the context of:

- poor memory recall,
- low intelligence,
- high emotionality and anxiety,
- high social desirability,
- fear of negative evaluation, and
- low assertiveness and self-esteem.

Compliance is the tendency to go along with propositions, requests, or instructions for some immediate instrumental gain, usually, within a police interview, to escape the immediate pressure being faced, and with the intention 'I can sort it all out later'. In contrast to those who are suggestible, the individual is fully aware that they are giving false information. It is associated with:

- eagerness to please,
- poor self-esteem, and
- the desire to avoid conflict.

A full psychiatric assessment is needed in order to identify any mental disorder that might render Mustafa more than normally vulnerable to either suggestibility or compliance, and to explain any identified abnormal suggestibility or compliance. It should include focused consideration of any of:

- learning disability (which seems likely in Mustafa's case),
- mood disorder,
- psychosis, and
- personality disorder or relevant traits (especially dependent and avoidant).

A detailed psychological assessment is also essential, usually including cognitive assessment, to supplement the Gudjonsson Suggestibility Scale (GSS) and the Gudjonsson Compliance Scale (GCS)[7] that have already been completed.

In this case, it may be important that the experts have experience of working with learning disability, as well as understanding, and experience of the influence of Pakistani culture. Other issues to consider in the assessment concern the reliability of the psychometric measures used and the cultural appropriateness of these. Although Mustafa has been in the UK for six years, his performance on some of the measures, in particular those assessing verbal skills, may under-represent of his true abilities. Compare the scores with his school reports and nonverbal measures of performance, and demonstrate awareness of this issue in your opinion.

As Mustafa has been shown to be both suggestible and compliant, you should scrutinise interview transcripts or recordings for evidence of Mustafa *acting* suggestibly or compliantly within the interviews, and of this appearing to influence his answers to questions.

Legal

Evidence of a defendant's confession having been influenced by suggestibility and/or compliance may result in the court ruling it legally 'unreliable', although not necessarily false, and to exclude it from the trial. The judge will make this determination within a *voir dire*: an investigation by the judge before trial into the admissibility of a witness's evidence.

If any contested material (e.g. part of the confession) remains admissible, then further expert evidence can be called later during the trial, in order to assist the jury in determining whether they should attach less weight than usual to the evidence.

---

[7] The GSS involves telling subjects a story and then seeing how they respond to leading questions, and then, after they are given critical feedback, whether they adjust their responses when asked the questions again. The GCS is a self-report questionnaire.

Clinico-legal

The prosecution is likely to want to introduce Mustafa's confession as evidence, as it constitutes strong evidence implicating him in the commission of the offence, and it may be the only strong evidence that they have.[8] However, the defence will seek to argue that his account is not reliable because he has psychological disabilities that made him both suggestible and unduly compliant with authority.

At the *voir dire*, the prosecution will point out that the police followed proper interview procedures and provided Mustafa with an 'appropriate adult', as well as his solicitor being present, and that any suggestibility and compliance were therefore mitigated. So you will need to be able to demonstrate evidence of his answers being influenced by these traits. You must not express an opinion on the confession being either unreliable in law or false.

If the confession remains in evidence, then you will be required to give evidence again (see above).

Mustafa's difficulties are also likely to impact upon how reliable he might be as a witness in court. It will be helpful to recommend adjustments, such as ensuring statements and questions are clear and concise, nonleading, open, and that language used is simple and explained clearly. Explain that Mustafa may respond badly to difficult and hostile questioning, and the judge may need to consider the risk of adverse inferences being drawn from this.

You might also conclude that Mustafa's difficulties render him unfit to plead (see criminal law cases 3 and 4 for a discussion of this).

Ethical

Although the court will often allow, within a *voir dire*, the expert to opine upon the reliability per se, in doing so you will be taking a view on the nature of the exchanges within the interview. And if the judge were to allow you to opine upon reliability at trial (less likely) you could seem then to usurp a function of the jury.

Describing Mustafa's mental disorder plus relevant traits, and its impact upon his likely responses during a police interview, will, for example, fall one side of the line; but giving a clear opinion that what he said *should* (as opposed to could) therefore be viewed as unreliable is likely to be on the wrong side of that line. Although there is variability in what courts will allow the expert to address, you should yourself take great care to keep the proper boundary for yourself.

---

[8] In Scotland criminal conviction can only occur if there is 'corroborative' evidence of guilt.

3 Fitness to plead–intellectual disability plus psychosis

Themes: *intellectual disability (p.110), paranoid schizophrenia (p.73), and cross-cultural psychological test validity (p.130) [C]; fitness to plead and stand trial (p.602) [L]; assessing for fitness to plead (p.604) [CL]; and clinical disabilities versus legal ability (p.354) [E]*

Case description

Nasir is a thirty-two-year-old man charged with two counts of fraud. He was born and raised in Bangladesh. He attended school until age fourteen years, when his parents withdrew him. He had learnt to read and to write Bengali to a limited degree, and had learned to speak basic English. He then worked on his father's land.

Nasir came to the UK at the age of twenty-nine years after an arranged marriage. His wife found him employment as a night security guard in an immigration centre. This lasted several months until he resigned due to deteriorating mental health. He has since been unemployed for two years. He has no previous forensic history.

Nasir is under the care of his local CMHT and has been diagnosed with paranoid schizophrenia. He responded well to oral antipsychotics and has been free of psychotic symptoms since the initial episode that caused him to leave work.

It is now alleged that, before he left the company that ran the immigration centre, he was made a director of it, and that over £1million has been found in bank accounts that he set up. He has told his solicitors that the company owner had asked him to sign various forms, but he did not understand what they were. Since being charged, Nasir has become mentally unwell again.

His solicitor instructs you to assess his fitness to plead and stand trial. Working with a Bengali interpreter, you elicit paranoia, and persecutory delusions about the company owner being a 'devil' who is trying to have him killed in prison, as well as a preoccupation with whether his solicitor can be trusted, as he might be an agent of the devil. Nasir admits, when you ask directly, that in his distress about the impending trial, he has not taken his medication for six weeks.

A clinical psychologist assessed Nasir's cognitive functioning two months ago using the WAIS-IV, which showed that he is functioning in the 'borderline' range. He also highlighted Nasir's poor daily living skills, including his inability to look after himself, budget, and use public transport independently. His opinion is that, although Nasir has a rudimentary understanding of court proceedings, he may not be fit to plead. He has recommended adaptations necessary if the trial were to go ahead, including the use of an intermediary.

Questions

1. What are the clinical, legal, clinico-legal, and ethical issues in this case?

Clinical

You should delineate Nasir's psychotic symptoms, plus any other mental symptoms, such as low mood or anxiety, and their impact on functioning, but also his cognitive abilities insofar as you can assess them in the presence of psychosis.

You need to be aware that the majority of cognitive assessment tools, including the most commonly used WAIS-IV, have been standardised with Western populations and are not appropriate for use with non–English speakers, given the role that culture plays in test-taking attitudes and learnt cognitive abilities. Many of the subtests of well-known measures are based on language abilities. There is a Bengali version of the WAIS-IV, which attempts to overcome some of these problems, and you should check that the psychologist used this. He should be able to identify those abilities that are strongly affected by sociocultural factors which happen to characterise a particular ethnic group, such as cultural beliefs and behaviours, ecological demands, language, and level and quality of education, and, by contrast, those measures that are relatively culture-fair, in the sense that they reveal equivalence in performance regardless of sociocultural influences.

Also, if two months ago when the psychologist administered the WAIS-IV Nasir was already psychotic, you should ask him to consider readministering it after recovery.

Legal

Defendants are assumed fit to plead, unless they come within the terms of 'unfitness' as described in *R v Pritchard*, further developed in *R v M*.[9] That is: 'on the balance of probabilities ... one, or more of six things [is] beyond the appellant's capabilities: (1) understanding the charges; (2) deciding whether to plead guilty or not; (3) exercising his right to challenge jurors; (4) instructing solicitors and counsel; (5) following the course of the proceedings; (6) giving evidence in his own defence'.

Although the court will give weight to the psychologist's opinion on Nasir's fitness, the law in E&W and NI requires the judge to hear evidence from two doctors before it can make a finding of unfitness to plead.[10]

Clinico-legal

If your psychiatric evaluation of Nasir concludes that he is suffering from a mild learning disability, or schizophrenia-related cognitive decline, or both, the diagnoses alone do not render him unfit to plead; you must consider the impact of his symptoms upon the legal abilities required for fitness.

Some example questions for doing so are:

- What are you charged with? What does that mean? Can you explain what they say you did?
- Can you explain the difference between pleading guilty and not guilty?
- Do you know why they say you did it?
- What does the jury do in a trial?
- What would you do if you saw someone you knew on the jury?
- What would you say if they asked you [a question that pertains to his likely defence]?
- How would you explain [an issue likely to arise]?

In relation to each question you put, consider how Nasir follows your question and responds to it, and assimilates and responds to new information. Also ask the solicitor how well Nasir understands matters when they try to take instructions.

[9] *R v Pritchard (1836)* 7 C&P 303 and *R v M (John)* [2003] EWCA Crim 3452 respectively. Very similar tests are laid out in s53F Criminal Procedure (Scotland) Act 1995 and, for RoI, s4 Criminal Law (Insanity) Act 2006.

[10] In E&W and NI, two registered medical practitioners, one of whom must be approved under mental health law; in NI, one of the two must give oral evidence in court. In Scotland, the requirement for medical evidence was abolished in 2010; though the court retains a power to adjourn proceedings for an investigation of the person's mental or physical condition, and evidence from two medical practitioners is still required before the court can order treatment in hospital. In RoI, the provisions are the same as in Scotland, except that only one 'approved medical officer' is required to give evidence for compulsory hospital or community treatment.

Your report should include specific reference to each of the capabilities described above, and describe the specific impact of his symptoms (and any indirect impacts e.g. distraction, poor concentration, and anxiety). Wherever you conclude that an ability is impaired, you should describe how that impairment could be mitigated for Nasir, if possible.

Nasir's active psychotic symptoms, the content of some of which bears directly on issues relevant to the trial, plus impaired cognitive functioning, are likely to render him unable to understand complex concepts such as 'beyond reasonable doubt', or the financial details of the alleged offences given in evidence. They are also likely to impair his ability to follow the course of proceedings and to give evidence adequately.

However, given his good recovery after his first psychotic episode, and the fact that his deteriorating mental state is due to him stopping medication, as well as the stress of the impending trial, there is good reason to believe that at least some of his symptoms will be reversible within a reasonable period of time. You should therefore recommend that the court consider adjourning whilst he receives treatment, if necessary as an inpatient.

Assume the court accepts your recommendation and then instructs you to reassess Nasir, which you do six weeks later. You find that Nasir has recovered from psychosis, but his cognitive deficits persist, to the same degree as the psychologist found before you first met Nasir. You express the opinion that Nasir's residual deficits do not, on the balance of probabilities, sufficiently impair his abilities to the extent that the court could find him unfit to plead. You note, however, that Nasir is likely to find it difficult to follow complex legal arguments in court, and state that he may need support to comprehend the discussions that are taking place in the courtroom, for example through the use of an intermediary. Be clear in describing in detail what an intermediary should do, and relate his use to the impairments described. You should ask the psychologist also to advise on support measures.

Ethical

Keep in mind the distinction between clinical opinion about mental disabilities and symptoms that may interfere with required legal abilities, *and* those legal abilities themselves. For example, you might find no clinical reason why Nasir remained unfit to plead after treatment of his psychosis, but the court might disagree on the basis of nonpsychiatric evidence which it has weighed alongside yours.

4 Fitness to plead–psychiatrists using psychological test results

Themes: *psychological testing (p.130) and psychiatric and psychological assessment (p.122) [C]; fitness to plead (p.602) [L]; 'mapping' clinical assessment onto legal criteria (p.358) and reporting raw test data (p.136) [CL]; and consent to testing for court (p.660) and apparent disagreement between psychologist and psychiatrist (pp.312, 655) [E]*

Case description

Marcus is a twenty-three-year-old man who has been charged with a sexual offence against a child. This is his first alleged offence.

Marcus left school with no qualifications. Since leaving school he has largely been unemployed, undertaking occasional manual labour for his uncle. He lives with his mother and younger sister, who wash his clothes, cook his meals, and manage his finances. He has no friends and has always been socially isolated. He rarely leaves the home. His mother describes him as always having been 'odd'.

His solicitors are concerned about his understanding of the charge, and about the impact of his personality and his intellectual functioning on dealing with the case. They request an opinion on his fitness to plead.

Lucas has been assessed by a clinical psychologist, and they concluded that he was functioning in the 'extremely low range of intellectual ability' and had schizoid and avoidant personality traits.

Questions

1. How should you incorporate or otherwise use the psychometric test results in your own assessment and reporting?
2. What other clinical, legal, clinico-legal, and ethical issues are relevant?

Clinical

Psychiatrists may include psychometric test results and interpretation as part of their assessments, depending upon the nature of the case. If the psychologist does not provide a report to the court in their own right, you should summarise the psychologist's qualifications and experience, state under whose supervision they carried out the tests (if they were a junior psychologist), state the methods used, and then summarise the findings. Where you rely upon the test results in your opinion, you should make clear how you have done so, and how the test results relate to findings from your own clinical examination and investigation.

Clinical psychologists and neuropsychologists apply psychometric tests to obtain a measure of individual's general intellectual functioning (intelligence quotient, IQ). These tests utilise normal-distribution statistical models, and the individual's scores are then compared to the known 'norms'. Hence, the test has to be relevant to the person's age, culture, and language background. Adaptations of the tests have been published worldwide including along with the relevant norms.

The Wechsler Adult Intelligence Scale-IV (WAIS-IV) is the most widely used clinical instrument to assess intellectual functioning. It is an individually administered psychometric assessment that is designed to assess intellectual functioning of adolescents and adults aged sixteen to ninety years. The test provides general intellectual functioning (full-scale IQ) and four index scores, namely Verbal Comprehension, Perceptual Reasoning, Working Memory, and Processing Speed. The mean IQ is 100; an IQ of 69, which is more than two standard deviations below the mean, is considered to indicate intellectual impairment.

Importantly, factors such as poor effort, intoxication, fatigue, and low mood, or other symptoms of mental illness, can negatively influence the individual's performance on the test; you will need to know the circumstances in which the psychological assessment on Lucas was conducted.

Finally, because of the suggestion of the defendant being 'odd', the psychologist administered personality tests which could be relevant to your assessment.

Legal

Fitness to plead is determined by the court, but with reference to expert psychiatric, and/or psychological evidence. Tests vary in detail between jurisdictions, but are all tests of cognitive ability.[11] In E&W and NI addressing fitness to plead requires evidence from at least two medical practitioners, albeit a clinical psychologist can also provide an opinion. In Scotland there is no longer a requirement for medical evidence.

Clinico-legal

Forming an opinion requires 'mapping' of any findings concerning disabilities onto all of the legal criteria, in order to determine whether the defendant's condition will affect their ability to meet one or more of the legal criteria for fitness to plead.

Often, psychologists will have been separately instructed, in which case their report should be available to the court. However, it may still be helpful for you to summarise their findings in your report and say how they relate to your own findings (do not attempt your own independent interpretation of them unless you possess adequate training in the specific tests used).

Ethical

Experts have a duty to ensure that they obtain consent from the individual assessed for the use of any instruments, which should be scientifically validated and evidenced as reliable.[12] Experts should not administer a psychometric tool for which they have not been properly trained, and you should be able to provide evidence of training if requested. In practice, an expert who uses a published instrument or tool should be prepared to be cross-examined on its validity and reliability.[13]

There is some debate about whether raw test data should be disclosed in legal proceedings.[14] The American Psychological Association's ethical standards state that psychologists involved in legal proceedings have the responsibility to create and maintain documentation in detail, of sufficient quality to allow reasonable scrutiny in court proceedings. There are numerous experts other than clinical psychologists who are qualified to interpret test data, depending upon the test and context. However,

---

[11] See criminal law case 3 for details of the test in each jurisdiction.

[12] This is especially the case in relation to risk-assessment tools.

[13] International Test Commission. (2014). The ITC Guidelines on the Security of Tests, Examinations and Other Assessments. Online. Available at: https://www.intestcom.org.

[14] See for example Lees-Haley P R and Courtney J C (2000) Disclosure of tests and raw data to the courts: A need for reform, *Neuropsychology Review* 10(3): 169–174.

the British Psychological Society recommends[15] that raw scores should not generally be communicated to test takers or other parties who have an interest in the results of testing, as they are not usually meaningful in themselves. Raw scores need to be placed in context through norm referencing, criterion referencing, or similar, and it is these contextualised scores that should be communicated. Furthermore, test results should not be used in isolation, and it is important to reference the context of the assessment.

The expert evidence of psychiatrists and psychologists is often mutually reinforcing: for example, the clinical diagnosis of a personality disorder may be strengthened by the results of a personality test.

However, the converse is also true: for example, a psychiatrist stating that there is no 'functionally significant' personality disorder, despite the patient scoring above a statistical threshold on a psychometric testing. If such conflict arises, all involved must keep within their own field and methodology of expertise, and explain to the court the difference of approach to diagnosing personality disorder, seeking to explain what is apparently conflicting evidence. This may be assisted by provision of a joint statement.

[15] The British Psychological Society (2017) *Psychological Testing: A Test User's Guide*. The British Psychological Society..

5 Diminished responsibility–psychosis

Themes: *schizophrenia (p.73) and homicide (p.46) [C]; diminished responsibility (p.624) and legal and medical constructs (p.354) [L]; substantial impairment (p.625); refusal to discuss the act (p.628) [CL]; and boundaries of expert evidence (p.686) and, expressing uncertainty (p.304) [E]*

Case description

Ben is to stand trial for murder, following an incident in a night pharmacy in which a security guard was killed.

He is thirty-nine years old, with a history of schizophrenia. He has had five admissions, the first at age twenty-three years, when his father took him to A&E because he was rambling about a conspiracy and was 'addicted' to marijuana. When unwell, he becomes dishevelled, develops grandiose and paranoid delusions, and sometimes assaults others, including staff. Each time he responds to antipsychotics, but does not gain insight into his condition. He continues to use cannabis.

He last took medication a year before the alleged homicide. In the days before it, he was seen wandering the streets, looking unkempt. He often visited the pharmacy to beg for snacks or soft drinks. On the day of the alleged offence he returned to the shop around 5pm, carrying a metal bar. The owner asked him repeatedly to leave, then asked the security guard to escort him out. Ben laughed at the guard, and when he put his hand on Ben's arm, Ben struck him forcefully with the bar on the head, killing him. He ran away and was soon arrested a few streets away.

He was transferred to hospital whilst on remand, with paranoia and florid persecutory delusions. When questioned about the alleged offence he said that the victim had, in fact, murdered the pharmacist.

You are asked by his solicitor to prepare a psychiatric report on diminished responsibility.

Questions

1. Given your instructions, what factors in Ben's history and recent mental state are likely to be important?
2. What factors in his case tend to support, and what factors go against, the partial defence of diminished responsibility?
3. How will you deal with Ben's denial that he did the act?
4. How would you respond if he acknowledged doing the act but refused to discuss it?
5. How should you express any uncertainty in your conclusions?
6. What other clinical, legal, clinico-legal, and ethical issues arise in the case?

Clinical

Ben has a well-established diagnosis of paranoid schizophrenia, severe enough to have required inpatient treatment several times. For over a year leading up to the alleged offence, he was without antipsychotic medication, making a relapse likely.

His behaviour at the time of the killing, evidenced by witness statements, strongly suggests he was psychotic, being consistent with previous relapses.

Ben's behaviour appears to have been disorganised in the pharmacist's shop; this again being consistent with his behaviour when psychotic historically. He made no attempt to conceal himself after the alleged offence. And he required treatment in a psychiatric hospital shortly after the alleged offence, which is again consistent with him being psychotic at the time of the killing; albeit you should at least consider the possibility in cases such as Ben's that the act of exhibiting severe violence, especially homicidal violence, might have itself caused a psychotic relapse, or have worsened a pre-existing psychotic state.

However, such a clear history creates a risk of overconfidence, resulting in insufficient assessment, and confirmation bias ('surely the case is obvious?'). Your assessment will need to consider any factor that might have contributed to the killing, psychotic or otherwise.

Legal

The partial defence of diminished responsibility, which reduces murder to manslaughter, is relatively similar across many common law jurisdictions. In E&W and NI, prior to its amendment, it required proof of there having been an 'abnormality of mind' that 'substantially impaired the defendant's mental responsibility' in doing the killing. This still applies in E&W to trials and appeals relating to any killing that occurred before 4 October 2010.[16]

For later killings, the defence has been amended substantially, arguably making it more congruent with medical constructs. So the defendant must have been suffering from a 'recognised medical condition' that gave rise to an 'abnormality of mental functioning', which 'substantially'[17] impaired his ability to understand his own actions, or form a rational judgement, or exercise self-control', and where such abnormality of mental functioning 'provides an explanation for (meaning, 'was a significant contributory factor in causing') the killing'.

Clinico-legal

Given the strong evidence suggesting that Ben was suffering from a relapse of the schizophrenia, proving he had a 'recognised medical condition' seems straightforward. The more difficult questions are whether that condition gave rise to an 'abnormality of mental functioning' at the time in terms of one or more of the relevant abilities (to exercise self-control e.g.), and if so, whether that was 'a significant contributory factor' in causing the killing (where there are other potential 'ordinary' contributory factors, e.g. a desire for money).

The disorganised thinking, inappropriate affect, paranoia, and persecutory delusions certainly amount to abnormalities of mental functioning. However, your assessment should look for evidence of him exercising, or failing to exercise, self-control, (mis)understanding his actions, or forming (ir)rational judgments (e.g. about the intentions of the security guard). Note that there was nothing in his behaviour at the time of the killing to suggest he was experiencing delusions or hallucinations at the time, and certainly none that appeared clearly to relate to the victim, nor anything to suggest that he would not have understood the consequences of hitting the guard with the metal bar.

If you find evidence of substantial impairment of one or more of these abilities because of psychosis, and you think this crosses the threshold of being 'a significant contributory factor', you should still avoid directly stating whether he satisfies diminished responsibility, since this is the ultimate issue for the court to determine, not you. However, the jury cannot ignore undisputed medical evidence supportive of diminished responsibility unless the prosecution challenges it 'on some rational basis'.[18]

---

[16] And in NI to any killing that occurred before 1 June 2011. The old and new legal criteria are explored more fully in criminal law case 6, along with the corresponding rules in Scotland & RoI.

[17] Concerning the meaning of *substantial*: *R v Golds* [2016] UKSC 61, and criminal case 6.

[18] See R *v Brennan* [2015] 1 Cr App R 14.

Denial of an offence is understandable, especially in the context of a mandatory sentence for murder. And, on the face of it, denial might appear to preclude raising the defence of diminished responsibility, since you will not be able to gain an account from Ben of his thinking when he killed. However, his likely mental state can be inferred from other evidence, particularly contemporaneous witness statements. A refusal to discuss the act should not therefore inhibit you from expressing an opinion, if the court finds him to have done the acts, upon the relevant legal elements of diminished responsibility.

Ethical

The primary duty of any expert is to the court, whether instructed by the defence or the prosecution. You must provide an opinion that is balanced, honestly held, and which acknowledges all of the relevant evidence, including evidence that goes against your opinion.

As always, you should keep a strict boundary between 'matters medical' and 'matters legal'. This means only commenting on the availability of the partial defence on medical grounds, not on whether the test is ultimately met.

There are clearly arguments on both sides in the present case. You should acknowledge any weakness in your conclusions, but also make it plain why you have nevertheless reached your opinion. You will then be in a better position to explain your conclusions under cross-examination than if you are only confronted with contrary evidence during the trial. This is particularly relevant when, as here, the case initially appears 'obvious'.

6 Diminished responsibility–neurotic illness

Themes: *depression (p.94) and homicide (p.46) [C]; diminished responsibility (p.624) and loss of control and provocation (p.630) [L]; causation and 'woundability' (p.631) [CL]; and ethical boundaries with complex law (p.664) [E]*

Case description

Joshua, aged sixty, killed his forty-year-old wife in an explosive attack. They had been married for fifteen years, but increasingly unhappily so. He had occasionally hit her.

He had been suffering from moderate depression for four years, treated by his GP with an antidepressant. He became impotent, about which his wife complained repeatedly, and she called him 'too old' and 'always depressed'. Four weeks prior to the killing, she said she was leaving him, and he tried to kill himself by taking an overdose. He was admitted to hospital under the Mental Health Act for a week.

His wife then said that she would stay with him, and witnesses, including his GP, report that his mood then lifted substantially for a few days. She later recanted and Joshua's mood again deteriorated. His work colleagues noticed his withdrawn state; although some stated that, during the days before the offence, he could occasionally be seen laughing and joking.

You assess Joshua. He reports that in the days before he killed his wife, he experienced low mood, anhedonia, insomnia, agitation, anergia, feelings of worthlessness and guilt, impaired concentration, indecisiveness, weight loss, recurrent thoughts of death, and ideas of suicide. Although he was able to continue work as a lorry driver. His wife allegedly repeated her complaints about his age, depression, and impotence on the day of the killing, and immediately before he killed her, she had said that she was having an affair with a younger man and would leave the next morning. Joshua does not dispute that he killed his wife.

Questions

1. Is there a medical basis for the partial defence of 'diminished responsibility' to be available to Joshua?
2. Could he also plead 'loss of control' or 'provocation' (depending upon legal jurisdiction)?
3. What would your answers be if the killing had occurred in 2008; there had been no psychiatric evidence at the original trial, when he was convicted of murder; and you were now instructed in regard to a possible appeal?
4. What other clinical, legal, clinico-legal, and ethical issues arise in the case?

Clinical

If, having completed a thorough assessment of Joshua, and having gained a history from available informants, plus his employer, and having also read the GP records, you are confident that he was suffering from moderately severe depression, and that this affected his mood at the time, his resilience to his wife's taunts and threats of separation, and his interpretation of her and others' actions, then you can address the partial defences.

Legal

Diminished responsibility

The test for diminished responsibility, both before and after amendment in E&W, is laid out in criminal case 5. However, of note, 'substantial' was interpreted by English courts,[19] in the context of the una-mended test of 'substantial impairment of mental responsibility', to mean 'less than total and more than trivial'.[20] But in *Golds*,[21] in 2014, the Court of Appeal opined that the meaning of *substantial* is obvious and should be left to the jury—albeit that if asked specifically, the judge should explain that the relevant meaning is not merely 'having substance' but 'significant or appreciable'. The Supreme Court confirmed this approach, and added that 'more than trivial' was not adequate.[22] And this also applies to 'substantial' within the amended defence.

Recent case law[23] has determined that, other than in exceptional circumstances, if there is unchallenged medical evidence of diminished responsibility as an explanation, then the jury must accept this; it is not open to them to balance the psychiatric evidence against an alternative explanation for the killing and prefer the latter, as was possible under the unamended defence, if there is unchallenged expert evidence supporting causation by way of an abnormality mental functioning.[24]

Any trial or appeal relating to a killing before 10 October 2009 would apply the law as it stood at the time of the offence.

In RoI and Scotland, the elements of the law relevant to Joshua's case did not change after 2010,[25] and the position would be essentially the same: the case would turn on whether the jury accepted that the impairment was 'substantial', as above.

Loss of control and provocation

The law in E&W and NI of 'loss of control' and 'provocation' (the latter replaced the former) is described in detail in criminal law cases 10–12.

In brief, the 'loss of self-control' must have had a 'qualifying trigger', so the defendant must not have acted in a considered desire for revenge, and a person of the same sex and age, with a normal degree

---

[19] Courts in the other jurisdictions have consistently been content to leave the term undefined for the jury to interpret.

[20] *R v Lloyd* [1967] 1 QB 175.

[21] *R v Golds* [2014] EWCA Crim 748.

[22] *R v Golds (Appellant)* [2016] UKSC 61.

[23] *R v Brennan* [2014] EWCA Crim 2387.

[24] To be precise, the Court of Appeal in *Brennan* stated that if there was unequivocal, reputable, and uncontradicted medical evidence of diminished responsibility, then the charge of murder should be withdrawn from the jury; only if the evidence is tentative or qualified, or successfully challenged at least in part under cross-examination, or cast in a different light by other facts or circumstances—or there is a contradictory opinion from another expert—should the jury be free to consider a conviction for murder. If the prosecution contends that there are other facts or circumstances which might cast a different light on otherwise uncontradicted defence expert medical evidence, then they should discuss this with the judge, who should specifically identify those facts or circumstances to the jury in the summing-up as capable of providing a rational basis on which the jury could decline to accept the expert evidence.

[25] What did change in Scotland was that psychopathic disorder became accepted as a cause of abnormality of mind, and the partial defence became available even when the defence of insanity would also be available. The statute also clarified that, although intoxication alone would not qualify as a cause of an abnormality of mind, being intoxicated would not prevent another condition suffered by the defendant qualifying as a cause.

of tolerance and self-restraint, and in the same circumstances[26] as the defendant, might have acted in the same or a similar way.

The qualifying triggers allowed are 'a fear of serious violence' or 'extremely grave' acts or statements that gave 'a justifiable sense of being seriously wronged'. 'Sexual infidelity' is explicitly excluded as a ground for feeling 'seriously wronged'[27]; although it can be taken into account if it is integral to the circumstances as a whole.[28]

The earlier defence of 'provocation' is far from identical, and requires 'sudden loss of control' arising from 'something said or done' that would have caused such loss of control in 'the reasonable person'. So that there is both an objective and subjective test.

In Scotland and RoI, the partial defence of provocation similarly requires a loss of self-control. In RoI this must be 'sudden and temporary', but there is no equivalent term in Scottish law.[29] In RoI, the provocation would have had to have caused loss of self-control in any reasonable person; in Scotland the reaction to the provocation must have been reasonably proportionate.

Clinico-legal

Diminished responsibility

Under the E&W and NI current tests for 'diminished responsibility', depressive illness is clearly a 'recognised medical condition', and Joshua's moderately severe symptoms could likely have caused an 'substantial abnormality of mental functioning', in terms of 'impairment of self-control'.

There is also much case law supporting his condition and symptoms qualifying as an 'abnormality of mind' (the test current in Scotland, and in E&W and NI for killings before 10 April 2010), and depression is obviously a 'mental disorder' (the test in RoI).

The salient question, under current E&W law, is whether Joshua's condition in fact *substantially* impaired (or 'diminished substantially' in RoI) his:

- ability to understand the nature of his conduct, form a rational judgment, or exercise self-control (E&W, NI);
- ability to determine or control his conduct (Scotland); or
- responsibility for the act (RoI).

Joshua's cognitive and other depressive symptoms would appear likely to have impaired his 'ability to exercise self-control'; although not his 'ability to understand his own conduct'. If the test of 'forming a rational judgement' is interpreted broadly to take into account the effect of his abnormal mood, then that too could have been impaired.

So, although the evidence is not clear-cut, a jury could reasonably conclude that one or other/both these impairments was/were 'substantial'. Likewise, a jury could reasonably find in RoI that his depression substantially impaired his responsibility for his act.

In E&W and NI the partial defence requires an additional element: that the impairment 'provides an explanation' for Joshua's actions, meaning that it was at least 'a significant contributory factor'. However, two main, competing, explanations of the killing suggest themselves: the 'abnormality of mental functioning' itself and his sexual jealousy and fear of the loss of his marriage.

Provided that the jury accept that the impairment of his ability to exercise self-control was substantial, therefore, the requirement for the abnormality of mental functioning being 'a significant contributory factor in causing the killing would appear to be *potentially* met in Joshua's case'(even if he was also jealous and/or fearful of loss of his marriage). So much will depend upon whether both you and (an)other expert(s) in the case agree on the causation limb.

[26] Circumstances whose only relevance is that they relate to the defendant's general capacity for tolerance or self-restraint (e.g. mental disorder in this context) are explicitly discounted.

[27] A sense of being seriously wronged or a fear of serious violence is also explicitly discounted by the statute if it was caused by something incited by the defendant for the purpose of providing an excuse to use violence.

[28] *R v Clinton* [2012] EWCA Crim 2.

[29] In Scotland, moreover, there is no clear case law on whether the loss of control has to be sudden, or whether a 'slow burn' can qualify, for example in cases of killing in response to domestic abuse. The statute in E&W and NI explicitly states that it need not be sudden.

As regards an appeal from conviction for murder relating to the killing having occurred in 2008, in E&W and NI the position would be somewhat different. As an appellant Joshua would have to show that he had suffered 'an abnormality of mind'[30] that 'substantially impaired his mental responsibility for his actions'. While it would readily be accepted that his moderately severe depression qualified as an 'abnormality of mind', the jury would be free to find that, nevertheless, he was fully responsible for killing, based upon a conclusion that the killing was driven more by his sexual jealousy and fear of the loss of his marriage, albeit triggered in part by his wife's taunts, than by his 'abnormality of mind'. So that, ultimately, the appeal would turn on determining whether the jury's view of that alternative explanation for the killing would have been unreasonable, making the conviction 'unsafe' if not.

Finally, in relation to the killing having occurred either recently *or* in 2008, reduced resilience (fragility or 'woundability'), arising from the defendant's condition, to the impact of other causal factors can be taken into account. For example, a depressive illness might not in itself substantially impair a person from exercising self-control—but it might determine that he was impaired in his ability to exercise self-control in distressing circumstances when another person would not have been impaired. The analogy of 'fragile bone syndrome' perhaps best makes the point (see also under loss of control or provocation).

Loss of control or provocation

By contrast, the role of psychiatric evidence in a 'loss of control' or 'provocation' partial defence is much more limited and circumscribed.

In E&W and NI, the 'qualifying trigger' test almost certainly would prevent Joshua from pleading loss of control successfully. Since the prosecution would argue that another man of Joshua's age, with a normal degree of tolerance and self-restraint, would not have responded in Joshua's circumstances (which cannot include his mental disorder insofar as that affects his degree of tolerance or self-restraint) with fatal violence. Moreover, Joshua did not fear serious violence; his wife's acts and words (having an affair, stating that she intended to leave, and taunting him) were not circumstances 'of an extremely grave character', and his only ground for feeling 'seriously wronged', his wife's 'infidelity', is explicitly discounted by the statute.[31] And only if the essence of the defence is made out (as above) can the defendant invoke 'circumstances': here in terms of being particularly vulnerable to his wife's behaviour, for example, to feeling 'not valued', because depressed.

In Scotland and RoI, Joshua's explosive attack upon his wife would be likely to be accepted by a jury as suggesting sudden loss of self-control. However, Joshua would have a problem with the objective reasonableness element of the test for the partial defence. A reasonable person would not respond to news of their spouse's infidelity and intent to leave, and to their taunts, with fatal violence. The defence could seek to argue that the reasonable person should be a person as 'woundable' as is Joshua, because of his depression (or in Scotland that woundability should affect what is seen as reasonably proportionate), but courts have tended to reject such arguments.[32]

In E&W, if appealing based upon 'provocation', he might be perceived to have been more 'woundable' by virtue of his illness, whilst 'things said or done' would be interpreted more loosely, and sexual infidelity would not be excluded as a 'trigger' (but any increased 'irritability' arising from depression could not be invoked as part of the provocation defence).

Ethical

The need to keep tight boundaries on one's expert evidence is enhanced in clinico-legal circumstances where there is subtle and complex law in regard to what is admissible into a defence and what is the proper boundary between ethical expert comment and the role of the jury, as here.

---

[30] There were also rules about what had to cause the abnormality of mind: it had to arise from a condition of arrested or retarded development of mind or any inherent cause or be induced by disease or injury.

[31] Save 'where integral to the circumstances as a whole' (*R v Clinton* [2012] EWCA Crim 2).

[32] See for instance *HM Attorney-General for Jersey v Holley* [2005] UKPC 23.

7

Diminished responsibility– personality disorder

> **Themes:** *homicide (p.46), borderline PD (p.84), and childhood sexual abuse (p.58) [C]; diminished responsibility (p.624) [L]; and formulation (p.146) [CL], clinical and legal constructs (p.354), and irrelevance of opinion on sentencing (p.670) [E]*

Case description

John, a thirty-nine-year-old man serving a long sentence for robbery, is charged in 2017 with murdering a fellow prisoner. He garrotted him in a deliberate and drawn-out fashion; he was not intoxicated. He admits he intentionally killed the victim, and had planned the attack three hours earlier, on learning that the victim was a convicted homicidal paedophile.

John has an established diagnosis of severe borderline personality disorder (BPD). Against the diagnostic checklist of the DSM-5 he has endorsed a high proportion of the symptoms, and these have had a major impact upon his behaviour and social functioning. He has repeatedly harmed himself seriously since his early teenage years, risking his life on several occasions (e.g. when he hanged himself and when he jumped onto electrified railway tracks). He has experienced a number of transient psychotic episodes.

He has received some psychological treatment, mainly in prison, although he has previously had several brief hospital admissions.

John's solicitor instructs you to write a report on diminished responsibility and disposal.

Questions

1. How would you assess John for this report?
2. Can his BPD found a plea of diminished responsibility?
3. Would your opinion be the same if John had not been sexually abused as a child, *or* if the victim had not been a convicted child sex offender and murderer?
4. What other clinical, legal, clinico-legal, and ethical issues arise in the case?

Clinical

You see from John's voluminous records that his borderline PD has been typified by maladaptive ways of coping with stress, anxiety, unstable mood, poor impulse control, and severe self-harm. He calmly describes violent sexual assaults upon him as a child. including anal rape on two occasions.

People with BPD are typically less able to contain their distress, soothe themselves, or negotiate solutions; they act out their feelings rather than acknowledging and managing them.

Legal

In E&W and NI, the law on diminished responsibility[33] requires an 'abnormality of mental functioning' which:

- arises from 'a recognised medical condition';
- 'substantially[34] impairs one's ability to understand the nature of one's conduct, to form a rational judgment, or to exercise self-control'; and which
- 'provides an explanation' for one's acts and omissions in relation to the killing, meaning that it was 'a significant contributory factor to the killing'.

In Scotland, the test is an abnormality of mind (other than one caused solely by intoxication) that has the effect of substantially impairing one's ability to determine or control one's actions. In RoI, it requires a mental disorder that diminishes substantially one's responsibility for the act. *Substantial* here means 'significant or appreciable'.

Caselaw in the UK jurisdictions (or statute in Scotland) confirms that PD can found the defence; there is no direct caselaw on the point in RoI, but no reason to believe that PD generally would be excluded.

Clinico-legal

There are specific symptoms of BPD that increase the risk of violence to others, including altered perception of external reality (during transient psychosis or dissociation); paranoid cognitions; hyper-arousal; heightened threat perception; dysregulated mood states, especially involving anger; affective instability; and behavioural impulsivity. John exhibits many of these.

Hence, John's attack upon the victim can be understood in terms of his history of childhood sexual abuse and the symptoms of his personality disorder. However, such clinical understanding does not necessarily mean that diminished responsibility can be made out.

Severe BPD is a qualifying mental disorder in all four jurisdictions. What is less clear is whether in John's case it substantially impaired his relevant abilities (UK), or his responsibility (RoI).

There can be little doubt John was not substantially impaired in his ability to understand what he was doing: he described planning the attack. He also explained his reason for killing the victim (because he was the kind of man who had raped him), and the prosecution will assert that this infers rational judgment, whatever its morality, whereas the defence might argue that it does not, because it originated in pathologically distorted reasoning and abnormal emotion (although this is unlikely to be accepted by the jury).

A stronger argument is that his impulsivity, affective instability, and unmanaged anger all impaired his ability to control his own conduct. So that, depending upon your clinical assessment, you might find that the intensity and intolerability of John's emotions towards his victim (as a representative of his past abusers) overwhelmed his limited capacity for self-control. And, even given the evidence of premeditation, the argument has merit by analogy with the concept of the 'slow burn' approved of by the courts in cases where the victim of abuse kills their abuser.[35]

You should expect to undergo detailed cross-examination on this point, and possibly be asked to comment upon the evidence of other experts who might not hold the same view. And the jury could reject your expert evidence if they considered that it was negated by the ordinary evidence of planning, provided your evidence had been challenged on a rational basis by the prosecution.

In Scotland and RoI, this would probably be the end of the matter.

However, in E&W and NI, there is the additional requirement to show that the BPD and its symptoms 'provided an explanation' for John killing the victim. And you could argue that the BPD was the key factor that led him to act against a paedophile.

---

[33] Explored in more detail in criminal law case 6.

[34] See *R v Golds* [2016] UKSC 61.

[35] R *v Ahluwalia* [1992] 4 AllER 889.

Ethical

People with PD often elicit strong (often unrecognised) emotional responses in the professionals working with them, leading to the risk that professionals' opinions become polarised. So this should emphasise the need to re-examine your opinion and reasoning, and explicitly to consider alternative conclusions. You must be honest, and strive for objectivity.

Counter-factual questions can help in recognising emotions that may be influencing your opinion. In John's case, this could include asking yourself what your opinion would be if John had not experienced severe childhood sexual abuse (but had BPD nevertheless), and/or his victim had not been a paedophile. If changing these emotionally charged but nonmedical factors would change your opinion, you should review your reasons, and reconsider whether you have properly applied the medical evidence to the relevant legal construct of diminished responsibility.

Your view about disposal if convicted should make no difference to the opinion you express concerning a mental condition defence. You might not recommend a hospital order, but that should not influence your view on diminished responsibility.

8

Diminished responsibility– recognised medical conditions

Themes: *psychopathy (p.90) and paraphilia (p.102) [C]; diminished responsibility (p.624) [L]; formulation (p.146) [CL]; and values influencing expert evidence (p.674), and conflict in accepting instructions (p.680) [E]*

Case description

Prince is a twenty-four-year-old man charged with murdering two men whose bodies were found buried in his garden. The postmortem showed they had been bound, gagged, and tortured before they died, as well as beaten after death, and that the murderer had had anal intercourse with them. Prince confessed readily to killing the men, whom he had picked up in a bar, two days apart; he had intended to go on to kill others. Police later found videos of the torture and killing on his phone.

Prince says he is a Christian and vehemently opposed to homosexuality; he described the killings as 'necessary for the good of the country'. He says he has had sexual relationships with both men and women but is not homosexual. He uses cocaine regularly.

Prince was successful at school but dropped out of university after a year because he found it unstimulating. He travelled to the USA and stayed with relatives. He has never been employed.

Prince is now studying in prison and claims to have a very good relationship with all the prison officers. He asserts that he is 'of highly superior intellect' and that it is '(his) destiny to be in prison'. He sees his offences, which have become notorious, as very important in stimulating public debate about homosexuality.

A clinical psychologist has assessed him, finding strong narcissistic personality traits, as well as a PCL-R score of 26, with a very high score in factor 1. He also found that Prince has deviant sexual interests, including sexual sadism. You are asked to assess him and provide an opinion on diminished responsibility.

Questions

1. Is sexual sadism a mental disorder?
2. Can psychopathy or a paraphilia support a diminished responsibility defence?
3. Are there valid 'recognised medical conditions' that an expert might reasonably refuse to put forward as the basis of a mental condition defence?
4. How might your values influence your approach to this case?
5. When might you be conflicted in accepting such instructions?
6. What other clinical, legal, clinico-legal, and ethical issues arise in the case?

Clinical

You should conduct a thorough clinical assessment: to corroborate (or not) the psychologist's findings of narcissistic PD and psychopathy (the score of 26 is just above the cut off of 25 used in the UK, although below the score of 30 that is conventional in the USA), and check for the presence of other psychiatric conditions, particularly paraphilia and substance dependence.

'Psychopathy' is a collection of behavioural, emotional, and psychological traits strongly associated with criminal offending. In the PCL-R two-factor model, factor 1 refers to cold, unemotional and callous traits plus lack of empathy; factor 2 relates to antisocial behaviour. People scoring highly on factor 2 usually also have ASPD.

Paraphilia describes intense and persistent sexual interests other than those pursued with consenting adult human partners. Intense persistent sexual interest in violence inflicted on others would be considered a paraphilia. A paraphilia is considered a mental disorder when there is distress or harm to the individual exhibiting the sexual preference, or to others.

The specific paraphilic disorder of sexual sadism is diagnosed when there is a recurrent and intense sexual arousal in response to physical or psychological suffering of other people, and there is distress or harm caused to the person concerned or to others. It is included in both DSM-5 and ICD-11.

In assessing these conditions, consider in particular Prince's capacity for empathy, his self-control, his reasoning skills, and his reflective ability. In this case, clinically the most complex issue is not the diagnosis (albeit that this might be disputed), but how any symptoms of mental disorder might have operated at the time of the killing.

Legal

The inclusion or use of personality disorders and certain other behaviourally based disorders like paraphilias in legal tests for defences to crime has been controversial, in part because of the paradox that the more severe the pathology in such disorders, the more serious the crime that may be committed, but the more likely the defendant might be able to employ a mental condition defence.

Similar reasoning has led to intoxication being excluded as a ground for a mental condition defence[36] as a matter of public policy, despite it being a 'recognised medical condition' clinically.[37] That is, not all medically defined medical conditions are legally recognised.

However, PD and paraphilias are widely recognised as medical conditions, insofar as they are accepted by diagnostic manuals, and their symptoms suggest operation so as to limit the defendants' responsibility for their actions in some way (expressed in general terms as substantially diminishing responsibility for the act in RoI, and in more specific terms of substantially impairing the ability to control one's actions in the UK[38]).

Clinico-legal

The criteria above leave psychopathy in an ambiguous position: while it is widely accepted as a valid construct, and many courts recognise the value of the PCL-R in risk assessment, it is not a diagnosis in either DSM-5 or ICD-11 (although it is a 'specifier' of the severity of ASPD in DSM-5 and is listed amongst the synonyms for ASPD in ICD-11). So that, to avoid cross-examination on whether psychopathy is a qualifying mental disorder, abnormality of mind, or recognised medical condition, it is wise explicitly to make an underlying diagnosis of ASPD or narcissistic PD (or both, possibly with other comorbid PD traits), in addition to using the term 'psychopathy' to characterise the pattern of personality pathology.

The defence could argue that Prince's narcissism and sexual sadism fundamentally alters his understanding and perception of others, including potential victims, and that he was unable to reflect upon

---

[36] Unless it counts as 'involuntary' intoxication, explored in criminal law cases 9, 14, and 22.

[37] See *R v Dowds* [2012] EWCA Crim 28.

[38] Changes that began with the Homicide Act 1957 and *R v Byrne* [1960] 2 QB 396 in E&W, and continued more broadly with the Criminal Law (Insanity) Act 2006 in RoI, Coroners & Justice Act 2009 in E&W and NI, and the Criminal Justice and Licensing (Scotland) Act 2010. The tests are explored in detail in criminal law case 6.

his actions or to perceive them as others would. Further, it might reasonably be suggested that Prince's pathological sense of entitlement contributed to his offending, with him being unable fully to understand the moral codes of others, and thereby to recognise the need to exercise self-control. The difficulty would be demonstrating that he *could not* exercise self-control, rather than that he chose not to exercise a (perhaps limited) ability to control himself.

However, if the court were to accept this as a substantial impairment of the relevant ability, then in the absence of intoxication there would appear to be no competing factor in explaining the killing (a requirement in E&W and NI).

Ethical

Some forensic psychiatrists would, as a matter of personal morality, prefer not to allow PD or sexual sadism disorder to permit a defendant to 'escape' conviction. However, is this a valid position to take?

It can be argued that it is not if the consequence is distorting one's professional medical opinion. It is for the court, not the expert, to determine whether any medically described condition can or should meet a legal test. If you choose to accept instructions, you must perform a dispassionate assessment that is as objective as possible. If this is to unpalatable, you should not accept the instructions.

Full objectivity is impossible, but you can aspire to it with insight into and honesty about your own values and how they might influence your opinion. In an emotive case such as this, there is even more need that usual to examine your own views, and to engage in a self-checking process. Directly addressing possible alternative opinions in detail within your report will assist, as will the opportunity for peer review.

9 | Diminished responsibility—substance dependence and intoxication

Themes: *intoxication and dependence (p.76) [C]; diminished responsibility (p.624), involuntary intoxication (p.614), and medical versus legal constructs (p.354) [L]; avoiding addressing voluntariness (p.664) [CL]; and personal values impinging upon expert opinion (p.674) [E]*

Case description

Greg is a forty-nine-year-old man charged with stabbing his partner to death. Witnesses overheard a disagreement between them. Greg has only a patchy recollection of what happened and cannot remember what led to the argument.

Greg has been drinking since he was aged twelve, and has only ever had three weeks of abstinence since his late teens. He has worked on and off for his whole life. He would drink before work, and at times would not go to work because he had been drinking throughout the night. He has had blackouts, and five admissions to hospital for injuries sustained when drunk. He has thought about trying to stop drinking because he feels so guilty about it, but has not tried to stop.

Greg recalled drinking the night before the alleged offence. The following morning, he woke up and drank to manage the withdrawal he was experiencing. He then drank approximately sixteen cans of strong lager throughout the day as well as some spirits.

You have been asked to prepare a report considering whether Greg might have a partial defence of diminished responsibility, based upon alcohol dependence syndrome. There is no evidence of any other mental disorder.

Questions

1. What are the clinical, legal, clinico-legal, and ethical issues in this case?

Clinical

You should conduct a full clinical interview and consult the available papers, including all past medical records. You will need to determine whether the diagnosis of alcohol dependence syndrome applies, and whether any other mental disorder was present at the time of the killing.

It may be difficult to form a firm opinion upon whether Greg was intoxicated at the time of the killing, or his degree of intoxication, as the evidence is likely to be unclear. However you should still try to address this. There may be dispute over it, and it cannot be a wholly clinical issue—since the jury might prefer some other conclusion that your own from any inference to that you might make from his dependence and other available the evidence. And he may have been under the influence of alcohol but not severely intoxicated. Or he may have been withdrawing from alcohol.

Legal

A defence of diminished responsibility can only be founded on a mental disorder (RoI), abnormality of mind (Scotland), or recognised medical condition (E&W, NI).[39] Broadly speaking, mental disorders relating to substance use such as dependence, or psychosis due to withdrawal or longstanding use, can qualify[40]; but intoxication alone cannot.[41]

The legal logic for this is that Parliament (and by extension the Scottish Parliament and the Dáil), in passing the statutes that revised the laws on diminished responsibility, did not state explicitly that it intended to overturn the longstanding common law principle that voluntary intoxication is no defence, and that therefore the legislation had to be read as implicitly excluding voluntary intoxication as a recognised medical condition.

Nevertheless, if another cause of abnormality of mental functioning (in E&W) is operating, the presence of voluntary intoxication does not negate diminished responsibility[42]; if only because the condition must only be 'a significant contributory factor' in causing the killing.

Also intoxication can count within a defence if it was 'involuntary'. For example, within diminished responsibility, because of dependence; although there must have been an 'irresistible craving or compulsion' to use the substance.[43] Intoxication can also found a defence via prescription medicine taken according to a doctor's instructions, or because another person administered it without the defendant's knowledge.[44]

Clinico-legal

Your clinical opinion will be applied to the legal tests described above. Your report should consider the possibility of different states at the time of the killing if this is not agreed as fact, including intoxication and withdrawal, and should describe the implications of each of these states in relation to the legal tests. Did each possible state substantially impair Greg's ability to understand his own conduct, form a rational judgement, or exercise self-control (E&W, NI), or to determine or control his actions (Scotland) or his responsibility for the act (RoI)?

If you diagnose dependence, then describe the nature and degree of the defendant's compulsion to use the substance, both generally and leading up to the offence. Avoid language implying whether the substance use fell on the 'voluntary' or 'involuntary' side of the line; that is for the court to judge.

The diagnoses of alcohol use disorders vary in diagnostic manuals, which can cause confusion. Whereas ICD-11 retains a category of alcohol dependence (6C40), DSM-5 merges it into an overall 'alcohol use disorder' which can be mild, moderate or severe. The loss of the term *dependence* with which courts are familiar means that you may need to educate the court on the new DSM-5 in order to successfully translate your opinion into the legal context.

Ethical

This kind of case may induce strong opinions on the moral question of whether alcohol or drug intoxication, especially if driven by dependence, should be a reason to reduce culpability. Some other jurisdictions do allow such reduction (e.g. Germany). Psychiatrists therefore have a responsibility to reflect on their own opinions on the issue and to use this reflection to ensure that any opinion is as free of the influence of their own values as possible.

[39] The disorder must have operated at the time of the killing to limit the defendants' responsibility for their actions in some way; this is explained in detail in criminal law case 6.
[40] The court may rule that 'self-induced psychosis' cannot found diminished responsibility.
[41] *R v Dowds* [2012] EWCA Crim 281.
[42] *R v Dietschmann* [2003] UKHL 10.
[43] *R v Tandy* [1989] 1 WLR 350; see also *R v Stewart* [2010] EWCA Crim 2159, and *R v Wood* [2008] EWCA Crim 1305.
[44] For example by 'spiking' a drink with GHB or flunitrazepam (Rohypnol). Involuntary causes other than dependence are explored in criminal law case 22.

10 Loss of control or diminished responsibility?

> **Themes:** *depression (p.94)and sexual dysfunction as motivation to kill (p.34) [C]; loss of control and provocation (p.630) and diminished responsibility (p.624) [L]; 'woundability' (p.631) [CL]; and boundaries of expert evidence (p.686) [E]*

Case description

Bill is a fifty-year-old man charged with murdering his wife and brother. He had been married for thirty years and has two adult children who live nearby. He has no previous convictions, cautions, or arrests. He has been employed in various jobs over recent years, most recently as a skilled labourer. He has required antidepressant treatment four times in four years for depression, and was taking an antidepressant prescribed by his GP at the time of the killings; his mother also had anxiety and depression. His mental state had improved recently, and GP's latest note, made three weeks before the killings, states 'improved, without any significant symptoms of depression, although still worried about his relationship and his future, 'continuing to take paroxetine'.

Bill had also sought help for erectile dysfunction in recent years and was awaiting investigation of this. His wife was supportive and had repeatedly reassured him that it was a problem that they would get through together.

Bill came home on the day of the killings earlier than expected and found his wife having sex with his brother. His account is that he shouted at them, and he recalls his wife then taunting him and saying, 'you're no fucking use, you haven't been able to have sex for years'. He does not recall the killings themselves; his last memory is hearing his wife's words. Forensic pathology evidence suggests that repeated blows to the head with a blunt object killed both victims; there is no evidence to suggest in which order they were killed.

On assessment you find Bill to be depressed. He acknowledges that the day he saw his GP he had been feeling better, and more hopeful, and that, because he had been feeling less depressed, he had been more optimistic about his erectile dysfunction being success-fully treated. However, he adds that, during the week before the alleged offences, he had again been feeling 'despondent' about his impotence.

You are asked by Bill's solicitors to provide a report on loss of control and diminished responsibility.

Questions

1. What clinical, legal, clinico-legal, and ethical issues does Bill's case raise?

> **Clinical**
>
> Consider whether at the time of the killing Bill was suffering from any mental disorder, including depression. In addition to interviewing him, you will need his medical records, plus any witness statements that report relevant things he said or did prior to the alleged offences. You should also ask

informants[45] about Bill's personality, history of mental symptoms, and state leading up to the time of the killings, as well as the nature of his relationships with his wife and brother.

It will be particularly important to determine whether any depressive symptoms had again developed since he had last seen his GP, and were likely to have been present at the time of the killings, or whether any depressive symptoms had occurred, or had significantly worsened, only since the killings.

You should also explore (and if necessary, have formally tested) his personality, his self-esteem, and his sexual interests and activities. This should include a history of any lack of self-esteem or a tendency towards anxiety that had previously borne adversely upon his sexual functioning (including factors relating to any mental illness or its treatment).

Lastly, you should explore with Bill what he recalls was the effect of finding his wife and brother having sex, and of the taunts he alleges his wife made. That is, you should 'formulate' the killings, including in regard to the effects of symptoms of mental illness and his history of sexual dysfunction, in the context of the nature of his personality.

Legal

The legal test for diminished responsibility in each jurisdiction, and for loss of control or provocation, are set out in criminal law case 6.

In regard to the defences of loss of control or provocation, the core of the legal test in all four jurisdictions is the combination of 'a qualifying trigger', or 'provocation', with an actual loss of self-control. Beyond this:

- In E&W and NI, the qualifying triggers are fear of serious violence,[46] and acts or words that constitute circumstances of 'an extremely grave character and give a justifiable sense of being seriously wronged' (but not including sexual infidelity alone). It must also be the case that a person of the defendant's sex and age with a normal degree of tolerance and self-restraint, *and in the circumstances of the defendant*, might have reacted in the same or a similar way; and the defendant must not have acted in a considered desire for revenge. The loss of control need not have been sudden.
- In Scotland, there must have been a reasonably proportionate relationship[47] between the provocation and the defendant's reaction to it, even if an ordinary person would not have acted in the same way.[48]
- In RoI the provocation must have caused a sudden and temporary loss of self-control, or of 'mastery over the mind',[49] and would have been expected to do so in any reasonable person.

Clinico-legal

The two proposed defences of diminished responsibility and loss of control, or provocation, are distinct, but the same clinical information and your formulation of the killings will be relevant to both, in different ways.

Loss of control and provocation

Loss of control and provocation are clearly not medical defences, and it follows that no medical diagnosis is required to argue that these apply to the defendant. However, medical evidence can still be relevant; albeit there are limits placed upon the role of expertise in regard to either defence (so that it is important to ask for detailed instructions, including the specific questions on which your opinion is sought).

[45] If any are prosecution witnesses (e.g. his children), you will need permission to interview them, on the basis that you will only ask clinically relevant questions, not explore legal issues.

[46] The feared violence must be from the victim, to the defendant or another person. It will not count (and nor will a sense of being seriously wronged) if the defendant incited it in order to have an excuse for violence.

[47] *Robertson v HM Advocate* [1994] SC(JC) 245.

[48] *Gillon v HM Advocate* [2007] SC(JC) 24.

[49] *R v Duffy* [1949] 1 All ER 932.

Psychiatric evidence cannot relate to any illness or personality aspect which may have made the defendant more likely to lose control in general. Rather, any mental aspect must be relevant to the circumstances of the killing, including 'circumstances' (in E&W) within the defendant. Hence, the depression and impotence might have made Bill more 'woundable' by his wife's taunts, or by seeing her cuckolding him, than would be someone with healthy sexual function who was not depressed. Although in E&W and NI the sexual infidelity cannot be a trigger in its own right, it can be taken into consideration as integral to a wider set of circumstances that caused the defendant to lose control.[50] And the required 'qualifying triggers' set a high objective bar before 'circumstances' can be considered.

You can assist the court by describing how any symptoms or other mental characteristics (such as low self-esteem, or depressive cognitions such as catastrophisation) would have affected Bill's experience of his wife's words, and of seeing her and his brother having sex. This could be considered more relevant to him killing her than to him killing his brother, and it is conceivable that they jury might therefore convict him of the manslaughter of his wife, but of murdering his brother.

Diminished responsibility

In relation to diminished responsibility, first consider whether the defendant was suffering from depression or another mental disorder at the time.[51] If you conclude that he did have a mental disorder, then the severity of his symptoms leading up to the killings will be of great importance in determining whether there was an 'abnormality of mental functioning' that resulted in 'substantial impairment of his ability to exercise self-control'[52] (given that depressive illness can render a person more irritable and even aggressive) or to form a rational judgment (if he had very distorted cognitions[53]).

In E&W and NI, you also need to consider whether the abnormality of mental functioning 'provides an explanation for' ('was a significant contributory factor to') each killing, considered separately. This includes not just the direct impact by way of his reduced ability to exercise self-control, but also the effect of his depression in making him more 'woundable' by his wife's taunts and by the sight of her having sex with his brother.[54]

Clearly this is a case where there is the possibility of multiple narratives. If the prosecution suggests, and the jury accept, that the killings were born primarily out of jealousy, or revenge, then neither partial defence will succeed.[55]

Ethical

Ethically, this kind of case challenges the boundaries of expert psychiatric evidence and emphasises the importance of having a detailed understanding of the relevant law, so as to ensure, for yourself, that you do not step beyond proper expert opinion expression (do not assume that the court will always properly 'police' your evidence). And there may be a tendency to stray from giving proper expert evidence within the two defences towards opining on the ultimate issue, especially in regard to loss of control or provocation, which must be resisted.

---

[50] *R v Clinton* [2012] 1 Cr App R 26.

[51] In E&W, NI, or RoI. It may still be possible to suggest in Scotland that he had some form of abnormality of mind falling short of the diagnostic threshold for depression.

[52] In E&W and NI; in Scotland, that the abnormality of mind substantially impaired his ability to determine or control his conduct; in RoI, that it substantially diminished his responsibility.

[53] For example that he believed *because of his depression* that such serious social opprobrium would have resulted from knowledge of his wife's and his brother's infidelity, that it was better for him to kill them, to spare them intolerable suffering. However, this is unlikely to be accepted by the court.

[54] This is very similar to woundability in the context of the defendant's 'circumstances' for the defence of loss of control, or provocation. However, there woundability is the sole relevance of the depression, and there is no role for enhanced 'reactivity'; whereas reduced ability to exercise self-control represents the core of diminished responsibility.

[55] With the proviso that it is not open to the jury to ignore *unchallenged* medical evidence of diminished responsibility. See criminal law case 6.

11

Loss of control or diminished responsibility—'slow burn'

Themes: *impact of violence (p.32) and motivations for homicide (pp.34, 46) [C]; self-defence (p.410), diminished responsibility (p.624), and provocation and loss of control (p.630), [L]; 'battered person syndrome' (pp.625, 632) [CL]; and citing disputed medical literature in reports (p.668) [E]*

Case description

Vena is a thirty-six-year-old woman charged with murdering her partner Angelo, by throwing petrol on him and setting him alight. He gave police a statement when in hospital, but died a week later from his extensive burns.

Angelo told police he had been sitting smoking, when he felt liquid being poured onto him from behind. He then saw Vena throwing a lighted match at him, and felt the heat of the flames. He ran outside, where a neighbour put out the fire with a hose. He told paramedics that Vena had said, 'I will kill you, boy.'

In her police interview, Vena said that earlier Angelo had woken her, demanding money; when she said she had none, he became angry and threatened her with a knife. They argued again downstairs, and he made a throat-slitting motion to her. He then sat down to smoke. She said she believed he would kill her with the knife.

Vena described Angelo as a drug addict who had been in and out of prison. She claimed he had beaten, raped, and threatened to kill her many times over the past ten years, and had also assaulted their son. Once he choked her to the point of unconsciousness. He was very jealous; he would often attack her for imagined flirtations with men. He frequently checked where she was, and demanded to see her mobile phone. She was often unable to sleep for fear when he was at home; when she did sleep, she had nightmares about him attacking and raping her.

Vena explained that she had often tried to leave him, but whenever she threw him out, he begged to be forgiven, and she would relent. She had no friends and little contact with her family because he became angry if she did. She never reported him to police or sought medical care because she feared his reaction.

Vena said she had also been a victim of physical abuse as a child and had been raped by an uncle at the age of fifteen.

Her solicitor instructs you to write a report on whether Vena suffers from 'battered person syndrome', and, if so, whether it could be used as a defence.

Questions

1. Can battered person syndrome be used in a defence of loss of control or provocation, or of diminished responsibility?
2. Is the justification of self-defence open to Vena?
3. What other clinical, legal, clinico-legal, and ethical issues arise in the case?

Clinical

Battered person syndrome (BPS), originally referred to as 'battered woman syndrome', as it was first described in women in the 1970s, is a well-described phenomenon. It is not a diagnosis in itself and is not listed in ICD-11[56] or DSM-5. However, it very often includes PTSD, anxiety, and depression.

BPS arises typically after the victim of violence in a relationship has experienced repeated cycles of violence and reconciliation, resulting in the abused victim:

- thinking that the violence is their fault;
- being unable to place the responsibility for the violence elsewhere;
- fearing for their life, and/or the lives of loved ones;
- believing irrationally that the abuser is omnipresent and omniscient; and
- experiencing a state of learned helplessness.

A three-stage cycle has been described in many cases of prolonged domestic violence. First, tension builds in the relationship, with the victim often trying to find ways to appease the abuser or otherwise avoid violence. Second, the abusive partner releases the tension through violence, while blaming the victim for having caused it. Third, the violent partner makes gestures of contrition, but does not change their behaviour, and the cycle repeats.

The feeling of being responsible for, yet helpless to stop the violence leads to depression and passivity, often alongside posttraumatic symptoms. Such learned helplessness makes it difficult for the abused partner to marshal the resources to leave the abuser, which seems impossible because they are perceived as all-powerful. This is exacerbated by the lack of friends or family who could assist, often because the abuser has deliberately isolated the victim from them.

The assessment of BPS in criminal proceedings is unusual, in that it involves consideration not only of the alleged perpetrator of the offence (the victim of abuse, i.e. the allegedly 'battered' person), but also the victim of the alleged offence (the abuser) and the relationship between them. The latter two will usually have to be assessed indirectly, via descriptions from witnesses and others. The abuser is very commonly insecure and dependent, and uses control, including violence, in order to shore up their position within the relationship.

On assessment, you find that Vena shows many of the features of BPS, and you diagnose her with PTSD plus depressive symptoms.

Legal

The legal criteria for diminished responsibility in each jurisdiction are described in criminal law case 6, and for loss of control or provocation in criminal cases 6 and 10. Diminished responsibility requires the presence of a recognised medical condition (E&W, NI), abnormality of mind (Scotland), or mental disorder (RoI).

Loss of control and provocation are not psychiatric defences, and no evidence of mental disorder (or behavioural syndromes) is required. However, it can be relevant to the 'circumstances' or 'woundability' of the defendant in the face of provocation, if the defendant is shown to have then lost control.

- In Scotland, the test is that the defendant's reaction to the provocation was still reasonably proportionate, even if an ordinary person would have reacted differently.[57]
- In E&W and NI, assuming the victim's behaviour amounts to a 'qualifying trigger',[58] such as a fear of serious violence, and the defendant does not act in deliberate revenge, the test is that a person of the same age and sex, with a normal degree of tolerance and self-restraint, 'in the same circumstances', might have reacted in a similar way.
- In RoI the test is drawn more tightly: the provocation must have caused a sudden and temporary loss of self-control ('mastery over the mind'), and would have been expected to do so in any reasonable person.

---

[56] Although it is mentioned in ICD11 as an 'entity' within PTSD.
[57] *Robertson v HM Advocate* [1994] SC(JC) 245; *Gillon v HM Advocate* [2007] SC(JC) 24.
[58] See criminal law case 10 for details.

Clinico-legal

Loss of control or provocation

The court will have to determine whether Vena's partner's violence and threats amounted to a qualifying trigger or provocation, and whether she lost control (despite her reaction to his violence being a delayed 'slow burn' rather than a sudden response[59]). These are subjective tests, relating to the defendant and the victim personally. Neither is generally a matter for expert comment. However, in RoI or Scotland, the defence might struggle to convince the court that she did indeed lose mastery over her mind, and might call upon you for expert evidence (e.g.) that her perception of her options was profoundly distorted by her BPS (or depression or PTSD)—but this might not be accepted by the court as falling within the legal definitions.[60]

The other element of the test relates to what a reasonable or ordinary person might have done in the situation, introducing a degree of objectivity. In E&W and NI, this means a person in Vena's circumstances (an abused woman suffering from BPS); in Scotland, the comparison is with an ordinary person not necessarily in her circumstances, but her different reaction can still fall within the defence provided that it was 'reasonably proportionate'. In RoI caselaw has long held that 'any reasonable person' includes people with the specific characteristics of the defendant.[61]

This allows the court to consider expert evidence that Vena's circumstances included being more fragile, or 'woundable', in the face of Angelo's threats than a person without BPS would be.

Diminished responsibility

Here, as BPS is not a diagnostic entity, the underlying diagnosis of PTSD and depression must be made explicit (in Scotland it is more likely to be accepted as an 'abnormality of mind'). If you go on to refer to BPS, you should make its medical status clear and refer to it in 'formulation' terms.

Self-defence

A lawyer for the defendant might suggest that Vena could have available to her the 'justification' of self-defence, based upon her belief 'in the moment' that only by killing him could she avoid him killing her. And evidence of her mental disorder and BPS would be accepted insofar as it helps the court understand how she would have perceived her circumstance; perhaps that she was in fear of imminent death (despite that not being objectively the case). However, for the justification to apply, the fatal force she used would have to have been 'necessary' in those circumstances, and both 'reasonable' and 'proportionate' to the threat she objectively faced. Neither of these requirements is met, in that she could realistically have left (even though she felt unable to), and as Angelo was not attacking her at that moment, even if unable to leave, killing him was not the only way to prevent him killing her.

Ethical

Being an expert witness relies upon your field of expertise being based upon a recognised body of scientific research or clinical knowledge, in this case of BPS. As with many areas of study, there are conflicting results in the literature that you may wish to rely on. You must nevertheless avoid selectivity in the literature you cite.[62] Referencing one study that backs an assertion that you make, without referencing competing literature, or without setting the study within the broader literature, is wholly unacceptable. Rather, what is reasonable and proper is to write, and say that there is a reasonable body of literature that describes and accepts, for example, the phenomenon of BPS.

---

[59] This is less of an issue in E&W and NI, where the law states explicitly that the loss of self-control 'need not be sudden', than in RoI, where it states explicitly that it must be sudden. Scottish law is unclear on this point.

[60] *R v Ahluwalia* [1992] 4 All ER 889; although this was an English case relating to earlier law.

[61] At the time of writing, the Irish Government is considering whether to reform the defence so as to reduce the degree to which a defendant's idiosyncrasies are taken into account.

[62] See for example *Squier v GMC* [2016] EWHC 2739.

12

Loss of control–woundability and malingering

Case description

Three years ago Edwin, then aged thirty-two, was convicted of murdering his girlfriend; no psychiatric evidence was introduced at the trial. Edwin claimed that his girlfriend had been killed by a man she met after they separated, and that he had seen the man running away from the scene of the killing. The police were called by a neighbour who heard 'a violent argument'. One officer gave evidence that, on arrest, Edwin said, 'I don't care what you do. I'd made up my mind to kill her.' Edwin accused the police officer of lying.

Before trial, Edwin attempted suicide on several occasions, including by cutting himself and taking an overdose of medication; he required short periods of treatment in the prison healthcare wing.

Edwin's lawyer gives you a recent statement, in which Edwin says, 'I now accept that I killed my girlfriend and that my previous account was false. We had separated a few weeks before ... I got really down, I lost my appetite, I was always crying, I couldn't sleep and I tried to kill myself ... on the day I killed her we met up; she told me she'd met someone else, and that I'd never been good enough, and our children weren't mine ... I lost it ... I saw red ... I had a knife in my pocket and I lunged at her and stabbed her'. Later in his statement Edwin describes being physically and sexually abused as a child, which left him with 'strong feelings of rage', and led to him repeatedly attempting suicide as a teenager.

You are instructed to prepare a report for an appeal based of loss of control.

Questions

1. How should you approach this case?
2. Should you consider whether Edwin may be malingering past symptoms?
3. How will you address the issue of loss of self-control in your report?
4. What other clinical, legal, clinico-legal, and ethical issues arise in the case?

Clinical

A careful and detailed clinical interview will be needed. This should include consideration of whether Edwin is currently depressed, or suffering from any other mental disorder including personality disorder, as well as pinning down his reported history of mental illness earlier in life.

You should also obtain collateral information from his GP and other medical records, such as when he attended A&E following self-harm, and if possible, interview informants such as family members, friends, or neighbours[63]. This should corroborate (or not) his history of symptoms of mental illness around the time of the murder.

The obvious potential motivation of escaping continued imprisonment, coupled with the fact that there was no prior suggestion of mental illness, means that you should also consider malingering: that is the intentional feigning or exaggeration of symptoms of illness. Determining whether appellants/ defendants are malingering can be challenging, especially if they have previously suffered from a mental illness and so have knowledge of possible symptoms. Clinically, it is important to consider the following factors, including addressing clinical 'plausibility', as distinct from 'credibility':

- Is he presenting with unusual symptoms of mental illness, or symptoms inconsistent with the inferred or claimed diagnosis? If so, their validity needs to be explored in depth.
- Is there internal coherence of his account?
- Has his account been consistent over time?
- Is his account consistent with the other evidence?
- What is, or was, his response to his symptoms, and is this typical of those with the claimed illness?
- How well does his account accord with the usual natural history of such an illness?
- Is there consistency between symptoms and behaviour?
- Are any of the symptoms or mental state signs difficult to feign?

Specialist psychological testing for malingering might well assist: for example, the SIRS,[64] a structured clinical interview for malingering, which checks for the internal consistency of a defendant's self-report and the typicality of symptoms, and the Test of Memory Malingering (TOMM),[65] a visual recognition test used in people potentially malingering memory problems (but potentially relevant to consideration of malingering of other symptoms). Although there can be 'false positive interpretation for malingering'. If you employ such tools yourself, you must be qualified to do so. Assessment will need to include a detailed account of any symptoms at the time of the killing, and of his mental response to what the victim said to him.

Legal

Psychiatric factors are only relevant to provocation or loss of control insofar as they relate to the 'woundability' of the defendant; that is, their vulnerability to the specific alleged provocation. This is taken into account in E&W and NI as part of the 'circumstances' of the provocative qualifying triggers, and included in RoI within the concept of the 'reasonable person' who would be expected to respond similarly. In Scotland, the woundable defendant's response must be 'reasonably proportionate' to the provocation.[66]

It remains unclear exactly what psychiatric or psychological factors are accepted as contributing to woundability in each jurisdiction: but there must be some specific link to the claimed provocation.[67] However it does not include a general tendency to loss of self-control.

Clinico-legal

If you think it more likely than not that Edwin had a mental disorder at the time of the killing, you should then consider whether any symptoms were in operation at the time of the killing, and if so, how they would have influenced his behaviour. Even if you have found evidence of malingering by exaggeration, you *might* still conclude that there was a sufficient level of genuine symptoms.

Edwin claims to have suddenly lost self-control after being hurt by his girlfriend's remarks that he was never good enough for her, and not the father of her children. Such taunts would be likely to have more of an impact upon someone who was depressed because of depressive cognitions such as catastrophisation, dichotomous thinking, and low self-esteem.

---

[63] You will need specific permission for any that were prosecution witnesses.
[64] Structured Inventory of Reported Symptoms.
[65] Test of Memory Malingering.
[66] These rules are explained in criminal law case 11, and the full legal test is set out in case 10.
[67] Where there are psychiatric factors indicating a generally reduced ability to exercise self-control, you (or the lawyer) should consider whether the defence of diminished responsibility is available.

Evidence of being affected by her abandonment of him, or jealousy about her cuckolding him, is not relevant. Likewise, any difficulty managing anger as a result of his abused childhood (if confirmed by your assessment) is not relevant, since it would relate to his general self-control and not to his 'woundability'.[68]

You should note that there is a strong piece of ordinary evidence against Edwin's claimed loss of control: his comment, when arrested, that he had made up his mind to kill his girlfriend. You should never assert that he met the full legal test in any case, as it is the ultimate issue, but your awareness of the likelihood that the court would conclude from that evidence that Edwin did not in fact lose control, despite any woundability you have found, should make you circumspect in the way you express your findings.

Ethical

The law of loss of control or provocation is a terrain within which the psychiatrist needs to be extremely cautious towards maintaining the boundary around what it is proper for them to address—especially when giving of oral evidence, where there is even greater danger of spontaneously overstepping the mark.

If you include reference to your assessment of malingering in your report, despite concluding that Edwin is not malingering, your instructing lawyer might ask you to remove it as disadvantageous to Edwin's case. You should not accede to the request since you considered it clinically relevant to assess for it.

---

[68] However, trauma following abuse might be relevant to woundability if his ex-partner had taunted him about that abuse (e.g. 'you're so worthless, you deserved to be beaten up by your uncle all those times').

13 Joint enterprise–encouraging or assisting

Themes: *intellectual disability (p.110) and autism (p.104) [C]; encouraging or assisting an offence in joint enterprise (p.408), diminished responsibility (p.624), and reliability of confession (p.608) [L]; misunderstanding within joint enterprise (p.408) and suggestibility and compliance (p.160) [CL]; and lack of clinical data (p.304) [E]*

Case description

Gregory is thirty-one years old. He and two co-defendants are charged with murdering a police officer. He has always lived with family: his mother and brother, until his mother's death three years ago, now just his brother. He was thought 'slow' and 'odd' at school, and left early to work for his uncle in a shop storeroom. He is single and has never had any intimate relationships. He has one conviction, for drug possession; he has never been imprisoned.

The police officer's car was blocked in by another car as he tried to leave the station, and three men then got out of the car. Two of the men shot the officer, who died at the scene. Gregory is not alleged to have had a gun, but to have been in the car as it blocked in the officer, and then outside it when the officer was shot. A witness saw all three men then get back into the car and drive off. There is no evidence of any conversation between the three defendants. They were each arrested, at separate locations, several days later.

After three days in custody, involving five interviews, Gregory confessed to taking part in the killing. He said he went with the other two defendants 'because they had some business to take care of'; and that they had told him they were going to 'deal with' the police officer in question, and needed him to accompany them. He said he had not known that they had planned to kill or seriously injury the officer.

You are asked by Gregory's solicitor to give an opinion on whether Gregory is mentally disordered, and, if so, how this would have affected his responsibility for involvement in the alleged offence. You are also asked whether his confession was reliable.

Questions

1. How could you assess Gregory clinically for any possible developmental disorder which might be legally relevant?
2. Are your instructions adequate?
3. Can developmental disorders be diagnosed without additional information?
4. How would you address Gregory's confession?
5. How might diagnosis of a developmental disorder be relevant to sentence?
6. What other clinical, legal, clinico-legal, and ethical issues arise in the case?

Clinical

The case history suggests possible intellectual disability and/or autism, each of which you should consider in your assessment.

The diagnosis of intellectual (or learning) disability is based upon clinical criteria, and not solely on IQ score (as lawyers commonly believe). There must be evidence of impaired intellectual function associated with impaired social or occupational function from childhood. You will need information from a range of sources, including a detailed developmental history from a primary caregiver, collateral information from family or friends,; school and employment records, and medical records. You will also need to arrange a psychometric assessment of intellectual function.

Autism spectrum disorder (ASD) is a[69] complex neurodevelopmental disorder characterised by deficits in reciprocal social interaction, communication and language, and flexibility of thought and behaviour. The condition is present from childhood, but many individuals with ASD without significant intellectual impairment fail to be diagnosed until they present with challenging behaviour, or come into contact with the criminal justice system in adult life. Assessment of suspected ASD requires the developmental history and other information listed above, plus a structured assessment[70] involving observation in different settings.

In a legal context, because of the nature of their deficits, individuals with ASD are more often suggestible and compliant, and they are likely to struggle to understand the police caution and to follow court proceedings. Additionally, because of their reduced understanding of interactions with others, they may not have the mental element for an offence that would ordinarily be implied by their behaviour (e.g. going along with what they think others want them to do without understanding the implications).

Legal

The law in this area is significantly different between the UK jurisdictions and RoI. In the latter, each defendant is considered separately: nobody is liable for the actions of others. However, a defendant who does not (for instance) strike the fatal blow can still be convicted of murder, because of the presumption[71] that they 'intended the natural and probable consequences of their conduct'. For example, a defendant who knew their co-defendant had a loaded gun and wanted the victim dead, and went along with them, nevertheless, would be presumed to have intended death to result and could be convicted of murder.

In the UK, by contrast, the actions of the various parties to the joint enterprise are analysed together. Following the Supreme Court's decision in *Jogee*, in 2016,[72] a person has secondary (or constructive) liability for the actions of their co-defendants if they intended to assist or encourage them, *and* had the requisite mental element for the primary offence. For example, if the offence that the co-defendant goes on to commit is unlawful wounding, in order to have secondary liability, the defendant must intend to assist or encourage the co-defendant, and be reckless as to the possibility of serious injury occurring.[73]

Clinico-legal

Your instructions as regards 'responsibility' are vague and do not set out the relevant legal tests to which your evidence should relate: so you should ask for more detailed instructions.

---

[69] ASD is commonly divided into a number of specific syndromes, such as classical autism, Asperger syndrome, semantic-pragmatic disorder, childhood disintegrative disorder, and so on. ICD-11 now groups them into a single ASD category; DSM-5 recognises autism spectrum disorder and social communication disorder.

[70] For example the Autism Diagnostic Observation Schedule 2 (ADOS2) or the Autism Diagnostic Interview—Revised (ADI-R). You must have specific training to use such instruments.

[71] Under s4 Criminal Justice Act 1964.

[72] *R v Jogee (Appellant)* [2016] UKPC 7.

[73] A more stringent test than the previous law that the defendant only needed to 'foresee what their co-defendant might do' *and* 'continue to remain involved'.

Assuming that it is an agreed fact that Gregory did not fire the shots that killed the police officer, for Gregory to be convicted of murder in the UK, he would have to be shown to have intended to assist or encourage his co-defendants, *and* either to have intended death or serious injury to occur, or been reckless (i.e. to have foreseen the possibility of death or serious injury and gone ahead anyway). In the RoI, only the latter element would be required, provided it was established that that the death of the police officer was a natural and probable consequence of going along with the co-defendants.

You will therefore need to consider whether, based upon your assessment of Gregory's developmental disorder and/or intellectual disability, he had sufficient ability to understand what was intended, so as 'to assist or encourage' the co-defendants,[74] or so as to form the intent[75] to kill or seriously injure (or be reckless). For example, you might consider that he may have adopted a concrete interpretation of the words, 'deal with', not realising that this could include harming or killing the victim, and that this was what he was going along with. Further, and less specifically, there may have been a more generalised dependence upon the other two defendants, so that he was unable to make his own judgment about what they were doing.

However, you must take note of any ordinary evidence which there might be that could suggest that whatever his disabilities, Gregory did, in fact, encourage or assist his co-defendants and form the relevant intent.

If the latter tests were met, Gregory might still be able to plead diminished responsibility to murder on the ground of any intellectual impairment, and/or ASD that you diagnose (see criminal case 6).

Beyond what may be undisputed evidence that Gregory exhibited an 'abnormality of mental functioning' (or 'abnormality of mind' or 'mental disorder'[76]), you would have to address whether there would be grounds for the jury to consider that his condition substantially impaired his ability to 'understand his conduct', to 'form a rational judgment', or to 'exercise self-control'.[77]

Separately, you will need to assess Gregory in relation to any vulnerability he might have exhibited under police questioning in relation to his confession to having taken part in the murder.

Ultimately, the reliability of a confession is a matter for legal consideration. However, if a defendant exhibits mental features that are likely to render his confession less than normally reliable, then expert evidence is admissible within a *voir dire* or prehearing. Hence, you will need to assess whether Gregory's disabilities would likely have had an impact upon his understanding of his situation and questioning within the police interviews. Further, it will be necessary to determine (almost certainly through instruction of a clinical psychologist) whether Gregory is abnormally 'suggestible' and/or 'compliant', since it is well recognised that these two 'traits' are more common in those of low intelligence.[78]

Ethical

There is no sense in prohibiting diagnosis because of an inability to interview relatives or because school records are not available. In legal terms, this might result in less weight properly being applied to your opinion, but there will always be circumstances where information is limited, and so you should give an opinion as best you can, and express a view as to the likely reliability and validity of that opinion, in light of any data that you would have wished to have and did not. And you can, and should, also include expression of what alternative opinions there might reasonably be, but why you favour your own opinion.

---

[74] If he lacked this ability, then in RoI his lawyers might seek to rebut the presumption that he intended the (objectively determined) natural and probable consequences of his actions, on the ground that he was not able to recognise the police officer's death as such a consequence.

[75] The test of this is explored in criminal law case 14.

[76] In non-E&W jurisdctions.

[77] In E&W and NI; in Scotland, substantially impaired his ability to determine or control his actions; and in RoI, diminished his responsibility for the act substantially.

[78] This is considered in more detail in criminal law case 2.

Capacity to form specific intent and intoxication

Themes: *serious violence (p.48) and role of intoxication (p.49) [C]; voluntary intoxication (p.616) and specific and basic intent (p.403) [L]; capacity to form intent (p.610) [CL]; and medical versus legal paradigms concerning intoxication (p.354) [E]*

Case description

Duncan has a long history of binge drinking, without alcohol dependence syndrome. He is charged with wounding with intent to cause GBH,[79] having, when heavily intoxicated, allegedly smashed a bottle, and slashed the victim's neck, causing serious injury.

Witnesses state that he left the pub very soon after the assault. He was arrested a few minutes later. He was seen by a forensic medical examiner at the police station; the alcohol level in a blood sample taken two hours after the alleged offence was 330mg/100ml. When he was interviewed under caution midmorning, by then twelve hours after his arrest, he described having drunk so much alcohol that he had no memory of the latter part of the evening, or of the alleged offence; he only remembered waking early in the morning in a police cell.

Duncan's solicitor has instructed you to produce a psychiatric report addressing his capacity to form the mental state required for the offence.

Questions

1. Can his likely severe intoxication at the time of the alleged offence negate the mental element necessary for a serious assault?
2. What other clinical, legal, clinico-legal, and ethical issues arise in the case?

Clinical

Your assessment should consider whether Duncan has had previous amnesic episodes when intoxicated, plus any history of violence, when drunk and when sober. You should assess for physical sequelae of long-term alcohol abuse, particularly brain damage, and for any possible personality disorder.

As regards his likely blood alcohol concentration (BAC) at the time of the alleged offence, it is generally accepted that, for the average non–alcohol-dependent man, BAC falls by around 15mg/100ml per hour,[80] allowing you to 'back-calculate' an approximate value of 510mg/100ml. However, you should look in the legal papers for an expert toxicology report giving the likely level of intoxication at the time of the alleged offence, and excluding any other substances having likely been present in the defendant.

---

[79] In E&W or NI; in Scotland, the closest equivalent would be 'assault to the danger of life', and in RoI 'causing serious harm'.

[80] For example Winston B B and Zunker M T (2010) How long does it take a person to sober up? Some mathematics and science of driving under the influence [of alcohol]. *Mathematics Teacher* 104(1): 58.

Legal

Amnesia for an offence or its circumstances is not relevant[81] unless it contributes to mental condition evidence that the defendant either did not have the required mental element for the offence, or had a mental condition defence available (e.g. automatism).

The doctrine of 'prior fault' means, as a matter of public policy, that voluntary intoxication is no excuse in law.[82] Duncan should have foreseen when he began to drink that intoxication might well make him more likely to commit an offence.

Nevertheless, if the offence charged is one requiring specific intent,[83] a defendant who was so intoxicated that they were incapable of forming such specific intent will be acquitted, according to the ruling in *Majewski*.[84] Wounding with intent to cause GBH is an offence of specific intent, requiring the intention that the assault will have the consequence of causing the victim serious harm.

The required degree of effect of intoxication upon mental functioning was set very high by the court in *Majewski*; in that the defendant is required to have been so intoxicated that he is unable to control his limbs effectively. In other words, it is not enough even to show that his judgment was severely distorted, or his ability to exercise self-control grossly impaired.

If, by contrast, the offence charged is one requiring only basic intent,[85] then the prior fault doctrine means that the voluntary intoxication cannot ground a defence, however intoxicated the defendant, and whatever the effect upon them mentally.

The categorisation of offences into those requiring specific as opposed to basic intent is not wholly rational, or philosophically robust, and has been widely criticised—for example, because of the varying degrees of sophistication of intention inherent to the offence. There is no reliable way to 'determine' whether an offences requires specific intent or not[86]; although, as a rule of thumb, offences which can be committed through recklessness alone are always offences of basic intent.[87]

Clinico-legal

In practice the role of medical evidence in applying the *Majewski* rule on specific intent is extremely limited, indeed usually nonexistent.

For example, any expert's 'back calculation' of BAC is prone to error, especially if over more than an hour or two. The metabolism of alcohol varies enormously between people, influenced particularly by their habitual level of alcohol consumption. Further, even if the BAC at the time of the offence could be known with confidence, the brain's response to that BAC is also highly variable between individuals. A frequent heavy drinker will be far more tolerant of high BAC.

The best evidence for whether the defendant was capable of forming the required specific intent will usually be CCTV or witness statements of the defendant's behaviour at the time. Hence, although medical and forensic science experts may be able to give evidence relevant to the *Majewski* rule, it will be set in the context of, and may well be dwarfed by, evidence of behaviour at the time.

Although intoxication is the most common reason for questioning a defendant's capacity to form specific intent, there can be other psychiatric causes, such as psychosis, or sufficiently severe depression (as in criminal law case 10).

---

[81] *R v Podola* [1959] 3 WLR 718.

[82] *A-G for N. Ireland v Gallagher* [1963] AC 349. Like all the rules in this case, it is followed strictly in E&W and generally in NI, whereas courts in Scotland and RoI retain far more discretion to deal with cases involving voluntarily intoxicated defendants as they see fit.

[83] That is, intent that a particular consequence will result from the defendant's acts or omissions, such as serious injury in this case. (The Scottish and RoI equivalents do not include the specific intent element.)

[84] *DPP v Majewski* [1976] UKHL 2.

[85] That is, presence of mind during the commission of the offence, which, depending on the offence, may mean intent to do the acts or omissions (e.g. in the case of sexual assault by penetration in E&W) or either intent or recklessness about whether the acts or omissions occur (e.g. in the case of unlawful wounding or inflicting GBH, or sexual assault by penetration in Scotland).

[86] Although it is notable that offences deemed to require specific intent generally have linked lesser offence of basic intent available, so that the prior fault doctrine remains in a weaker form.

[87] *R v Caldwell* [1982] AC 341.

Ethical

Although it might seem obvious that severe intoxication is an abnormal mental state within a medical paradigm, resulting in judgement and decision-making being severely affected, you must resist any temptation to import this into what is a strictly defined legal test, however unfair this may appear.

15 Capacity to form intent to kill—drugs and alcohol

Themes: *intoxication and dependence (p.76), drug-induced psychosis (p.72), and homicide (p.46) [C]; intent (p.402), capacity to form specific intent (p.610), and diminished responsibility (p.624) [L]; retrospective reconstruction of mental state (p.670) [CL]; and consent for interview (p.660) [E]*

Case description

Charles is twenty-five and charged with murdering a young woman, Jada. He spent much of the afternoon of the killing drinking strong rum and playing rock music. He picked up Jada and a male friend of his, and drove to a quiet location where he continued to drink and listen to music.

His friend stated that Charles started touching Jada's breasts, but she pushed his hand away. Charles told the police, 'a demon rose up inside me and I choked her for a minute. I blocked her mouth and slit her throat. I pulled her out of the car, and she fell to the ground. Then I stabbed her in the chest before driving off. I didn't intend to kill her: it was a demon inside my head. I didn't know what I was doing. I saw a dark object in front of me and I didn't know what it was. I didn't see or hear her in front of me; I didn't know I was stabbing her.'

He admitted smoking marijuana and crack cocaine before he met Jada, adding that he had never used crack before; he said he was 'very high' on alcohol and drugs by the time he killed Jada. Information from family included that he had drunk more and more heavily over the past couple of years, and had had blackouts on several occasions, although had had no withdrawal symptoms or other signs of dependence.

A postmortem showed that Jada died from a slash wound to her neck, which had cut through her trachea and carotid arteries. She also had multiple stab wounds and bruises on her face and chest. There was no evidence of sexual interference.

Charles' solicitor instructs you to assess whether his use of drugs and alcohol could have prevented him forming the intent to commit murder.

Questions

1. How should you approach determining Charles's capacity to form the specific intent for murder?
2. How should you take consent from Charles before you interview him?
3. What other clinical, legal, clinico-legal, and ethical issues arise in the case?

Clinical

A comprehensive psychiatric assessment is needed, involving a detailed interview and gaining collateral information, addressing amongst other things:

- Exactly what did he drink, and what drugs did he use and at what times?
- Is there a calculation of intoxication levels (e.g. BAC) at the time of the killing, worked backwards from a blood test after arrest (calculated by a specialist toxicologist)?
- When had he eaten? (This could affect the absorption of alcohol or orally ingested drugs.)
- What was his subjective perception of his degree of intoxication?
- What signs of intoxication were there in his behaviour (e.g. how well did he drive when travelling to the scene of the killing)?
- Does he suffer from any physical conditions that might exacerbate intoxication (e.g. diabetes, resulting in hypoglycaemia from insulin therapy or hyperglycaemia)?
- What is his usual pattern of drinking and of drug use?
- What previously unrecognised signs of dependence are there (e.g. tolerance requiring him to drink more heavily)?
- How does he usually behave when drunk or high (e.g. does he typically become violent or lose self-control)?
- Is he ever violent when not intoxicated?
- Has he ever exhibited possible psychotic symptoms when drunk or high before?
- Does he suffer from any other mental disorder? (Comorbid mental disorders are very common in people who use drugs and/or alcohol.)

Assume you come to the conclusion that he was intoxicated but also experiencing a transient drug-induced psychotic episode at the time of the killing, that he had never previously had psychosis, and that he often becomes aggressive when intoxicated, not when sober, but has never previously been seriously violent.

Legal

Murder requires proof of specific intent to cause death or serious injury: that is, either direct evidence that the defendant intended either to occur, or inference from their statements and/or behaviour that they foresaw that it was virtually certain[88] to result from their actions. (See criminal case 14.)

It used to be accepted that psychosis that was drug-induced could amount legally to a 'recognised medical condition', 'mental disorder', or 'abnormality of mind'[89] for the purposes of diminished responsibility. However, there is now caselaw in E&W that excludes transient psychosis that is induced by voluntary intoxication alone.[90] And this may be why the solicitor has not asked you to address that partial defence. (It is not clear whether in E&W the exacerbation of a pre-existing psychotic disorder by drug use would still be accepted as a recognised medical condition[91]; of whether the precedent will be followed in other domestic jurisdictions.)

[88] In RoI, a 'natural and probable consequence'. Such inferences are sometimes referred to as 'oblique intent'.

[89] The terms used in E&W and NI, RoI, and Scotland, respectively. The full tests for diminished responsibility in each jurisdiction are set out in criminal law case 5.

[90] *R v Lindo* [2016] EWCA Crim 1940.

[91] This is uncertain because, in *Lindo*, the defendant was accepted to be in a prodromal state for schizophrenia at the time he had the intoxication-induced transient psychotic episode. So was the *ratio decidendi* that a prodrome is not a recognised medical condition, or that *any* drug-induced psychosis is not a recognised medical condition? Imagine a defendant with schizophrenia who had been well, but then killed during a month-long relapse triggered by drug use. Under the first *ratio* they would be able to plead diminished responsibility; under the second, they would not. A later case (*R v Kay and Joyce* [2017] EWCA Crim 647) clarified that a relapse in someone who had a dependence syndrome would qualify, but left open the case of an intoxication-triggered relapse without dependence.

Clinico-legal

Charles's account raises the possibility that he might have been incapable of forming the intent to murder. There might, however, be ordinary witness evidence (e.g. things he said to his friend) that demonstrates that he did in fact form that intent. It is crucial that you do not try to establish what Charles' intent actually was; that is an issue for the court. You should focus upon the impact of his mental state on his reasoning and decision-making abilities at the time.

If there is a back calculation of his level of intoxication, you may take that into account, provided you note that the interaction of the different drugs and his tolerance to alcohol make inferences from this about his mental state unreliable.

Finally, the threshold for a finding of incapacity to form specific intent as a result of voluntary intoxication, for whatever offence, is set extremely high: the defendant must have been all but unable to control his limbs as a result of intoxication.[92]

Ethical

Defendants who participate in a psychiatric assessment in the course of criminal proceedings are in an unusual and potentially difficult position: they are assessed by a doctor employing their usual techniques for engaging with a patient, and yet the information obtained will not be held confidentially, as is the case in an ordinary doctor-patient encounter. It will be shared with lawyers, and potentially far more widely (judge and jury, even the public if stated in open court and then reported by the media). Further it will be applied to a non-clinical, justice purpose. You must explain all this when seeking consent before the assessment commences.

If a defendant, with an understanding of the consequences, withholds consent, then the interview should go no further. Unless the defendant changes their mind after a discussion with their solicitor, a capacitous refusal must be respected.

The situation is more complicated if the defendant lacks the capacity to refuse to participate in an assessment; when you should act in their best interests, which may mean preparing a report based on the available information. However, it is particularly difficult in such cases to balance the overriding duty to the court to be impartial and frank with the medical prerequisite of doing no harm, and care will be needed only to include material in the report which it is necessary for the court to know for its purposes.

Finally, any matter relevant to the obtaining of consent, or failure to do so, including your reasoning, needs to be clearly documented, so that the court can decide how to proceed in the interests of justice.

[92] *DPP v Majewski* [1976] UKHL 2.

Capacity for reform and sentence of death

Case description

Idris was convicted two years ago in St Vincent of raping and murdering a young woman in Trinidad. He is now twenty-one years old. He is a businessman's son with no other offending history. He was successful at school. He has no close friends.[93]

The victim attended the same school. They were never friends nor in a relationship. For a year Idris had sent her messages on social media, and visited her home uninvited. She responded politely, then later asked him to stop. Her last note to him included, 'You will have to torture me before I love you.' Nevertheless he persisted, and his messages became more sexual; the last two indicating that he believed her to be sexually interested in being tortured by him. She did not respond. Her body was found on a beach; she had been raped, cut, and strangled. DNA testing showed Idris's semen in in her vagina.

After arrest, Idris stated, 'she said I'd have to torture her before she'd love me'. Beyond this, he has always refused to discuss what happened, including with his parents, his solicitors, and the police. He spends time in his cell reading.

Idris was assessed by a psychiatrist pretrial; he answered questions about himself but not about the victim or the offence. The psychiatrist also interviewed his parents in some detail, and formed the opinion that he likely suffered from autism, but no other disorder. She did not feel able to offer an opinion on diminished responsibility, having been unable to discuss the offence with Idris.

You are instructed by Idris's lawyer to give an opinion, which may be served on the Eastern Caribbean Appeal Court, on whether Idris has a mental disorder and, if so, what the prognosis is and whether he has the capacity for reform, as well as his level of remorse. He is appealing his death sentence. He says that he will not cooperate with more interviews as he has already spoken to a psychiatrist.[94]

Questions

1. Can you make a diagnosis without seeing the defendant?
2. How should you describe prognosis in a disorder such as autism?

---

[93] Concerning expert psychiatric practice and the death penalty generally: Eastman N, Krljes S, Latham R, and Lyall M (2018) *Handbook of Forensic Psychiatric Practice in Capital Cases*, Second Edition, Death Penalty Project; Eastman N, Krljes S, Latham R, and Lyall M (2018) *Casebook of Forensic Psychiatric Practice in Capital Cases*, Death Penalty Project.

[94] The death penalty is retained in a significant number of other Commonwealth jurisdictions, some of which, including St Vincent, still use the UK Privy Council as their final appeal court.

3. How should you address the capacity for reform?
4. What other clinical, legal, clinico-legal, and ethical issues arise in the case?

Clinical

You cannot diagnose a disorder without participating in an examination of the appellant. Unless and until that becomes possible, you can assist by gathering collateral information for the suspected diagnosis of autism,[95] including interviewing Idris's parents and prison officers, discussing him with the local psychiatrists, and reviewing school and GP records. This should enable you to shorten and focus the interview (while ensuring it remains sufficiently comprehensive), which might facilitate Idris taking part.

Likewise, you may be able to increase the chances of Idris consenting to answer your questions if you find a cool, quiet, calm, and dimly lit interview setting, and specifically ask Idris via his solicitor beforehand what he found distressing about the first interview in case you are able to mitigate it.

If he will not speak to you face to face, he might agree to respond to written questions—ideally with you present, so that you can observe his responses. Even if he decides not to answer questions about the killing, you may be able to glean useful information from such observation, and you will be able to combine what he tells you with what he told the first psychiatrist.

Assuming you conclude that you think it more likely than not that he has autism, you must make clear in your report that this is a provisional diagnosis, with a significant degree of uncertainty because of the inability to conduct a full clinical interview.

One of the intrinsic difficulties in assessing the prognosis of people with autism is that despite it being a lifelong and relatively stable disorder, it is neither unchanging nor untreatable. For example, patients can learn new behaviours that enable them to adapt better to specific social situations. A further difficulty is that the data on people with autism as a group do not relate specifically to prison inmates, and there is a high likelihood that the prognosis for someone with autism living for a long period in prison will differ from the typical prognosis. You should describe what the best currently available evidence suggests about management, and how this might lead to changes in functional ability or recovery, and then attempt to set out what of this might be possible in prison.

Legal

In St Vincent, and most other West Indian jurisdictions, the death penalty can only be applied for an offence carrying the nonmandatory death sentence if there is evidence that the offence is 'the worst of the worst' *and* the defendant 'shows no reasonable prospect of reform'.[96]

The legal test of capacity for reform has not been defined, but courts appear to have interpreted it chiefly in terms of reduced future risk of offending, including through 'social readaptation'. Expert psychiatric or psychological evidence is required before the court can determine this.[97]

Although not relevant here, in some other jurisdictions (e.g. some US states), psychiatric evidence is relevant to fitness for execution in terms of whether the offender has the capacity to comprehend the rationale for death penalty being applied to them.[98]

Clinico-legal

Psychiatric or psychological evidence might assist the court in determining capacity for reform by considering:

- the risk of further violence associated with Idris's mental disorder;
- the prognosis;
- any treatment, and its likely effect (including on risk of violence); and
- the additional effect (if any) on risk of violence through risk management in prison or hospital.

---

[95] The process of diagnosing autism spectrum disorder in a criminal context is set out in criminal law case 13.
[96] *Trimmingham v the State (St Vincent and the Grenadines)* [2009] UKPC25.
[97] *Pipersburgh & Robateau v R* [2008] UKPC 11.
[98] *Ford v. Wainwright* 477 U.S. 399 (1986), relevant to the fitness to be executed.

You must take care not to address the ultimate issue of 'reformability' itself.

Particularly with conditions such as autism, treatment and risk management are not just about enabling the individual to change; altering their context can also lead to significant changes in behaviour (including reduced risk of violence).

Remorse is not a psychiatric concept, and you should avoid commenting on it directly, even if the court expects to hear about it. Moreover, it is not at all clear that remorse is either a robust construct or has any predictive value in regard to reform or future offending.[99] However, it may assist the court if you have an opinion on whether the defendant's condition affects how or whether they would *express* any remorse. Many individuals with autism in particular may fail to show the emotional response and social interaction that others expect when someone is remorseful, and you could advise the court against drawing any adverse inferences from such factors in Idris.

People with autism characteristically also have deficits in empathy. A clear explanation of how this can manifest itself, and may have been manifested in Idris, is likely to be of assistance. The related concept of 'theory of mind' might also assist, in that people with autism are prone to concrete interpretations of words and actions (e.g. written to Idris by his victim) which might be relevant to Idris having committed his offence, evidence which the court would apply in mitigation of sentence.

If you think that any such evidence as above could have founded a defence of diminished responsibility at trial, you should discuss this with his solicitors, in case they and Idris wish to appeal the conviction.

Ethical

The gravity of the case, and the potential consequences for Idris, mean that it is your duty to try your utmost to give Idris and the court the most comprehensive psychiatric evidence possible. This means taking considerable time and effort to facilitate Idris's participation in a thorough interview, despite his reluctance.

[99] Research suggests that, at least in relation to sexual offending, there is little or no correlation between expressed remorse and future risk, and that more limited constructs that are capable of being operationalized, such as blame attribution (i.e. who the offender deems responsible for their predicament—themself or their victim, society, or others) have much better predictive value.

17 Insanity–appeal against verdict and death sentence

> **Themes:** *delusional disorder (p.73), folie à deux (p.74), and cultural congruence of symptoms (p.149) [C]; insanity (p.620) and capital sentencing criteria (p.450) [L]; retrospective reconstruction of mental state (p.670) and mapping onto defence (p.358) [CL]; and inadequacy of data (p.304) and impact of personal values (p.330) [E]*

Case description

Ten years ago Anthony, then aged thirty-two years, was convicted in Guyana of double murder, and sentenced to death. He was not assessed psychiatrically pretrial.

He and his co-defendant entered a cathedral where a large congregation was celebrating mass. They lit torches with petrol and sprinkled petrol over the congregation, beating those who attempted to stop them. A frail elderly priest approached them carrying a silver cup, as if to offer communion. Anthony threw petrol over him, said 'don't do that!', then set him alight. He then turned to an elderly nun near him, repeated 'don't do that!', and struck her with a stick, causing fatal head injuries. Both men were arrested at the scene.

He stated, 'I wanted to burn the Vatican and the demons there ... I wanted to destroy the cathedral ... I thought this would destroy the Pope and the Queen of England ... a punishment for crimes against Black Africans ... I told people what my plan was, I don't know why they were shocked.'

A presentence probation report noted an abusive childhood, and disruptive behaviour and defiance at secondary school, as well as fighting with knives, for which he was expelled.

Anthony has appealed against his conviction and sentence. His new lawyers instruct you to give an opinion on insanity at the time of the offence,[100] and on his fitness for the death penalty.

Questions

1. Can and should you try to reconstruct Anthony's mental state ten years ago?
2. How will you address the defence of insanity?
3. How will you address the capital sentence?
4. What other clinical, legal, clinico-legal, and ethical issues arise in the case?

---

[100] The partial defence of diminished responsibility was not available at the time.

Clinical

There is no recorded history of mental illness, so determining whether Anthony was mentally ill at the time of the killing will be complex and time-consuming.

Before the interview, gather as much background information as possible with the help of his lawyers and family, in order to piece together his life story from childhood. You need to know about his personality, his relationships, and his propensity for violence. School and social services records might explain the nature of the abuse he suffered. Given the nature of the offence, his religious views will be important to understand, as well as his previous criminal history. Any material that bears on his mental state during the months preceding the offence will be useful.

Read his GP and hospital records for possible unrecognised symptoms of mental disorder, and the witness statements likewise (his remarks to the victims and police hint at possible mental disorder). Put these in the context of his usual beliefs, activities, and involvement with the church.

When interviewing Anthony, take a detailed history of any mental symptoms or distress from childhood onwards. Examine his pattern of drug and alcohol use, if any. Gain a picture of his usual mental functioning, and any association of symptoms with violence in the past. Follow-up any suggestion of psychosis meticulously. Even if he offers nothing suggestive of illness, ask direct questions about possible symptoms you consider relevant. At the same time, consider the possibility of him now malingering past symptoms.

Only after doing this, and coming to a provisional view on possible diagnoses, should you start asking him in detail about his mental state at the time of the offences. Establish from him a detailed timeline of events prior to the offences:

- Was there any change or development of his mental functioning during the weeks and days prior to the killings?
- Was any change associated with use of drugs or alcohol?
- When did he first think of committing the offences, and why?
- Why did he purchase the petrol the evening before?
- Why target the cathedral?
- Why the two particular victims?
- Why that day?
- Why not flee the scene afterwards?

Ask questions in such a way that any information gained can, if relevant, be mapped onto the potential psychiatric defence of insanity (see below).

An added issue to address with Anthony is the relationship between him and his co-defendant, who appears to have taken a lesser role in the offending. How did they come to offend together? Was there any evidence that his co-defendant was mentally ill, and if so, did that relate to any symptoms in Anthony (i.e. could he have been suffering an induced delusional disorder or *folie à deux*?). Ideally, you would interview the co-defendant about Anthony and their relationship, but he is unlikely to be available to you.

Legal

The defence of insanity, unlike the partial defence of diminished responsibility, is not limited to murder. In most jurisdictions it is narrowly drawn, with a high threshold, since a successful plea of insanity leads to a verdict of not guilty (or as in Guyana, 'guilty but insane'), with no mandatory sentence.

Although the definition of insanity varies between jurisdictions, the essence of it is abnormality of cognition due to a medical condition, with a consequential threshold (e.g. not knowing what you are doing is wrong); meaning that severe psychosis or affective disorder can potentially qualify, but generally not disorders of emotional regulation or expression. Defendants who experienced intense persecutory delusions, passivity phenomena, and command auditory hallucinations are on the strongest ground.[101] Interpretations of the threshold can sometimes be flexible: for example, someone who would be capable of knowing their actions were wrong if they stopped to think about it, but who was

[101] Provided these are not due simply to drug-induced psychosis arising from voluntary intoxication. This is the same rule as for capacity to form intent: see criminal law case 15.

too preoccupied through psychotic drive to appreciate such knowledge, would fall within the test in some jurisdictions but not others.

In Guyana, the specific test is that the accused 'was labouring under such a defect of reason, from disease of the mind, as not to know the nature and quality of the act he was doing; or, if he did know it, that he did not know that what he was doing what was wrong'.

The criteria for imposition of the discretionary death penalty are that the offence must be 'the worst of the worst', and the defendant 'beyond reformation'.[102] This will only be relevant if the court accepts that he is 'guilty but insane': if he is found straightforwardly guilty, the mandatory sentence in Guyana is death.

Clinico-legal

If you have been instructed as an expert in a jurisdiction that is not your own, ensure that your instructions explain the exact legal test for insanity that applies, and the local criteria for the death sentence.

Read all the legal (and medical, if any) papers in the trial, including relevant sections of the transcript: certainly the appellant's evidence and that of key witnesses, the judge's summing up and sentencing remarks.

If you have come to the conclusion that Anthony harboured religious, persecutory, and grandiose delusions relating to priests and nuns at the church, for example, his evidence might be that he believed he was acting in self-defence because he thought the priest and nun were attacking him in some way. Bear in mind the possibility of ordinary evidence showing other causes of his behaviour unrelated to mental disorder.

In this case, the lack of prior medical evidence of mental illness is likely to be emphasised, as is Anthony's antisocial behaviour as an adolescent. The defence will also need to explain why medical evidence was not offered at trial: if you are able to offer reasons relevant to this (e.g. evidence that he was not fit to instruct his solicitors at the time), inform the defence solicitor.

You should also produce a formulation of Anthony's mental disorder, its likely response to treatment, and the prognosis overall. Evidence that he is likely to recover from mental disorder and that this would reduce the risk of harm he poses, would be of use to the defence in showing that he is not 'beyond reformation' and therefore ineligible for the discretionary death penalty. You cannot comment on whether his offence was 'the worst of the worse'.

Any inconsistency between Anthony's accounts on different occasions, and between others' accounts and his, will be closely examined at appeal, as will anything unusual about his presentation of the mental disorder you have diagnosed. The prosecution may suggest that he has misled you into wrongly believing him to have been mentally unwell. The proper response to this, both technically and ethically, is to explain how you have reached your diagnosis, not just on the basis of what he has told you, but also on observation of behaviour and symptoms he would be unable to control, and the contemporaneous reports of others (none perhaps sufficient alone to show that he was unwell, but all pieces of the jigsaw that you have assembled).

Ethical

What is the proper threshold of confidence for expressing a clinical or clinico-legal opinion? Withholding your opinion from the court because you are not sure could deny Anthony justice. A proper approach is to give your opinion, while being clear about your degree of confidence (without letting your personal values influence your expression of confidence, e.g. if you disagree with the death penalty in principle). You should explicitly express your opinion on the validity of reconstructing a long-ago mental state.

Working in a foreign jurisdiction can be challenging. The context of clinical assessment, the availability of records, and the cultural presentation of symptoms and information may all be very different from what you are used to. You should seek the advice and support of others familiar with the country.

---

[102] Explored further in criminal law case 16.

18 Insanity or infanticide—by an adolescent

Themes: *psychotic depression (p.94), mother killing baby (p.46), and diagnosing adolescents (p.154) [C]; infanticide (p.414) and diminished responsibility (p.624) [L]; insanity test (p.620) [CL]; and raising new issues (p.690) and minimising bias (p.674) [E]*

Case description

Radhika is a seventeen-year-old girl charged with murdering Rayane, her ten-month-old daughter, by drowning her in the bath. Her mother discovered the child's body. Radhika then said she had taken an overdose; she was admitted to hospital but suffered no ill-effects. She has only patchy memories of what happened.

Radhika had been treated for postnatal depression, from which she recovered fully. Eight weeks before the killing, she again began to feel low in mood. She stopped going out, and her mother was concerned that she was not feeding Rayane regularly. She also started to say odd things, such as that she and Rayane were both dead. Her mother tried not to leave them alone.

Afterwards, she was diagnosed with psychotic depression and given antipsychotics and antidepressants in hospital. She said she drowned Rayane and attempted suicide because they were already dead, and should be together in heaven.

Radhika was sexually abused by an uncle between the ages of five and eight. She cut her arms from the age of twelve years, but stopped two years ago, and had never seriously harmed herself before the overdose. She has never used any drugs. Her mother has a history of depression.

You are asked by the CPS to assess Radhika and give an opinion on whether she was suffering from a mental disorder at the time, and was legally insane.

Questions

1. To what should you pay particular attention when assessing someone under the age of eighteen years?
2. Are there any diagnoses that cannot be made in children and adolescents?
3. What weight should you give the diagnosis made by the treating clinicians?
4. How should you approach the issue of insanity?
5. Should you raise with the CPS the possibility of diminished responsibility, and/or infanticide?
6. How can you best approach a case such as this objectively and minimise bias?
7. What other clinical, legal, clinico-legal, and ethical issues arise in the case?

Clinical

Depression is characterised by low mood, loss of interest or pleasure, feelings of worthlessness, poor sleep, poor appetite, poor concentration, low energy levels, thoughts of lack of self-worth, plus sometimes suicidal thoughts. When severe, it can be accompanied by psychotic symptoms that are usually mood-congruent, such as nihilistic delusions or derogatory second-person auditory hallucinations. It is particularly common after childbirth, and is strongly associated with increased risk of infanticide (especially psychotic depression, and especially if the mother has a history of childhood sexual abuse).

This case involves a seventeen year old with a presentation almost indistinguishable from an adult; it would be equally reasonable for an adult or a child psychiatrist to be appointed as an expert, provided in either case they have sufficient training or experience of working with adolescents. You should pay particular attention to issues arising from Radhika's youth, such as that minor self-harm is very common at this age and of less diagnostic weight than in a twenty-seven year old, say. Moreover, as personality is not fully formed at this age, any evidence of persistent emotional dysregulation or of impulsive or oppositional behaviour (e.g.) can only support diagnoses of emotional or related disorders, and not of personality disorder.

Do not simply assume that the diagnosis of the treating clinicians is correct. Give your opinion based upon your own assessment, using all the data available, rather than seeking to confirm (or refute) the diagnosis already made.

Legal

Defendants are presumed to be sane, and the defence of insanity requires them to show, on the balance of probability:

- that they were suffering from a mental disorder[103] or disease of the mind,[104]
- and that this made them incapable[105] of appreciating the nature[106] or wrongfulness of their conduct (or in RoI, of refraining from committing the act).

The defence, prosecution and judge can all raise the possibility of insanity.

You might properly ask the CPS whether you should also address diminished responsibility, a partial defence that would reduce the conviction from murder to manslaughter (the test is set out in criminal law case 5).

Many societies treat the killing of a child under one year by its mother differently from other homicides because of the effect of the stresses of childbirth and child-rearing on the mother's state of mind. In E&W, NI, and RoI, infanticide is both an alternative charge and a partial defence to murder,[107] with the same range of penalties as manslaughter; in Scotland, it is charged as culpable homicide. The court must be satisfied that 'the balance of the mother's mind was disturbed by the childbirth or lactation'. If you think this could apply to the defendant, you should inform the CPS.

Clinico-legal

The role of an expert is to describe the defendant's likely mental state at the time of the killing, and its likely causal relationship to the killing, and not to opine definitively upon whether the insanity defence is satisfied, since to do so could infer taking a view on the ultimate issue.[108]

[103] In RoI and Scotland (excluding personality disorder in Scotland, if it is characterised solely or principally by abnormally aggressive or seriously irresponsible conduct).
[104] In E&W and NI.
[105] 'Unable', in Scotland; 'labouring under such a defect of reason as' in E&W and NI; and 'ought not to be held responsible' in RoI.
[106] 'The nature and quality of the act' in E&W, NI, and RoI.
[107] Unlike other partial defences to murder, other elements of the offence of murder do not need to be proved, as infanticide covers a wider range of circumstances and (in particular) does not require an intention to kill or cause serious bodily harm: *R v Gore* (2007) EWCA Crim 2789.
[108] Many psychiatrists, and courts, do not hold to this principle, with the expert being allowed to address directly the legal question of insanity.

Break down the insanity test into its individual components, and describe the way in which any mental state abnormalities present at the time of the killing map onto each component. For example, describe Radhika's delusions and how they affected her ability to recognise she was drowning Rayane, or to recognise that killing her was legally wrong.[109]

Ethical

The nature of the relationship between lawyers and psychiatric experts is that the former instruct the latter. However, lawyers may lack familiarity with psychiatric issues, wrongly inferring for example that someone who is psychotic must by definition be legally insane. They may also overlook a psychiatric issue by focusing on the binary outcome of conviction versus acquittal (e.g. in this case, the CPS might have overlooked the option of charging with infanticide).

An experienced expert witness psychiatrist will be aware of subtleties at the interface between psychiatry and law, and should tactfully raise such issues with the instructing solicitor.

Cases involving the death of children can be emotionally highly affecting and difficult to comprehend, making objectivity especially difficult to achieve. For example, the apparent horror of a case might invoke anger or retribution or an attempt to make sense of an 'unnatural' killing might lead to an assumption that the mother must have been abnormal in some way.

Attempt to anticipate your own likely responses to it, and actively consider alternative explanations of the killing, plus alternative opinions that might properly be offered to the court, so as to minimise the impact of your personal values.

---

[109] As required in E&W and NI. Not knowing that an action was morally wrong is insufficient (*R v Windle* [1952] 2 QB 826).

Duress–drug importation

Themes: *posttraumatic stress disorder (p.96), anxiety (p.98), and depression (p.94) [C]; duress (p.412) [L]; 'battered person syndrome' (pp.625, 632) and 'reasonable fortitude' (p.635) [CL]; and sympathy for the defendant (p.674) [E]*

Case description

Wanda is a twenty-one-year-old woman charged with drug importation for allegedly trying to smuggle 6kg of cocaine into England. The drugs were found by airport security in her false-bottomed suitcase when she arrived on a flight from the Caribbean. Her boyfriend is a co-defendant.

Wanda was sexually abused from age five years by a paedophile ring. Her foster father, the instigator of the abuse, died before he could be charged. She confided in her older foster brother when she was nine; he responded by abusing her too. The sexual abuse eventually ended when, aged thirteen, she told her best friend, who then told a teacher. She received no therapeutic input. She attended a 'special school' for her secondary education due to problems with literacy.

Wanda met her first partner aged eighteen years, when he was twenty-six. He was violent to her throughout their two-year relationship, causing her black eyes and bruised ribs. He eventually left her for another woman.

Nine months ago, she began a new relationship, during which she experienced even more severe violence. She said, 'it was okay at first ... but I didn't know he used cocaine ... he attacked me twice ... raped me ... put a gun in my throat and almost strangled me ... he tried to drown me'. Her boyfriend forced her to smuggle the cocaine, threatening to kill her if she refused. He remains in Jamaica.

You are asked by her solicitor to prepare a psychiatric report commenting upon her vulnerability, and its relevance to her defence that she acted under duress.

Questions

1. What aspects of Wanda's mental condition are important to assess?
2. How can mental symptoms be relevant to the defence of duress?
3. How should you respond to sympathy you may feel for the defendant?
4. Should you take account of any bias against the defendant that you expect judges and juries to hold, based on their cultural beliefs and stigma?
5. What other clinical, legal, clinico-legal, and ethical issues arise in the case?

Clinical

The assessment should focus upon whether Wanda developed a mental disorder in response to the abuse she suffered, and if so, how this has affected her behaviour. Given that she suffered sexual abuse as a child, and two partners have been violent to her, consider in particular PTSD related to her abusive experiences as a whole, as well as anxiety and depression.

In addition, her history and time at a special school suggest she may suffer from intellectual impairment; so you should assess for this.

Consider 'how did any symptoms of mental disorder affect her relationship with her co-defendant boyfriend, in particular?' Consider also how (un)empowered she felt in the relationship, how (un)equal the relationship was, and how (un)able she was to exert her wishes. You should also address her psychological response to abuse.[110]

Legal

Duress by threats,[111] or coercion in Scotland, if proved by the defendant, results in acquittal for any offence other than murder, attempted murder, or treason. Its essence is that the will of the defendant was overcome by the threats of another person (a subjective test), and that the same would have happened to a person of ordinary courage or fortitude (an objective test). The threats must presage immediate death or serious violence,[112] and there must be no reasonable alternative way of avoiding the threatened harm.[113]

The ordinary person of the objective test is deemed to be of the same age and background as the defendant, and this can include a mental disorder that impairs their fortitude. 'Background' has also been held to include pregnancy and serious physical disability—but not (by contrast to the defence of 'loss of control' or 'provocation') other characteristics or 'woundability', such as timidity or emotional instability unless it amounts to a diagnosed medical condition.[114]

Clinico-legal

Like many other defendants pleading duress, Wanda has been traumatised by abuse by the co-defendant and others, and she shows symptoms of 'BPS'. However, her symptoms will only support a defence of duress if they amount to a mental disorder such as PTSD, anxiety, or depression.

You should consider whether Wanda's mental disorder and symptoms were such as to reduce her fortitude below that of the ordinary person in response to the threats to which she describes being subjected. You should not opine on whether the treats, in fact, overwhelmed her will. And you should be aware of any ordinary evidence suggesting other explanations of her behaviour that the court may take into account (e.g. evidence of being a willing participant motivated by money).

Assuming that Wanda suffered from diagnosable depression and/or PTSD at the time of the alleged offence, you should then consider:

- her dependence on others in relationships;
- whether she developed 'learned helplessness' within the relationship, such that she did not take opportunities to leave;

---

[110] Mental responses to abuse are explored in criminal law case 11 on 'battered person syndrome'.

[111] As distinct from duress of circumstances or necessity, which amount to committing an offence in order to avoid imminent death or serious injury. The offence must be proportionate to the circumstances, and the danger not brought about by the defendant, and a 'sober person of reasonable firmness' should have responded in the same way.

[112] In E&W and NI, to the defendant, their immediate family or someone else close to them; in Scotland & RoI, it is not clear which threatened victims other than the defendant would count.

[113] *R v Hasan* [2005] UKHL 22; in addition, the defendant must not voluntarily have run the risk of such threats. In Scotland, the wording is 'inability to resist or avoid' the immediate danger: *Thomson v HM Advocate* (1983) JC 69. In RoI, the duress must be operating at the time of the offence, with no opportunity for the defendant to escape: *AG v Whelan* [1934] IR 518.

[114] *R v Bowen* [1996] 2 CrAppR 157.

- any heightened (mis)perception of risk of violence, and associated fear of death or injury resulting from her experience of violence and learned helplessness;
- whether her boyfriend's threats were therefore more 'powerful' than they would otherwise have been; and
- to what extent these factors arouse from her mental disorder.

Generally, Wanda seems to be fragile in her self-esteem, with little sense of self-worth. Possibly, she has an ingrained sense of not expecting to be believed after her experiences of reporting being sexually abused as a child. Provided that you can relate this to her mental disorder, you might find that this means that she would be more easily coerced than the ordinary person.

Lastly, address the specific behaviour of her boyfriend as she described it, and her reaction to it; the court will need to see evidence of her reaction demonstrating her lack of reasonable fortitude.

There may be disputed facts that would affect your opinion, in which case you should give conditional opinions, along the lines of, 'If the facts are as claimed by the prosecution, then my opinion on the relevance of her mental disorder would be ... ; if, however, it is true that the co-defendant said X, as claimed by the defendant, my opinion would be....'

Ethical

Wanda's story would evoke sympathy from many, especially a doctor, whose temperament and training likely predisposes them to care for others. It is therefore important to monitor your own reaction to her story and to think solely of her as a defendant, and not as a patient. Indeed, this emphasises why it is often ill-advised to give expert evidence on defendants you have treated as patients. You must ensure you give a fair and balanced opinion as to whether she exhibited a relevant recognised mental disorder at the time of the alleged offence, and not address the ultimate issue of 'duress' per se (note there may be ordinary evidence that points to her guilt).

20 Vulnerability short of duress— personality disorder

Themes: *personality disorder (p.78) [C]; robbery (p.426) and duress (p.634) [L]; inadequate instructions (p.680) and expert witness boundary (p.686) [CL]; and being confident you are 'expert' (p.654) [E]*

Case description

Ferdinand, charged with robbery, is twenty-six years old, homeless, and unemployed. He had left a bar intoxicated with alcohol and drugs and walked for some time before allegedly punching a woman in the head from behind and stealing her jewellery. She was found unconscious six to ten hours later and has made only a partial recovery.

Ferdinand's mother used crack cocaine from when he was a small child. He has never known his father. His mother died when he was aged fifteen, and he knows no other relatives. Since then, he has been homeless most of the time.

Ferdinand attended school until age eleven; his reports indicate behavioural problems from an early age. His IQ was measured as 79. He has never worked. He has a record of theft and burglary, but no convictions for violent offences. He has used cannabis and crack cocaine since childhood but does not drink regularly.

He has been admitted to hospital three times after suicide attempts, two by hanging and one by cutting his throat. He has many other scars from self-injury. He rarely attended outpatient appointments.

Ferdinand was arrested the day after the robbery. He admitted to punching the woman and taking her jewellery, but said he only did it because of threats from a creditor. This man had seen him in the bar and grabbed him by the throat, saying that if Ferdinand did not pay some of the debt that night he would cut off his hand. Ferdinand said that he went straight from the bar and committed the offence 'in a dreamlike state', as 'if I wasn't himself'. He claimed that he then gave the man the jewellery. The man has since denied ever meeting Ferdinand.

Ferdinand has cut himself at times on remand in prison, but is largely drug-free and relatively mentally well; he describes feeling better than he has for years.

You are asked for an opinion by his solicitor on whether Ferdinand has any mental disorder, and if so, whether it rendered him particularly vulnerable to threats, making his actions 'not wholly voluntary'.

Questions

1. How might the conditions you may diagnose impact his vulnerability?
2. How should you respond to your instructions to assess 'voluntariness'?
3. Do you require specific expert qualification to diagnose personality disorder?
4. What other clinical, legal, clinico-legal, and ethical issues arise in the case?

Clinical

There are various diagnoses that might be considered, including personality disorder, substance use disorders, mood disorder, and developmental disorder, such as intellectual disability. The latter seems possible, given his relatively low IQ, but still requires formal assessment, for which you may require the assistance of a psychologist.

The diagnosis of personality disorder, whilst being based upon clinical interview, requires additional information of the consistency and longevity of Ferdinand's patterns of emotional experience and behaviour in their social and cultural circumstances, from informants, school records, work records, and witness statements. A structured personality assessment[115] provided by a clinical psychologist should augment the clinical interview. The diagnosis is ultimately based upon clinical judgement, based upon all of the data that can be gathered.

Personality is defined as characteristic pervasive patterns of thought, emotion, and behaviour that govern the way a person sees and relates to themselves and to the world. *Personality traits* are prominent features of personality that are present consistently across time and different situations. *Personality disorder* is defined as traits that deviate markedly from cultural expectations, are pervasive and inflexible, arose in adolescence or early adulthood, are stable over time, and lead to distress or impairment.

A good assessment will include formulation of any personality disorder: its developmental origins (e.g. early life trauma or neglect), as well as predisposing, perpetuating, and protective factors relevant to the individual's presentation and offending.

Legal

The only potentially relevant defence is that of 'duress by threats'. As described in criminal law case 19, the basis of the defence is that another person's threats overwhelmed the defendant's will, and would have overwhelmed the will of a person of ordinary courage or fortitude.

The potential relevance of psychiatric evidence to a defence of duress is that evidence of a recognised medical condition (not merely a mental vulnerability)[116] may be accepted as reducing the degree of fortitude to be expected from the defendant.

Clinico-legal

Your instructions are inadequate. They imply that the legal issue to be considered is duress, but do not give the correct legal test, which is not, 'Were Ferdinand's actions wholly voluntary?'[117] Ask for them to be amended.

You will need to consider carefully how far you should go in following your instructions. Addressing the presence or absence of mental disorder is clearly within a psychiatrist's remit, as is the effect of any mental disorder upon Ferdinand's behaviour in relation to the alleged offence. This is likely to include specific consideration of the impact of any threats Ferdinand received.

There may be dispute between prosecution and defence about whether Ferdinand really was threatened. If so, express your opinion conditionally: 'if there were threats of X then the Ferdinand's mental disorder would have affected his response as follows ...'.

Questions about the voluntariness (or not) of his actions go beyond valid expert evidence. The court's determination of whether Ferdinand acted voluntarily is more likely to turn on ordinary evidence of his speech and actions than on psychiatric evidence of mental disorder. Moreover, as the legal test does not refer to voluntariness, it is not clear how your opinion on this will assist the court. So, if you do accept instructions to comment on 'voluntariness', you should proceed with great care. Your role can only be in addressing whether Ferdinand is of 'less than normal fortitude'.

---

[115] For example questionnaires such as the Millon Clinical Multiaxial Inventory (MCMI-IV) or the Minnesota Multiphasic Personality Inventory-2-Restructured Form (MMPI-2-RF), or interview tools like the International Personality Disorder Examination (IPDE).

[116] *R v Bowen* [1996] 2 CrAppR 157.

[117] For full details of the legal test, see criminal law case 19.

On the facts given, it is unlikely that the court will find the defence of duress by threats to apply to Ferdinand, despite evidence you might give of vulnerability due to personality disorder and intellectual disability: he had ample opportunity to report the man to police and seek protection, or to move to another town to avoid him; moreover, he could be said to have run the risk of such threats by taking on the debts in the first place. Even in this situation, though, your evidence may be useful to the court when considering mitigation in sentencing.

Ethical

Personality disorder is a diagnosis that can be controversial, particularly in legal settings, because it is not conventionally perceived as 'illness' and therefore as relevant to culpability. A psychiatrist diagnosing personality disorder should explain in clear terms what it is, and why it is classified as a mental disorder. This could include explaining its developmental nature and its identification by comparison with the normal population, rather than an earlier state of health.

Personality disorders are common, and all psychiatrists should be capable of assessing and diagnosing them. To be accepted as an expert for legal proceedings, though, you would be expected to have particular training, knowledge, or experience, and/or to work in a service that includes patients with personality disorder.

Before accepting instructions, consider whether you are expert in the relevant clinical area, and whether you are sufficiently familiar with expert witness work in a case of this nature, with adequate understanding of the relevant law.[118] You do not have to be 'a leader in the field', but you should be prepared to answer questions about your clinical and expert witness experience.

[118] See *Kennedy v Cordia (Services) LLP* [2016] UKSC 6 re 'who is an expert'.

Self-defence in attempted murder

Themes: *mania (p.92) and violence (p.26) [C]; justifications (p.410) and insanity (p.620) [L]; self-defence (p.410) [CL]; and inadequate or ill-informed instructions (p.680) [E]*

Case description

Daniel, aged sixty-five, is charged with attempting to murder a policeman by hitting him over the head with a stick. He has no past history of violence or mental disorder.

You interviewed him at his lawyer's request. He told you that during the weeks before the incident, his neighbour 'pulled up his carpet and dropped paper clips and marbles on the floor to create noise' to disturb him—because she was 'jealous of [his] special powers' and 'close relationship with God'. He slept much less than usual, and often found it hard to concentrate. He said, 'I was so upset … thoughts were falling on top of each other'.

His daughter reported that her father had become difficult to understand. She called the police to his flat because she was concerned about his behaviour.

Daniel said he remembers little of what happened when the police arrived, but said 'the police weren't able to deal with me … it felt like I was going to be treated cruelly'. He thought that one policeman, the victim, was 'sneering' at him. He said, 'it's like a nightmare … I thought I was going to be killed … I shouted out the names of the people I loved'. He has no memory of the alleged assault.

The police witness statements describe Daniel taking hold of a stick and swinging it wildly. They say he stepped forward and said something like 'now you're going to get it!', and then hit an officer on the head, causing serious injuries.

You are asked to advise whether Daniel had a mental illness at the time of the alleged offence, and if so, about its relevance to a claim of self-defence.

Questions

1. How should you approach this case?
2. Could psychiatric evidence be relevant to Daniel arguing self-defence?
3. What other clinical, legal, clinico-legal, and ethical issues arise in the case?

Clinical

There is a strong suggestion of mental illness; you should explore in detail the nature of Daniel's symptoms, and how they developed, as well as any history of altered mental functioning or odd behaviour. Consider drug and alcohol use, and possible organic causes of mental disorder. The relationship between his symptoms and the alleged offence should be meticulously explored as best you can, given Daniel's apparent amnesia for the event.

Legal

Self-defence is a justification[119] that excuses conduct that would otherwise be unlawful (and is therefore not technically a defence, although it is commonly called one). It can apply to any offence. Acts of self-defence must be both 'necessary' (there must have been no reasonable alternative, such as running away), and 'proportionate' (e.g. any force used must have been reasonable in the circumstances).

This test of 'reasonable force' is both subjective and objective:

- What were the circumstances that the defendant believed[120] to exist?
- Would a reasonable person have acted similarly in such circumstances?

In deciding what a reasonable person would do, the courts allow a considerable margin of appreciation for the difficulty of judging force in the heat of the moment. They also take account of any offence the defendant or victim was committing at the time (e.g. burglary), whether the defendant was provoked or struck the first blow or acted in revenge, and whether the acts took place within the defendant's home.

The role of psychiatric or psychological evidence is limited to the impact of mental disorder on what the defendant might have believed the circumstances to be. Courts have repeatedly refused to allow such evidence to alter the interpretation of what the reasonable person might do,[121] in cases involving paranoid personality disorder and depression,[122] and even florid psychosis.[123] This appears to be on grounds of public policy, to avoid situations in which people who may be at high risk of assaulting or killing others are acquitted, which would mean that the state had no power[124] to contain their risk of harm to others (e.g. by imprisoning them or sentencing them to treatment in hospital).

Clinico-legal

The instructions you have been given are vague: ask the solicitor to explain the legal test to which your evidence will be applied, as well as any other defences that may be applicable.

Daniel was irritable, paranoid, and disinhibited because of his illness, and he may have misinterpreted the intentions of the police officers as a result. In his own mind, he may well have been acting in self-defence. Evidence from you that he believed himself under threat would be admissible, but unless the imminence and magnitude of the perceived threat were so close or great that a reasonable person would also have attempted to kill the police officer (which seems unlikely), his claim of self-defence will fail.

He may, however, be able to plead insanity, on the ground that he misunderstood the nature and quality of his actions (he believed he was attempting to kill a deadly attacker, rather than a police officer trying to help him).[125] If successful, he would be found not guilty by reason of insanity, and liable to treatment in hospital or community supervision.

[119] The others are public defence (defending others), preventing an offence, apprehending an offender, and preventing serious damage to property.
[120] Whether or not the defendant's belief is reasonable, provided that it was not induced by voluntary intoxication. This rule applies by statute in E&W; it is unclear whether courts in Scotland, NI or RoI would accept unreasonable mistaken beliefs as sufficient for self-defence.
[121] In contrast to loss of control (or provocation) and duress: see criminal law cases 10 and 19.
[122] *R v Martin (Anthony)* [2002] 1 CrAppR 27. Mr Martin shot and killed a burglar who broke into his isolated farmhouse at night. He was convicted of manslaughter; his depression and paranoid personality disorder were accepted as grounds for diminished responsibility, not self-defence.
[123] *R v Jason Cann* [2005] EWCA 2264. Mr Cann killed a nurse whom he believed was going to rape him. He too was convicted of manslaughter on the grounds of diminished responsibility. Had his claim of self-defence been successful, he would have been acquitted.
[124] Under criminal law. Civil powers to detain and treat in hospital are of course available (and in Scotland, directly available to the court at the moment of acquittal, using the order for the urgent detention of acquitted persons under S60C Criminal Procedure Scotland Act 1995).
[125] See criminal law case 17.

Ethical

A psychiatrist instructed to prepare an expert report should aim to offer an opinion focused upon the relevant legal questions. Hence, taking instructions should be a two-way process, especially given that lawyers are often unaware of what a psychiatrist can validly comment upon clinically and what they cannot, or may misunderstand how particular clinical opinions could be legally relevant.

You should decline inadequate instructions or instructions that require you to go beyond what is proper. Clinico-legal skill and understanding what legal questions are in play in a case will help you to recognise the proper scope of medical evidence and assist you in staying within the limits of medical expertise.

22 Automatism–intoxication

Themes: *intoxication and dependence (p.76) and drug-induced psychosis (p.72) [C]; automatism (p.612) and insanity (p.620) [L]; intoxication and prior fault (p.618) and capacity to form intent (p.610) [CL]; and commenting on the ultimate issue (p.664) [E]*

Case description

Oliver is forty-one years old and charged with the attempted murder of his girlfriend, with whom he lived. He has convictions for theft and burglary, but none in the last five years. Both Oliver and his girlfriend had drunk alcohol, taken a stimulant pill, and used crack cocaine at the beach. Oliver had also chewed khat.

Oliver has used crack and heroin most days for twelve years, with his longest period of abstinence being one year, three years ago. He does not drink alcohol regularly.

He does casual work, and has had no consistent employment for over ten years. His parents are both dead. One of his brothers died from a heroin overdose, and a sister from hepatitis C. He has no contact with other relatives.

Oliver recalls going to the beach, and that they both 'smoked some crack and took the tablet' and were getting on well and not arguing. He also recalls an experience of the sky starting to open up, but has no memory after that until in the police station after his arrest. He was injured and does not know how.

Oliver's girlfriend recalled hallucinating and lying on the beach. She is not sure how much time passed but she awoke to find Oliver throwing rocks at her head. She was only conscious briefly. She suffered a skull fracture, and was hospitalised for eight weeks. She emphasised that Oliver has never been violent before, and the attack was out of character.

Oliver and his girlfriend were observed by three witnesses, who described Oliver as 'wild and out of control', suddenly attacking his girlfriend. They restrained Oliver until the police arrived, when he continued to be very disturbed according to police witness statements.

You are asked by his solicitor to assess whether Oliver was insane or whether he acted in an automatism when he attacked his girlfriend.

Questions

1. How should you approach this case?
2. How do insanity and automatism relate to each other?
3. Should you comment upon the ultimate issue?
4. What other clinical, legal, clinico-legal, and ethical issues arise in the case?

Clinical

Your opinion will depend upon you having a clear understanding of the common effects of various substances Oliver may have taken, including patterns of use, typical effects of intoxication, and risks of precipitating psychosis. You also need to consider whether Oliver exhibits, or exhibited at the time, any kind of mental disorder, particularly any drug or alcohol use disorder. The nature and effect of any such disorder(s), and your determination of Oliver's likely mental state at the time of the alleged offence, will then inform your opinion.

Take a detailed history of his drug use, and the effects of various drugs upon him in the past. Ask about any previous episodes of unexplained behaviour, memory loss or violence, including, if possible, information from informants (his girlfriend may be an obvious and key source of such information, if you are allowed to interview her[126]). Enquire carefully about Oliver and his girlfriend's memories of the incident on the beach. If the precise substances that were taken cannot be verified, then your opinion will need to explain this.

The medical diagnosis should be accompanied by an opinion on his likely mental state at the time, the likely effects of the substances consumed, and possible causes for his claimed amnesia.

Legal

An automatism is 'an unwilled action', such as when one person's arm is moved by another person's hand, or they perform actions while asleep or in a fit. Various forms of physical and mental disorder have been accepted as causing automatism,[127] but voluntary intoxication cannot legally cause it.

Some forms of automatism are regarded as having been caused by a physical or psychological 'external blow', examples of which have included a bee stinging a lorry driver, a head injury, an injection of insulin without food (*R v Quick*), and dissociation precipitated by sexual assault following a past rape (*R v T*[128]). If accepted by the court, these forms of automatism result in a complete acquittal.

Other automatisms are described as 'insane', and if proved, result in a verdict of 'not guilty by reason of insanity'[129] because they are caused by a legal 'disease of the mind'; defined as being 'intrinsic to the defendant's mind', with no physical or mental 'external blow'[130]—but also as due to 'any cause that resulted in violence and is prone to recur' (*Bratty*[131]). The latter appears illogical, incoherent, and potentially unjust; the sole 'logic' appearing to be that if the public will be at risk from the defendant, the state should be able to manage that risk through (e.g.) treatment under mental health law following a finding of insanity.

Clinico-legal

The relationship between intoxication, insanity, and automatism is complicated clinico-legally, and your opinion must be based on a good understanding of the relevant law. The instructing lawyer should explain the relevant legal tests to you.

In Oliver's case, the posited cause of automatism was the combination of alcohol, crack cocaine, and the stimulant tablet. If this were accepted by a court as causing automatism, it would be a non-insane one, as the drugs that caused it were an external factor (by analogy with the insulin in *Quick*).

However, the court is almost certain to reject this under the doctrine of 'prior fault': in choosing voluntarily to become intoxicated, the defendant should foresee (and will be held responsible for) what they might do when intoxicated. So any intoxication is only a valid basis for a defence if it is involuntary—for example, because the defendant had been drugged by another person. Taking a substance that is not 'dangerous' and does not normally cause intoxication can also be accepted as

[126] You will need the permission of the prosecuting lawyer, after undertaking only to ask questions of solely direct clinical relevance.

[127] Such as epilepsy, hypoglycaemia, parasomnias, dissociation, and concussion.

[128] *R v T* [1990] CrimLR 256.

[129] In E&W and NI. In Scotland and RoI, the courts apply the criteria of the ordinary defence of insanity to situations which in E&W and NI would be analysed as insane automatisms.

[130] *R v Quick* [1973] 1 QB 910.

[131] *Bratty v AG NI* [1963] AC 386.

valid,[132] but this would not apply to alcohol, crack cocaine, or (perhaps) the stimulant pill, where in the language of the court, it is 'common knowledge' that the user 'may become aggressive or do dangerous or unpredictable things'.

If the intoxication rendered Oliver incapable of forming the intent to kill, he could be acquitted because attempted murder requires specific intent.[133] However, the threshold for incapacity to form intent through intoxication is extraordinarily high, and if even Oliver were acquitted of attempted murder on this ground, he would almost certainly be convicted of a lesser offence requiring only 'basic intent', such as unlawful wounding.

If you believe that Oliver met the criteria for drug dependence then, if this were so severe that he experienced an 'irresistible impulse' to use the drug,[134] then his intoxication might be considered involuntary, and a possible basis for automatism. In the unlikely event that a court accepted this plea, it would, on the logic of *Bratty*, and also the 'intrinsic' nature of dependence, regard it as an insane automatism. However, the MHA in E&W excludes 'dependence' as 'mental disorder' basis for detention, and so this outcome seems highly unlikely on the logic of *Bratty*.

You might consider instead that Oliver was not simply intoxicated, but suffered a drug-induced transient psychotic episode. This will be a tricky clinical distinction to make on the evidence available, but if you are able to diagnose psychosis with confidence, this could meet the criteria for insanity or an insane automatism. However, a psychosis solely precipitated by drugs would likely not qualify in E&W, given that it has been excluded as a 'recognised medical condition' within diminished responsibility.[135]

In summary, therefore, in the great majority of cases, intoxication or drug use will not found a defence; although it may be taken into account as an aggravating or mitigating factor in sentencing, where the rules are less binary and more capable of reflecting medical reality.

Ethical

In cases such as Oliver's you should restrict yourself to commenting upon the nature of any mental disorder, its likely cause, the way in which his mental state was related to intoxication, and the relationship with his behaviour. You should not interpret the legal test for yourself, even if the court invites you to do so (as some judges will).

---

[132] Intoxication resulting from the nonreckless use of diazepam was held to be involuntary in one case, for example: *R v Hardie* [1985] 1 WLR 64.

[133] *DPP v Majewski* [1977] AC 443; this is explored in criminal law case 14.

[134] *R v Tandy* [1989] 1 WLR 350; *R v Wood* [2008] EWCA Crim 1305; *R v Stewart* [2010] EWCA Crim 2159.

[135] *R v Lindo* [2016] EWCA Crim 1940; see criminal law case 15.

23 Automatism–brain injury

Themes: *acquired brain injury (p.112) and epilepsy (p.114) [C]; attempted murder (p.415) and insanity (p.620) [L]; traumatic brain injury (TBI) and epilepsy in automatism (p.612) [CL]; and clarity of expression (p.682) and experts reaching different conclusions (p.655) [E]*

Case description

Jamal is a twenty-six-year-old man charged with the attempted murder of his mother. Three years ago, Jamal had a meningioma (a benign form of brain tumour) removed; this left him with frontal lobe damage causing cognitive impairment.

Jamal reports having had no problems at school. Before having the meningioma, he had a calm temperament, was well liked, and had many friends. He was close to his parents but lived separately. He had never been violent.

After the operation Jamil was cared for by his family. They soon noticed he had become impulsive and irritable, and his personality was different. He suffered seizures, and sometimes acted oddly just before one, such as by threatening his parents incoherently with a knife, with no memory of it after the seizure.

Jamal allegedly attacked his mother with a knife in his parent's garden, where the family had been enjoying lunch. His mother suffered multiple stab wounds in the attack, which was not witnessed by anyone else. Jamal's father came out of the house in response to his wife's screams. He saw Jamal with blood on his hands; Jamal seemed disorientated, vague, and perplexed. He told the police he could not remember what happened. The parents subsequently reported that Jamal had had two bottles of beer during the lunch.

You are asked by defence lawyers whether Jamal had a mental disorder at the time, and whether it could amount to a legal automatism.

Questions

1. How should you assess him clinically?
2. How should you address the issue of legal automatism?
3. How should you address the legal relevance of 'frontal lobe syndrome'?
4. What other clinical, legal, clinico-legal, and ethical issues arise in the case?

Clinical

This is a complex case involving the possible effects of brain injury arising from a tumour and then surgery, plus the possibility of organic psychosis associated with epilepsy, plus the additional factor of the effects of a relatively small amount of alcohol on the functioning of a damaged brain. A key question will be whether, at the time of the attack, Jamal was ordinarily conscious, experiencing a seizure, or within a peri-ictal period.

The long-term effects of brain injury are highly variable and depend upon the severity, nature, and location of the injury.[136] A frontal (especially orbitofrontal) location commonly results in 'frontal lobe syndrome': disinhibition, mood changes, perseveration, apathy, and executive dysfunction, shown by poorly planned and disorganised behaviour.

Neurocognitive disorders are diagnosed when there has been significant cognitive decline in one or more cognitive domains. Initial clinical assessment is based upon the subject's account, plus that of a reliable informant, followed by straightforward 'bedside' tests. This is accompanied by a battery of standardised neuropsychological tests administered by a qualified clinician (almost always a clinical neuropsychologist), plus brain imaging (usually an MRI and CT scan, depending on the suspected pathology).

There is an association between significant TBI and impulsive violence and disinhibition, both of which are more frequent when the person also uses substances or has a pre-existing antisocial personality disorder.[137]

Any opinion on the possibility of Jamal's seizure already having begun when he attacked his mother (or him being in a peri-ictal state) will require the input of a neurologist. They will consider his past brain injury, his history of seizures, and his typical behaviour around the time of seizures. The account by his father of his presentation immediately after his violence towards his mother, the lack of any history of violence, and the lack of any clear precipitating event (e.g. an argument between Jamal and his mother) all suggest that epilepsy might have played a role.

Voluntary intoxication will need to be considered as a factor. However, if Jamal truly drank only two bottles of beer, which on their own in a person of normal nonviolent propensity would be unlikely to precipitate serious violence, then what will be needed is careful consideration of whether the effects of such mild intoxication either were enhanced by his brain damage or precipitated a seizure.

Finally, psychosis can occur before, during, and after seizures; such psychotic episodes tending to be intense and relatively short-lived. Post-ictal psychosis is the most common, seen in 2%–8% of patients. Ruling this out, or in, will depend upon careful history-taking, including from the parents (bearing in mind that they will be prosecution witnesses whom you will need specific permission to interview).

Legal

An automatism is 'an unwilled action': when someone behaves without any conscious awareness or control. If the cause is intrinsic to the mind (e.g. a peri-ictal state or psychosis), the result is a finding of not guilty by reason of insanity; if it is external, the result is acquittal. This is explored in detail in criminal law case 22.

In E&W and NI, insanity is a separate defence with a narrower definition, the criteria for which are set out in criminal law case 18. In Scotland and RoI, by contrast, the narrower insanity criteria must be met for a person to plead insane automatism successfully.

If neither of these defences applies, the prosecution will still need to show that the defendant had the required mental element for the offence. For an offence requiring specific intent, such as attempted murder, this means that psychiatric evidence that the defendant could not have formed such intent can result in an acquittal, provided it is not contradicted by ordinary evidence of them forming that intent. See criminal law case 15 for details.

Clinico-legal

In a case like Jamal's, your evidence is likely to rest in part on the opinions of others (e.g. a neurologist and a clinical neuropsychologist), and on specific tests they or you have performed. You should satisfy yourself that all the evidence you have incorporated is based upon sufficient facts or data, and the product of reliable principles and methods, reliably applied to those facts.[138]

[136] Severity after a head injury can be estimated from the duration of posttraumatic amnesia, with anything longer than twenty-four hours indicating severe injury. Other markers of severity include more than thirty-minutes' loss of consciousness, open brain injury, skull fracture, cerebral contusion, and haemorrhagic contusion.

[137] Conversely, patients with ASPD and psychopathy can be shown to have signs of executive dysfunction on psychometric testing, in the absence of brain injury.

[138] This is a simplified version of the *Daubert* standard in the USA (*Daubert v. Merrell Dow Pharmaceuticals, Inc.*, 43 F.3d 1311, 9th Cir. 1995), and is broadly the standard followed in the UK and RoI, though it is worded differently in each jurisdiction. Practice Direction 19A.5 (linked to Chapter 19 of the Criminal Procedure Rules) sets this out in detail for E&W, for example.

If Jamal's mother had died from the attack, then Jamal's brain injury (even without any peri-ictal state) would have founded a partial defence of diminished responsibility. However, on a charge of attempted murder, the only potential defences are insanity, automatism, and lack of capacity to form intent.

It is possible that Jamal's cognitive disabilities could have deprived him of the capacity to form the specific intent required for conviction of attempted murder. However, frontal lobe syndrome most typically disinhibits behaviour (i.e. making the patient more likely to act on their intent), rather than removing the capacity to form an intention. Hence, Jamal is unlikely to be able to plead lack of capacity unless there is clear evidence of a peri-ictal state.

It is similarly unlikely that his cognitive disability alone would allow him to plead insanity; even people with severe cognitive impairment are usually able to explain what killing is, and that it is legally wrong. Again, though, if Jamal were in a peri-ictal state or psychosis, this might well mean that he was insane because he did not know the nature and quality of his actions, or (more straightforwardly) to have amounted to an insane automatism.

Even if convicted of attempted murder, Jamal's cognitive impairment (and any peri-ictal state or other vulnerability) will be relevant in mitigation of sentence, or in providing grounds for a mental health disposal.

Ethical

The psychiatric issues and potential defences in Jamal's case are highly complex, and you should expect very clear instructions setting out the relevant legal tests, and their relationships, in detail.

The same complexity will determine that clinical opinions may legitimately vary. This is no cause for concern so long as all witnesses express their genuine opinions, give clear reasons for them, acknowledge their limitations, and appropriately change their opinion if presented with new evidence. The court may ask the experts to prepare a joint statement summarising areas of agreement and difference, in order to narrow the range of issues that need to be explored at trial.

All experts will need to behave professionally and with courtesy. However, it is reasonable not only to explain the basis of your opinion but also to highlight any weaknesses in other experts' opinions, which will properly be explored in cross-examination.

Automatism–dissociation

Case description

Harley is a twenty-eight-year-old man charged with attempted murder. He allegedly attacked another driver after a minor car accident. The fifty-seven-year old victim suffered severe head injuries, fractured ribs, and a fractured humerus. He had driven accidentally into the rear of Harley's car. Harley got out, picked up a lump of concrete from beside the road, and attacked him; witnesses described him as 'crazy' and as ignoring their shouts to stop. They said the victim simply covered his head, and had done nothing to provoke Harley.

Harley was still at the scene when the police arrived, and did not resist arrest. One officer recorded him growling and muttering when they arrived. Harley was initially disbelieving when he was told why he had been arrested. He does not remember the alleged offence; his last memory before arriving in the police station is of driving calmly.

Harley served in the Army for four years, and since then he has worked as a night security guard. He is married and has two children. He has twice been treated for depression by his GP; he attended five of eight sessions of cognitive-behavioural therapy. He does not use drugs, drinks moderate quantities of alcohol, and has no convictions.

Harley served in Afghanistan, where his patrol was ambushed. He was uninjured but witnessed two colleagues being killed. However, no clinician has found symptoms of post-traumatic stress disorder.

You have been asked by his solicitor for an opinion on whether his amnesia is genuine, and whether he could have experienced an automatism.

1. What are the clinical, legal, clinico-legal, and ethical issues in this case?

Clinical

The clinical interview will be limited by Harley's claimed lack of memory for the alleged offences. Include in your assessment information from the witness and police statements about his mental state at the time.

Amnesia (often valid) for a violent offence is common. Dissociation could explain his reported presentation, and has been linked to both PTSD and stress.

Consider the long-term impact upon him psychologically of any trauma that he had previously experienced, plus any history of past dissociative episodes (e.g. during battle) and of factors that might predispose him to dissociate (e.g. childhood abuse, cluster B personality traits).

Note that dissociation can occur as a result *perpetrating* violence; albeit it is usually impossible clinically to be sure whether any dissociation preceded, or occurred during, or rapidly followed the violence.

Dissociative symptoms include disruption of consciousness, memory, identity, emotion, perception, body representation, motor control, and behaviour. Acute dissociative reactions to stressful events can last a few hours and can include amnesia.

Dissociative amnesia (failure to recall events experienced during a normal mental state), also termed *psychogenic amnesia*, is characterised by inability to recall autobiographical information, usually of a traumatic or stressful nature; it is more commonly 'patchy' rather than dense. It is to be distinguished from amnesia arising from being dissociated during the time that cannot then be recalled.

You should also consider the possibility of malingered amnesia, and incorporate relevant psychological tests into your assessment.[139]

Legal

The basic requirement for a finding of automatism is that there is a total lack of control over one's actions (see criminal law case 22). If the automatism arises from an intrinsic cause, which is likely to recur, it results in a finding of not guilty by reason of insanity; if from an external cause, it results in acquittal.

Intrinsic causes are not necessarily mental disorders. For example, someone who experiences automatism during a hyperglycaemic episode caused by diabetes would be found insane; the same person with hypoglycaemia caused by accidentally taking too much insulin would be acquitted, as the insulin constitutes an 'external blow'.[140]

The external blow can even be psychological in nature. For instance, an automatism during dissociation precipitated by the unusual external stressor of rape is not insane[141] (whereas dissociation in a susceptible individual precipitated by 'ordinary stresses and disappointments' *is* insane[142]).

Clinico-legal

Set out in your report any underlying diagnosis; say whether there is a basis for opining that Harley was in a state of dissociation when he offended, and if so, whether this explains the claimed amnesia.

Dissociation can be difficult to explain: in particular, the fact that the person is still conscious, but may not be in conscious control of their actions. Using the self-descriptions of some people who have experienced dissociation might help, such as 'like watching a video of myself' or 'having an out-of-body experience'.

If your opinion is that the accident triggered dissociation, the court will need you to explain how such a minor event could have such consequences, by reference perhaps to specific traumatic events Harley suffered in Afghanistan which shared some characteristics with the car accident.

Address also the alternative opinion that his amnesia, though likely genuine, is 'psychogenic', and whether it is likely malingered.

Ethical

Providing an opinion in this case will involve careful explanation of the rationale for your opinion and the degree of (un)certainty with which you hold it. The role of dissociation in violent offences is not well understood, and you must acknowledge this, and the range of opinions on the topic, in your report.

You should consider whether the offence and the defendant evoke any particular response from you: For example, are you sympathetic to his experience in Afghanistan? Do you have a personal view about whether dissociation should be a defence? Scrutinising yourself and your values when you have produced your report may assist in achieving the most balanced and objective opinion.

139   Such as the Test of Memory Malingering: see criminal law case 12 for details.
140   *R v Quick* [1973] 1 QB 910.
141   *R v T* [1990] CrimLR 256. (T was still convicted: the jury did not accept the defence.)
142   *R v Rabey* [1980] SCR 513.

25

Ability to understand the police caution–dementia

Themes: *dementia (p.116), child sexual assault (p.58), and interpreting clinical tests (p.131) [C]; police caution (p.572) [L]; ability to understand caution (p.573) [CL]; and mapping onto unclear law (p.358) [E]*

Case description

Uriah is seventy-five. He is charged with sexually assaulting a fourteen-year-old girl two years ago.

Uriah cannot recall the name of his secondary school or his university. He went on to serve as a Naval officer, and then worked in a bank, for twenty-two years as a branch manager. He is married and has two children. There is no family history of mental or neurological disorder. Uriah has always been a light drinker.

He has suffered two head injuries. In the Navy, a hatch fell and fractured his skull. He thinks he lost consciousness and was hospitalised for two to three days. Three years ago, he tripped and fell, injuring his head, cheek, and shoulder, and again lost consciousness briefly. He was not admitted to hospital. He experiences frontal headaches most days. He has no psychiatric history.

Over the last twelve months his memory has worsened significantly; his wife puts appointments on the calendar to prompt him. She first noticed changes in his behaviour last year. She now manages their finances. She said Uriah sometimes repeats himself in conversation, cannot recall events of the previous day, and leaves the shower running two or three times a week. He also falls asleep at the dinner table, and has lost weight recently.

Uriah cannot remember being interviewed by police six months ago. He says he has no memory of ever meeting the alleged victim. Police recorded, however, that when interviewed he said, 'Oh no! I knew I shouldn't have done it, but I thought she liked me.'

His lawyer hopes to exclude this and other evidence from his interview on the ground that he would not have understood the caution, and instructs you to give an opinion on this.

Questions

1. How should you investigate his mental condition?
2. How could you retrospectively assess his ability to have understood the police caution when arrested?
3. What other clinical, legal, clinico-legal, and ethical issues arise in the case?

Clinical

Given Uriah's memory loss, taking a detailed collateral history from a close relative is essential. Include questions about personality and behavioural change, the duration of any memory decline, the impact this has had upon his functioning, and how varied has been that impact, including any disinhibition.

Dementia assessment includes a thorough psychiatric history and physical and neurological examination, addressing both possible cognitive decline and functional impairment. Consider starting with a screening test of cognitive function, such as the ACE-III,[143] a one-hundred-point test that is valid for Uriah, though not for all cultural groups. This will probably confirm the need for detailed neuropsychological testing by a clinical neuropsychologist, including current and premorbid cognitive functioning, memory, language, and executive function.

Neuropsychological test results should be interpreted with caution, and can never found a diagnosis on their own. However, in a case where the issue of understanding the police caution is likely to be finely balanced, and to depend upon detail that can only reliably be assessed neuropsychometrically, you may need to emphasise that your opinion relies a good deal on such tests.

Also arrange blood tests, including thyroid function tests, Vitamin B12 and folate plus renal and liver function tests, an HIV test, and perhaps syphilis serology, since it is important to exclude any treatable form of dementia (should that prove to be the diagnosis) or some other cause of his cognitive impairment. Structural imaging with CT or MRI will show reversible causes such as hydrocephalus, or some other cerebral pathology, and help determine the dementia subtype.

People with dementia or other cerebral pathology commonly experience high levels of anxiety and mood symptoms, so consider comorbid mental disorder, such as depressive pseudodementia.

Legal

In almost all common law jurisdictions, when arrested a suspect is given a police caution. The wording of this varies: typically, it explains that the suspect has the right to remain silent, but whatever they say may be recorded and used in evidence against them. In E&W the courts can make adverse inferences from a suspect's silence, and the caution mentions this as well, unless he had some mental disorder that determines otherwise.

Unlike fitness to plead, there is no clearly defined legal test of understanding the caution. Moreover, a suspect who did not understand the caution should not be interviewed, but the criteria for reliability of interviews do not consider this (see criminal law case 28).

Finally, a police interview should not have gone ahead if likely to cause significant harm to the suspect's physical or mental state; although frequently police interviews do proceed without this having been considered.

Clinico-legal

Give your opinion on Uriah's likely mental state at the time of the caution (and later, if there is evidence of deterioration), plus its implications for his ability to understand it, and to retain the information during the interview process. You should also consider his fitness to have been interviewed, including his ability to understand the questions, the ongoing nature and significance of the caution, the nature and purpose of the interview, and the significance of questions and any answers he might give. You should also consider whether he was likely to have been able to make reasoned decisions about whether to answer questions, whether his mental state impaired his ability to be accurate or tell the truth, or whether the interview process might have caused a significant deterioration in his condition.

One UK study investigated comprehension of the caution among two groups, police station suspects (N = 30) and individuals attending a job centre in the same area (N = 24), matched for intellectual ability. In both groups, understanding was very limited and did not relate either to their situation at the time of testing or to self-reported experience of the criminal justice system. Even under optimal experimental conditions, only 11% (six) of the participants were able to demonstrate full understanding of its meaning. Even more worryingly, though, more than 96% (52) claimed to have understood

143 Addenbrooke's Cognitive Examination, version 3.

the caution fully after it had been presented to them, as it would be by the police, yet none of them actually did. The authors suggest practical measures to ameliorate the difficulties, but also emphasise the importance of devising a new, simplified, version of the caution.

Although Uriah will not now be able to give a reliable account of his state at police interview, it might be helpful to explore his understanding of the caution given to him *now*, and to test his recollection at intervals throughout your assessment. If he can explain the meaning to you now, he would be likely to have done six months ago, unless you have evidence that his condition has improved.

Listening to an audio recording or viewing a video recording of the police interview is likely to assist in forming a view on Uriah's mental state at the time of his arrest, which may, by inference, suggest a proper view of his likely prior understanding of the earlier caution. If neither is available, then read the transcript of the interview. The police custody record might also offer relevant evidence.

If he was assessed by a forensic medical examiner before the interview, then you should read their witness statement; although assessments by FMEs are commonly brief and usually not subtle or definitive in regard to understanding the caution or fitness to be interviewed.

If, as is likely, Uriah has dementia, then his cognitive function will probably decline further over time. His fitness to plead and stand trial is therefore also likely to be at issue, especially if there has been a substantial delay since the police interview was conducted.

Ethical

Given that the ability to understand the police caution is not clearly legally defined, great care should be taken not to 'make up' the law in giving an opinion. Rather, adopt the advice given above, and allow the courts to 'interpret' its legal significance.

26

Amnesia and brain injury– fitness for interview, interview reliability

Themes: *traumatic brain injury (p.112) and malingering (p.118) [C]; fitness for interview (p.573) and reliability of evidence (p.382) [L]; recognising signs of malingering (p.700) [CL]; and avoiding the ultimate issue (p.664) [E]*

Case description

Mark is a twenty-four-year-old man with an established diagnosis of acquired brain injury. He is charged with murdering a customer during a violent altercation outside the nightclub where Mark worked as a doorman. When interviewed by the police, Mark claimed to have no memory of the incident.

Mark had a stable childhood and had no difficulties at primary school. Aged twelve, he fell three metres from a tree and landed on his head. He lost consciousness for ten minutes. On arrival at hospital, his Glasgow Coma Score was 11/15. A CT scan showed that he had a temporal skull fracture and an extradural haematoma, which was evacuated during emergency surgery. He spent seven days in hospital, two in intensive care. He later reported posttraumatic amnesia lasting twenty-four hours after the fall, with no significant pre-traumatic amnesia.

Mark returned to mainstream school but found it hard to concentrate, could recall little new information, and failed his school-leaving exams. After leaving school he worked as a security guard in nightclubs and pubs. He has been able to live independently as an adult, but his parents have partly supported him financially.

He was assessed by a clinical psychologist instructed by his solicitor, who administered a trio of screening tests for malingered amnesia: these indicated a high possibility of feigning psychiatric disorder.

You are asked by the prosecution for an opinion on whether Mark's lack of memory is genuine and whether he has any psychiatric disorder.

Questions

1. How will you assess Mark specifically for malingered amnesia?
2. Should psychiatrists comment upon possible malingering?
3. What factors should be considered when assessing whether a defendant was fit to be interviewed, or the reliability of interviews?
4. What other clinical, legal, clinico-legal, and ethical issues arise in the case?

Clinical

You will need to consider the neuropsychological and psychiatric impact of his head injury, any other mental disorder, and the possibility of malingering.

Malingering is the deliberate fabrication or exaggeration of symptoms or deficits, by contrast with 'lack of effort' (where a defendant does not engage fully with an assessment e.g. because of poor attention, fatigue, depression, or anxiety) and with factitious disorder (a mental disorder in which a person adopts the sick role for internal psychological reasons rather than external gain). It is very difficult to assess with any certainty, in part because genuine symptoms and deliberate exaggeration can coexist.

Typically, malingering relates to memory or other cognitive deficits, or to symptoms of mental illness. However, true amnesia for violent offences is also common, especially after severe violence: 25%–70% of offenders claim amnesia for violence after conviction (when there may be no external incentive to lie).

True amnesia is associated with intoxication, alcohol or drug dependence, and some mental disorders such as dissociative disorders.[144] Amnesia is more likely to be genuine in offenders who are not habitually violent.

Clinical assessment of claimed amnesia requires a full medical history, including any evidence of sleepwalking, epilepsy, head injury (past or recent), and diabetes; look also for trauma and abuse, and use of psychoactive medication or drugs. Then take a detailed history of the episode of claimed amnesia (last thing remembered, islets of memory, length of amnesic gap, next thing remembered, and whether events unrelated to the offence but during the period of claimed amnesia can be recalled), and of the pattern of any previous or subsequent episodes, for example as recorded in depositions or police interviews.

Memory is a complex process, with fallibility at different levels. Look for:

- internal inconsistency in the defendant's account;
- inconsistency between accounts different at different times;
- inconsistency between the defendant's self-report and other information;
- inconsistency between symptoms claimed and observed behaviour;
- how the memory deficits are described at interview, compared to common and clinically coherent accounts of valid memory disability;
- absence of anxiety and concern (concern is to be expected except in certain organic or functional causes such as frontotemporal dementia);
- how well the account accords with the natural history of the likely pathological cause of the memory deficit; and
- likely motivations for a false claim of amnesia.

Overall assess clinical plausibility, distinguished from ordinary credibility.

Similar requirements apply to determining the likely validity of other mental symptoms complained of by a defendant: for example, psychotic experiences.

Individuals who have previously suffered from a given mental condition typically find it easier to fabricate symptoms on a further occasion than those who have not. And, in such cases, psychological testing can particularly assist, as in Mark's case, where there is strongly suggested at least an element of malingering.

A psychologist will look for:

- floor effect, a defendant performing very poorly on the majority of tests;
- below-chance responding on forced-choice tests, such as the TOMM and the Word Memory Test (WMT);
- exceptionally poor scores on a forced-choice test such as the 'coin in hand' test: such tests are in reality very easy and can be passed by people with severe cognitive impairment, but they are designed to appear difficult;
- better performance on harder than on easier tasks; and
- large errors in answers to questions (e.g. stating that it is 1908 when asked to identify the current year).

However, a person can 'fail' on malingering tests because of mental disorder rather than malingering. So that it is unwise simply to report TOMM or WMT scores, rather than placing them in context.

[144] See criminal case 24.

Legal

Amnesia is commonly claimed by defendants, and the justice system understandably views it with scepticism. It is not, for example, relevant to fitness to plead,[145] even though true amnesia for events directly relevant to an offence must often place the defendant at a substantial disadvantage.

However, it is relevant to the ability to understand the police caution (explored in criminal law case 25), fitness to be interviewed, and to the reliability of evidence. Further, expert opinion supporting claimed amnesia may reduce jurors' scepticism about claimed amnesia, which may otherwise colour views of the rest of the defendant's evidence.

Clinico-legal

Your report should consider the nature of Mark's claimed amnesia, and if it is genuine, its impact on his likely fitness to have been interviewed, and the reliability of his evidence.

There is no legal test for fitness to have been interviewed.[146] Ask Mark about his recollection of his arrest and the interview, as well as how he answered questions. If he does not remember the interviews, this will be relevant to his fitness. You might start by asking, 'Why were you arrested?'; 'What did the police want to find out in the interview?'; and 'Who, if anyone, did you feel able to turn to for help during the interview?'

Further, it is important to set any disability relevant to being interviewed in the context of the defendant's specific mental disorder, to make clear from what any possible unfitness arises.

If Mark has true amnesia, his evidence may be unreliable even if he was fit for interview. For example, he may have confabulated answers to questions in the interview, without realising it.

Ethical

Psychiatric experts should not state directly that a defendant is malingering: aside from the uncertainty inherent in the diagnosis, it implies that the defendant is being untruthful, which is a matter for the court. Focus instead on whether claimed symptoms are clinically coherent, and whether any incoherence can be explained by mental disorder.

There is a duty to be honest in giving your opinion, including about your degree of confidence, so that, if you genuinely cannot answer the question whether the defendant's claimed amnesia is clinically coherent, you should make this clear.

---

[145] *R v Podola* [1960] 1 QB 325.

[146] However, published clinical criteria are available: see Ventress M A, Rix K J,B, and Kent J H (200) Keeping PACE: Fitness to be interviewed by the police, *Advances in Psychiatric Treatment* 14: 369–381; Kent J and Gunasekaran S (2010) Mentally disordered detainees in the police station: The role of the psychiatrist, *Advances in Psychiatric Treatment* 16: 115–123.

27

Retracted confession– intellectual disability

Themes: *intellectual disability (p.110) and suggestibility and compliance (p.160) [C]; admissibility of interviews (p.382) and voir dire (p.383) [L]; retracted confession and interview reliability (p.608) [CL]; and keeping to expert boundaries (p.686) [E]*

Case description

Lee is arrested in connection with the death of a seventy-eight-year-old man during a burglary. They lived near each other and were passing acquaintances. He was interviewed by the police over two days and eventually said, 'yes, it was me'. He was then charged with murder.

Lee has been assessed by a psychologist, whose notes include: '28-year-old man, told by his mother that he nearly died *in utero*. Unable to describe any details of his early development or remember many childhood events. Beaten by his mother as a form of discipline, sometimes with a belt. Made friends at school and was close to teachers. Poor literacy and numeracy. Attended a special school for a while before returning to mainstream secondary education with support. Learned trades such as woodwork. Worked briefly as a security guard for his mother's firm. Since then has worked intermittently as a building contractor with a colleague; his wife assists with written records and a friend collects payments for his work. Ran a market stall selling clothes bought with the profits from his building work—described himself as a "good salesman". Victim of theft and robbery on four occasions; wife reported that the police "did nothing". Lived with wife for nine years, an older woman with children from a previous relationship. She did the cooking and much (but not all) of the family finances. He helped with childcare. Six years ago, suffered a head injury after falling 15 feet whilst at work; discharged after observation in hospital overnight.'

The report goes on to summarise the result of psychological testing: 'Lee has a reading age of between 6 and 7 years. Lee's performance on testing suggested an intellectual level within the least able 1% of the population.'

You are asked by his solicitor to prepare an expert report concerning the reliability of Lee's confession, given his intellectual disability.

Questions

1. What clinical, legal, clinico-legal, and ethical issues does Lee's case raise?

> **Clinical**
>
> Beyond the impact of intellectual disability, some accused persons and defendants can be additionally vulnerable because of their 'suggestibility' and/or 'compliance' when questioned. Interrogative suggestibility represents the extent to which an individual accepts messages or information communicated to them during formal questioning in a closed social interaction (e.g. a police interview, or

cross-examination); compliance is the tendency to go along knowingly with propositions, requests, or instructions for some immediate instrumental gain.[147]

These psychological constructs are known to be associated with intellectual disability, mood disorder, psychosis, and cluster C personality disorder, all of which you should assess for systematically. Given Lee's history of a head injury, a neurological examination, CT or MRI, and neuropsychometric assessment may be needed to rule out sequelae of TBI.

A detailed psychological assessment is also essential, including cognitive assessment and specific psychological tools such as the GSS and the GCS.[148]

Beyond these traits, there is research evidence that retracted confessions are more common in younger defendants, those with learning disability, and those under the influence of drugs and/or alcohol at the time.

Legal

Any retracted confession, or other aspect of a police interview that is deemed by the judge to be unreliable,[149] will be excluded from the trial: this will be decided during a *voir dire* prehearing, taking into account expert evidence. If such contested material is ruled admissible, then expert evidence can then be called during the trial itself to assist the jury in determining whether they should attach lesser weight to the evidence than they would otherwise.

In the UK jurisdictions, it will also be important to determine whether an 'appropriate adult' was present during Lee's police interviews.[150] Any absence of an appropriate adult where one should have been provided will be taken into consideration by the court, but does not automatically render evidence inadmissible.

Clinico-legal

If Lee is shown to be abnormally suggestible or compliant on testing, then the next step is to determine whether those traits likely operated significantly during the interview, by scrutinising interview transcripts (and recordings, if available). If there is evidence they did, this will both support the finding of suggestibility and/or compliance and identify parts of the interview that the court may later find unreliable.

An expert must always avoid commenting on whether a defendant or witness is truthful: that is a question for the court alone. You must be clear in your report (and in your own thinking) that you are addressing only whether there are psychiatric or psychological factors that infer the risk of unreliability. In cross-examination, keep strictly to description of clinical constructs, such as diagnosis, mental state, suggestibility, and compliance, plus their implications for reliability.

You might therefore properly comment upon Lee's:

- ability to understand the interview process, and the significance of making a statement (with reference to his mental disorder or characteristics);
- vulnerability to fear or influence (as a result of his mental disorder or characteristics);
- demonstrated suggestibility and/or compliance; and
- statements and interactions during interview that appear to represent abnormal suggestibility or compliance.

[147] Suggestibility and compliance are explained in more detail in criminal law case 2.
[148] Described in detail in criminal law case 2.
[149] On grounds that the evidence was obtained by 'oppression' (coercion, torture, or threats i.e.) or anything else likely to render it unreliable or to have too great an adverse effect in fairness. In Scotland and RoI there are no specific rules on excluding unreliable evidence, but evidence in Scotland must usually be corroborated to be accepted, and in RoI the court should be warned about the lack of corroboration for any evidence.
[150] The Police and Criminal Evidence Act 1984, and its associated Codes of Practice: Code C, and Code H in relation to suspected terrorists, are particularly relevant to interview procedure.

Ethical

Beyond keeping to the expert role and not opining on the truth or falsehood of Lee's confession, there is a further issue of whether you should even go so far as to express an opinion upon the reliability of the confessions. Because in doing so, you take a view of the nature of the exchanges within the interview, in order to determine whether Lee's abnormal suggestibility or compliance were affecting his responses—yet this is tantamount to taking on the role of the jury, determining what weight to give the interview evidence. So it might be argued that you should simply describe how, in the abstract, Lee's mental disorder and characteristics *might* affect his responses; yet this would deprive the jury of a proper understanding of how the defendant's characteristics should be viewed in the context of the actual interviews. Most would accept that a careful opinion on reliability is essential, therefore.

28

Reliability of witness evidence–borderline personality disorder

Themes: *borderline personality disorder (p.84); assessing a witness (p.156) [C]; witness reliability (p.382) [L]; report on a vulnerable witness (p.684) [CL]; and distinction between expert and treating doctor (p.298) [E]*

Case description

Barbara is a twenty-seven-year-old woman who claims she was raped by Jim, aged thirty years. They are both residents in a long-stay hostel for people with learning difficulties and mental health problems, and both have diagnoses of schizophrenia and substance misuse. Barbara and Jim used to be in a relationship; they separated a year ago, but have stayed friends.

Jim claims the sex was consensual, and he honestly believed she had consented. Barbara says she screamed and shouted, 'No, no', but Jim ignored her. Her friend Ann, who lives in the room next door, supports her account. Ann is a thirty-year-old woman with BPD who frequently harms herself. She has been arrested previously for fraud and shoplifting.

You are instructed by the prosecution to provide an opinion on the reliability of Ann's evidence. They hope you will be able to interview Ann, although she is currently in hospital (she took an overdose of aspirin after she made her statement to the police). The prosecution have indicated that they are reluctant to prosecute the case because both prosecution witnesses (Ann and Barbara) have 'mental health issues' that reduce the chances of successful conviction.[151]

Questions

1. What clinical, legal, clinico-legal, and ethical issues arise in this case?

> ### Clinical
>
> This case requires you to consider the impact of mental disorder upon reliability in giving evidence. The issue is clearly distinct from the unreliability of eye-witness testimony, the influence on memory of emotions and cognitive prompts from others, and the evidence base on suggestibility and confessions.

---

[151] In E&W, the CPS has a duty only to prosecute when there is a realistic (more than 50%) probability of conviction, and prosecution is in the public interest. Similar considerations are made by the Procurator Fiscal in Scotland, the Public Prosecution Service in NI, and the Office of the Director of Public Prosecutions in RoI.

There are powerful social stereotypes of the impact of mental illness or disorder on reliability, but there is no evidence base to support a general claim that mental disorders impair reliability. Every case has to be considered on its own merits.

Clearly disorders that impair reality testing are relevant, as are intoxication, withdrawal and substance dependence, and neurocognitive disorders that may influence memory, perception, and interpretation. You may wish to consider formal neuropsychological and cognitive tests (by a psychologist).

In this case, there is no prima facie reason to assume that Ann's testimony will be unreliable, solely on the basis of a diagnosis of BPD. However, Ann's postinterview overdose suggests that she is a vulnerable witness who, at the very least, may need additional support to give her testimony. You will need access to her medical records, and will want to interview her carefully.

Legal

The Crown Prosecution Service has produced guidelines on assessing the reliability of vulnerable witnesses. They advise that any expert must have access to all relevant material, including copies of all accounts given to police, the prosecution bundle and defence statements, and any available medical records. And instructions be clear as to the questions to be answered. Prosecutors should additionally consider holding a conference with the expert where this might assist in the presentation of the issues for resolution.

An underlying concern in such cases is that sound prosecutions may be abandoned because mentally disordered witnesses are unjustifiably seen as unreliable; an issue compounded by the unwillingness of many people with mental disorder to make statements to the police for fear of being dismissed. For example, where the trial of 'Mr FB's attacker' for assault was dropped because FB was not seen as a credible witness, solely on the grounds of his mental disorder. He successfully sought judicial review of the CPS decision to offer no evidence at trial, which was ruled unlawful. The CPS changed its guidance to prosecutors in response.[152] In another case, a motorcycle mounted the pavement and caused injury to the female victim. The prosecution abandoned the case of dangerous driving because the victim had a history of attempted suicide, and it was argued that she may have put herself in harm's way. Moreover, it is not uncommon for barristers to ask witnesses irrelevant questions about their history of mental disorder.

Clinico-legal

The CPS can advise the police to seek to obtain the past medical records of vulnerable witnesses, but they are advised to consider whether they need to 'disturb confidentiality'. The witness must give informed consent to disclosure. If she or he refuses, the police can apply for a court order to gain disclosure of the records.

The expert assessment should address:

- the nature and extent of the witness's mental disorder;
- how its symptoms have manifested themselves in the witness;
- whether they could affect the witness's understanding, perception, or recollection of an incident (and if so, to what extent compared to someone without mental disorder);
- the likelihood that this might undermine the credibility or reliability of the witness's evidence;
- any factors which increase or decrease that likelihood;
- what measures could be taken to reduce that likelihood; and
- how the mental disorder might affect their ability to give evidence and withstand cross-examination, particularly with reference to concentration and attention, ability to communicate, and interaction with other people.

If Ann were to refuse to see you, then you could potentially provide a very limited expert opinion about BPD *in general*, provided you have sufficient expertise, but this would probably be inadequate for the prosecution's purposes.

---

[152] See *R (B) v DPP* [2009] EWHC 106 (Admin).

If you are granted access to Ann's medical records, then provided they contain sufficient detail this might allow an opinion about the manifestation of BPD *in her*; although again, you might not be able to answer all of the questions above.

If you were Ann's treating psychiatrist, you might instead be approached simply for factual information about her history and treatment. Here the usual principles of confidentiality apply: if Ann gives informed consent, you can assist the police, but if she refuses, you can only disclose the minimum information necessary for the prosecution of a serious offence (which alleged rape certainly is). However, in this situation you might prefer to ask the police to obtain a court order for the disclosure of records, thus protecting your therapeutic alliance with Ann.

Ethical

Psychiatrists have duties to respect and support the justice process, and to do what they can to undermine stigma and discriminatory treatment of people with histories of mental illness and disorder. However, you should take great care in expressing any opinion based upon limited data. Moreover, you should offer an opinion *relevant* to reliability, not purport to *determine* her reliability.

As Ann's treating psychiatrist, you would also have a duty of care to support her psychiatrically through any legal process.

29

Extradition and autism

> **Themes:** *autistic spectrum disorder (p.104) [C]; extradition (p.558) and human rights (p.516) [L]; 'unjust or oppressive' extradition (p.648) [CL]; and maintaining clinical objectivity (p.674) and use of supervision/mentoring (p.308) E]*

Case description

Joseph is a thirty-seven-year-old British citizen, alleged to have killed his mother in the USA. He has lived independently for the last twelve years, although he sees one of his siblings every day. His father died five years ago. Last year, he visited his mother in Delaware; three weeks after he returned to Britain, her body was found at her home. She had been hit over the head with a blunt instrument. The USA has applied for his extradition, giving an assurance that he will not be charged with capital murder.[153]

Joseph was once admitted to hospital for depression, six years ago; he had stopped eating and drinking after the death of his father. He has not had any further psychiatric treatment. He worked for ten years in a DIY shop, stacking shelves and helping with deliveries, with a good work record.

He has been diagnosed with ASD based on clinical assessment and informant interviews. He is currently anxious, low in mood, and has harmed himself by scratching his arms, although he does not describe any intention to kill himself. He has been readmitted to hospital under the Mental Health Act, and transferred to a medium secure unit because of the charge against him. He said that he 'just lost his temper with his mother' on the day he was leaving.

Joseph's solicitor has instructed you to give an opinion on whether he would be fit to plead if tried in England, on the risk of damage to his health if extradited, and on whether extradition would be 'oppressive or unjust'.

Questions

1. What clinical, legal, clinico-legal, and ethical issues arise in the case?

> **Clinical**
>
> You should fully reassess Joseph's mental disorder, jointly with a specialist in autistic spectrum disorders if you do not have that expertise yourself. This must include reconsideration of records and information relating to his early development.[154]

---

[153] The Extradition Acts 2003 (in the UK) and 1965 (in RoI) prohibit extradition for offences that carry the death penalty abroad but not in the UK/RoI, unless such an assurance is received.

[154] Failing to do this has been criticised in extradition judgments.

You should also assess Joseph's risk of self-harm and suicide, and (based upon information provided by the State and solicitors) consider whether the treatment available in the country seeking his extradition would be adequate. This will be difficult if it relates to a country with whose health and prison system you are unfamiliar. But you may well be provided with expert reports on relevant hospitals and prisons by Joseph's solicitor, or documents from those institutions.

Legal

Medical evidence is relevant to the legal tests of whether extradition would breach the suspect's human rights, particularly their right to life, right to freedom from inhuman or degrading treatment, and right to a family life.[155]

Even if extradition would not breach their human rights, if it appears that the physical or mental condition of the person is such that it would be 'unjust or oppressive' to extradite them, the judge must either order discharge of the proceedings or adjourn them[156] until the circumstances appear such that it would no longer be so.

The terms *unjust or oppressive* are not clearly defined, and will be interpreted by the court on a case by case basis.[157] A high threshold has to be reached in order to satisfy the court that a requested person's physical or mental condition is such that it would be unjust or oppressive to extradite him, since 'there is a public interest in giving effect to treaty obligations', with a 'substantial risk of suicide', whatever steps are taken. And there must be a link between any mental disorder and the risk of suicide, whilst it must be such that the disorder 'removes his capacity to resist the impulse to commit suicide'.

Being 'unfit to plead'[158] does not automatically mean that extradition would be unjust or oppressive. In *Dewani*, for example,[159] it was ruled that, where a defendant was unfit to plead, there would be an expectation that the receiving government undertake to return the defendant to the UK if he remained unfit for a year, and give assurances of adequate safeguarding and treatment in the meantime. Such expectations are in practice often impossible to enforce.

Clinico-legal

Your assessment should include the risk of deterioration in his mental health, the nature of any deterioration that you suspect may occur, and specifically the risk and 'cause' of suicide. You cannot state per se whether Article 3 is breached, of course.

You will need to consider the likely conditions in which Joseph will be kept, and the impact upon his mental health and risk of suicide of those conditions; also whether, in your view, he would be likely to receive the medical treatment you deem necessary, in sufficiently safe conditions, bearing in mind your assessment of his risk of suicide or self-harm.

Other factors might include the extent to which he has any ties in the USA (other family members who might visit), that could mitigate the potential harm caused by his detention.

You should also assess Joseph's fitness to plead under English law, but he is very likely to be found fit. The case will likely turn mainly on whether Joseph would be 'at substantial risk of suicide'.

Ethical

The court's ruling will depend in large measure upon your risk assessment, and the high stakes create a risk of your personal values influencing your opinion. You should reflect on your values, as part of ensuring that your opinion is as objective as possible. Appropriate peer mentoring may help.

---

[155] Under articles 2, 3, and 8 of the European Convention on Human Rights respectively, applied by s21, s21A, and s87 of the Extradition Act 2003 in the UK.

[156] Under s25 and s91 of the Act in the UK. There is no direct equivalent in RoI.

[157] *Turner v USA* [2012] EWHC 2426.

[158] Using the E&W criteria for fitness (perhaps illogically: the fitness to plead provisions of the country wishing to try the individual would seem more relevant).

[159] *Republic of South Africa v Dewani* [2014] 1 WLR 3220.

30

Appeal against murder conviction—emerging psychotic depression

Themes: *mental illness and homicide (p.36) and psychosis (p.72) [C]; appeal based on new evidence (p.372) and professional versus expert evidence (p.652) [L]; report on mental condition post trial (p.694) [CL]; duty to the court and justice (p.660); and reporting versus treating (p.678) and bias (pp.298, 305) [E]*

Case description

You are an MSU consultant and the responsible clinician for Howard, a sixty-one-year-old man recently transferred from prison. He has developed agitation, paranoia, and irritability and now neglects himself and refuses treatment, food, and water. He is often awake all night, muttering and shouting.

Last year, Howard was convicted of murdering Jane, his wife of thirty years. She had started divorce proceedings a few months earlier, alleging domestic violence and relationship breakdown. Howard had by then been diagnosed with depression by his GP, but may not have taken the antidepressants prescribed.

The day before the killing Howard received a letter from Jane's solicitor requiring him to leave their home. He packed his belongings. When Jane returned, he stabbed her repeatedly, then held her in his arms as she died. Afterwards he killed their pets, rang the police to say what he had done, and then stabbed himself in the stomach and neck. Howard's adult children say this was totally out of character.

At trial, a defence psychiatrist provided evidence of depression in support of his plea of diminished responsibility, but the prosecution expert gave conflicting evidence. The jury preferred the prosecution narrative that he was a violent man who could not tolerate his wife leaving him, and convicted him of murder. The judge noted Howard's degree of remorse and, in passing the mandatory life sentence, imposed a reduced minimum term of fifteen years.

Howard is now recovering gradually on antipsychotics and antidepressants, and explains how he had become impotent and then paranoid and suspicious of Jane over two years, believing without evidence that she was having an affair with her boss; he had hit her only because she would not 'confess' to the affair. This evidence of the severity of his depression was not given in evidence at the trial.

Howard's solicitor asks you to write a report for an appeal against conviction.

Questions

1. Should you write a report?
2. What other clinical, legal, clinico-legal, and ethical issues arise in the case?

Clinical

In E&W, 60%-70% of homicide victims knew their attacker, and were frequently in a relationship with them. Close attachments generate strong emotions, which can lead to violence. And high emotional arousal can distort cognitions and reality testing, whilst severe affective disorders can generate psychotic symptoms. A 'crime of passion' is committed in a state of distress and affective arousal, often with patchy psychogenic amnesia. However, such violence does not necessarily imply the presence of mental disorder.

Legal

Howard's lawyers will have to obtain leave to appeal, and set out a skeleton argument suggesting that his conviction of murder is 'unsafe', and that he should have been found guilty of manslaughter on the grounds of diminished responsibility. They will need to convince the court that there is sufficient new (medical) evidence to render the conviction unsafe.

The Court of Appeal may hear such new evidence if it is capable of belief, could give grounds for allowing the appeal, would have been admissible at trial, and is relevant to the reason for the appeal, and provided there is a reasonable explanation for the failure to adduce it at trial (e.g. the reason was not 'tactical').[160]

Clinico-legal

This is a case with high stakes. As Howard's treating psychiatrist for some months, you have followed your duty to care for him in the interests of his welfare. It could well be argued that you are therefore insufficiently objective to be an expert witness. However, you could still provide factual evidence as a professional witness of Howard's current condition and treatment, alongside an independent expert, even if you do not accept instruction as an expert. And his records will suggest he was psychotic when he killed.

Expert opinion that Howard had psychotic depression not merely after his conviction, but at the time of the killing, would represent relevant new evidence. If accepted by the court (perhaps corroborated by a prosecution psychiatric expert), it could render the conviction unsafe, and provide grounds for a retrial because a jury, knowing he had been psychotic, might well have given to a different verdict. Alternatively, the Court of Appeal might substitute a manslaughter verdict.

Howard's motive for killing will be central to any appeal, as it was at trial. This is strictly an issue for the court, but psychiatric evidence may help to offer a narrative of the killing which incorporates the role of his psychotic disorder.

You will have to advise Howard at all stages of the need for you to have his consent to disclosure of all relevant materials. including perhaps material from his therapy sessions in which he disclosed his thoughts about his wife. You should prepare Howard for what will be a long process. If family members do not support the appeal, there may be anger, distress, and even threats to Howard and those supporting him.

Ethical

The main ethical issues here are the duty to respect the justice process, the scope of the psychiatrist's duty to the court, and awareness of possible bias. Some clinicians might feel that, after conviction by a court, it is not appropriate for treating clinicians to help in challenging the verdict, especially as they may not be impartial because of their therapeutic relationship with the appellant. There can even be a kind of hubris in thinking that one knows better than other professionals did when the trial took place. However, it is reasonable to take the position that, perhaps especially in psychiatry, new evidence relevant to diagnosis may often emerge when people are admitted to hospital and treated.

---

[160]   *R v Erskine; R v Williams* [2009] EWCA Crim 1425.

31 Request to alter court report for sentencing

Themes: *personality disorder (p.78) [C]; expert witness rules (p.656) [L]; changes to reports (p.690) [CL]; and managing conflicting duties (p.298) and anticipating court use of report (p.670) [E]*

Case description

You have submitted an expert psychiatric report concerning Fiona, a woman found guilty of killing her two young children. Fiona was suffering from postnatal depression and cluster B personality disorder, with prominent borderline and histrionic features.

She was transferred from prison on remand and is receiving treatment in hospital from another psychiatrist. You recommended that this continue, under a restricted hospital order. Mindful of the judgment in the UK[161] that courts must consider alternatives to hospital sentencing, you noted that treatment in hospital could alternatively be provided under a hospital direction[162]—being careful not to recommend it, as it contains an element of punishment.

Fiona's solicitor asks you to amend your report. He explains that now that she has recovered from depression, there is a good chance that Fiona will be imprisoned—and that the judge might use the evidence in your report on prognosis and future risk to others as grounds to impose an extended sentence. He also asks you to add an opinion on the likely psychiatric effects of terminating the psychological treatment she is currently receiving in hospital, and of a prolonged period of imprisonment.

Questions

1. Should you amend your report to remove the sections on Fiona's prognosis and risk assessment related to her personality disorder?
2. Should you include a section on the effects of imprisonment and termination of current psychological treatment?
3. Had you anticipated the request, would you have written your original report any differently?
4. What other clinical, legal, clinico-legal, and ethical issues arise in the case?

---

[161] *R v Vowles* et al [2015] EWCA Crim 45. The case only sets a precedent for E&W, but may come to have persuasive authority in NI and Scotland.

[162] A hospital and limitation direction ('hybrid order') under s45A MHA in E&W, or a hospital direction under s59A CPSA in Scotland or s174 MCANI. No equivalent is available in RoI.

Clinical

The clinical assessment informing the expert opinion is not likely to be followed by any further clinical involvement. The clinical encounter should always have included discussion with the defendant of the nature of your role and duty, and the limits of confidentiality, with emphasis upon the difference between your role and that of the doctor who is treating her.

Legal

Sentencing to prison by the court will take mitigating and aggravating factors into consideration. The psychiatric report you provide may well form the basis of evidence for these factors (even if that is not what was intended by you), which is why the solicitor is concerned.

You are expected to abide by the rules governing the conduct of all expert witnesses.[163] These rules emphasise that you have a legal duty to the court, which requires (amongst other things) that you be truthful, and that you give your whole opinion. Your duty to the court overrides any obligation to the instructing solicitor. In E&W, the full expert witness declaration includes the statement: 'I have not, without forming an independent view, included or excluded anything which has been suggested to me by others including my instructing lawyers.' You are required to form your own view on what should be included, based upon relevance to the issues you have been asked to address. Continuing relevance will go against any decision to amend (or not amend) your report.

Clinico-legal

Generally, this means that nothing should be removed from a report unless it is information that is either legally privileged or irrelevant to your opinion. Removing relevant unprivileged information may breach your duty to the court.

You can change your opinion or correct factual inaccuracies; however, this must be done in a way that makes clear what you wrote originally, what you are writing now, and why you have changed the text.

The information you have set out on the prognosis and risk associated with Fiona's personality disorder forms part of the grounds for your opinion that she requires continued treatment in hospital, in the interests of her health and safety, and for the protection of others (some of the legal criteria for a court order for mental health treatment). You should not remove it, despite the risk of it being used for other purposes.

There is no problem with you adding information about her vulnerability to the effects of terminating current psychological treatment, or to the effects of imprisonment, provided that you make clear that your report has been amended by way of such addition, and why. Indeed, adding this information may balance the potential impact on sentencing of the prognosis and risk assessment. One easy way of doing this is to set out the additional paragraphs in a part of the report headed 'addendum', with an explanatory paragraph setting out the additional instructions received from the solicitor.

Ethical

Your ethical duty as a psychiatrist is to make the care of your patient your first concern. This means that you should not write anything that goes directly to the issue of punishment, without therapeutic benefit, for instance. However, this cannot override your legal duty to the court.

It is always worth anticipating how information you provide in a report may be used in court, as this may not be how you intended it to be used. If your instructions and your opinion do not require you to set out a risk assessment, for instance, then it may be better to omit it, so that it is not used for an alternative purpose, and to preclude any request for removal. However, in this particular case, the risk assessment was essential to your opinion and recommendations.

---

[163] For example, part 19 of the 2015 Criminal Procedure Rules (E & W).

B.4
Civil law cases

1 Clinical negligence– prison suicide

Themes: *suicide risk assessment (p.176) [C]; negligence (p.550) and rights to life and freedom from torture (p.516) [L]; inquests (p.560) and inquiries (p.598) [CL]; and difference between ethical and legal duties of care (p.290) [E]*

Case description

You are a prison psychiatrist. An officer asks you to see Riley, a thirty-four-year-old single man with few friends inside the prison, who is estranged from his family.[1] Last week, he was sentenced to life imprisonment for attempting to murder his boyfriend, and today he has learned that after he has served his minimum term[2] of twenty-one years, he will be extradited to Germany to face trial on a further murder charge.

A specialist nurse in your team saw him two weeks ago, shortly before sentencing, and was satisfied that he was not depressed, although he was highly anxious about the outcome of the hearing. You see him briefly on the wing and—while noting his distress about the very long period of imprisonment he now faces, plus the uncertainty of what will happen in Germany, and his reports of low mood, anhedonia, and hopelessness—you conclude that he is suffering from an adjustment reaction, and that he can be managed safely without transfer to the prison healthcare unit or to hospital. You ask the nurse to review him in a few days' time in case his mental state has worsened, and to offer problem-focused counselling. The nurse goes on sick leave the following day, and your instructions are not handed over to anyone else.

Ten days later, Riley is found dead in his cell, having hanged[3] himself using his bed-sheets from the hatch of his cell door.

Questions

1. What duties to Riley did the prison and its staff have?
2. What duties to Riley did you and your healthcare employer have?
3. Is your ethical position or professional responsibility different from your employer's?
4. If sued for negligence, could you be said to have caused Riley's death?
5. What is likely to happen next and before any possible legal claim from his family?
6. What would you do differently in future?
7. What other clinical, legal, clinico-legal, and ethical issues arise in the case?

---

[1] See the wide range of critique paradigms dealt with in detail in Part C.
[2] The punishment part of the sentence in Scotland, or the tariff in NI (and formerly in E&W too).
[3] Strictly speaking, this is a 'partial hanging' or even simply a death by asphyxiation and venous congestion because part of Riley's body would have remained in contact with the ground, and there was no sudden drop to fracture his cervical vertebrae.

> **Clinical**
>
> You should read all relevant records, reflect on the clinical care you and your team have provided, and address areas which may be the focus of the forthcoming investigations.

> **Legal**
>
> Riley was your patient: as a doctor, you owed him the same duty of care as you would in any other healthcare setting, as does your NHS or other employer.
>
> There is no question that prisons in the UK and RoI, and individual officers, owe inmates a duty of care. This has been confirmed in several UK legal cases[4] and before the European Court of Human Rights,[5] and is also set out in Prison Service rules.[6] Breaches of the duty of care may result in a negligence claim against the prison and individual officers, plus healthcare staff, as well as internal disciplinary proceedings.
>
> In addition, the State has further duties under human rights law. It has a positive duty to take appropriate steps to safeguard the lives of detainees under its control, under article 2 of the European Convention on Human Rights and Fundamental Freedoms; in the event of a death in its custody, it has an additional duty to investigate and to provide a 'satisfactory and convincing explanation'[7] for the events leading to death. If the prison, as the agent of the State, is found to have breached the inmate's article 2 right to life, or their article 3 freedom from inhuman or degrading treatment or punishment (e.g. by failure to transfer a severely mentally ill person to hospital for medical treatment), the European Court of Human Rights can award compensation directly, or if the finding is in a British or Irish court, it is highly likely to lead to a finding of negligence and subsequent award of damages.

> **Clinico-legal**
>
> In law, your duty is to practise in accordance with a responsible body of medical opinion.[8] Professional and ethical guidance goes further: in the case of assessing and treating detainees in prison and elsewhere in custody, this makes clear that you should consider not only the inmate's current condition, but also the likely effect of continued detention and the risk of deterioration in mental state.[9]
>
> Obviously, you did not directly cause Riley's death: his own actions led to his death. Legally, however, you can be said to have caused the death if it would not have resulted if you had not acted as you did.[10] For instance, if your diagnosis of an adjustment disorder was incorrect and any responsible psychiatrist would have diagnosed him with depression with suicidal ideation, or if your management plan of follow-up several days later (with no checking that this was done) would not have been supported, as it may well not have been, by a responsible body of medical opinion, then you could be found to have breached your duty of care and caused (in the sense of unreasonably failed to prevent) his suicide. A court would also examine the acts and omissions of others (including the system of management of the prison) that could have contributed to causing Riley's death.
>
> As soon as his death is reported, several processes will be set in train. There will be a coroner's investigation leading to an inquest. There will be an internal inquiry by the Prison Service, and either an internal inquiry by your health employer or an external inquiry commissioned by another NHS/HSE body. If any of these results in serious concerns about your practice, you could be referred to your regulatory

---

[4] For example *Knight v The Home Office* [1990] 3 All ER 237.

[5] *Keenan v United Kingdom* [2001] ECHR 242; *Edwards v United Kingdom* [2002] ECHR 303.

[6] For example National Offender Management Service (2015) *Adult Safeguarding in Prisons* PSI16/2015. London: NOMS at p.4

[7] For example *Velikova v Bulgaria* [1998] No. 41488/98, 18.5.00, para 70; *Salman v Turkey* [1993] No. 21986/93, 27.6.00, paras 99–100

[8] The *Bolam* test; the body must have a logical basis (*Bolitho*), and there is a further test if consent is required (*Montgomery*).

[9] RCPsych (2007) *Council report CR141: Prison psychiatry: Adult Prisons in England & Wales*. Royal College of Psychiatrists; RCPsych (2015) *Council Report CR199: Psychiatric Reports: Preparation and Use in Cases Involving Asylum, Removal from the UK or Immigration Detention*. RCPsych.

[10] Provided also that the harm was not too remote from your actions, and there was no subsequent intervention by a third party that changed the course of events.

body (GMC or IMC) for fitness to practice proceedings. In the UK, the suicide will also be examined by the National Confidential Inquiry, a research body that looks for patterns in suicides by patients. You should consult your medical defence body immediately, and follow its advice.

If faced in future with a patient whose circumstances (not just imprisonment, but the lack of social support and the very recent very bad news) could place them at high risk of suicide and of mental disorder that might further increase the risk of suicide, then you may wish to consider a more intensive care and support plan. Your initial assessment that he was not depressed may well have been correct, but symptoms of illness can emerge rapidly, and you should perhaps have reassessed the situation on a much more frequent basis. If you delegate this to someone else, you should ensure this is followed up. You should also ensure that your unit operates a safe system of work in which, for example, the work of staff who are absent is discussed, and where necessary reallocated temporarily.

Ethical

Your duty of care to any patient arises not only from law but also from your professional ethics. In many cases, the ethical standard to which you are held is higher than the minimum legal standard (e.g. to provide the best care you reasonably can in the circumstances, not merely to not provide care unsupported by responsible medical opinion).

2

Right to disclose clinical information to third parties

Themes: *bipolar disorder (p.92) and risk assessment (p.163) [C]; hospital order (p.500), hybrid order (p.504), and duty of confidentiality (p.690) [L]; bases for disclosure (p.320) [CL]; and breach of confidentiality (p.320) [E]*

Case description

You agree to write an independent psychiatric report on Lara, a thirty-five-year-old woman detained in an MSU under an interim hospital order. She was convicted of maliciously administering poison to her girlfriend; the girlfriend survived, but with long-term neurological damage. She has no other forensic history, or any previous psychiatric history. The treating team have diagnosed bipolar disorder, and regard her mania and delusions as having caused the offence. She has responded well to olanzapine, and is now symptom-free.

You concur with the treating team on her primary diagnosis, and their treatment plan. You note that she has capacity and consents to this plan. During your interview, Lara discloses that for the previous couple of years she had thought about fatally poisoning her girlfriend, to end the relationship (her girlfriend frequently assaulted her, and she felt dominated and controlled by her and unable to leave). Lara explains that she had been too scared to act until her manic disinhibition 'allowed' her to. You conclude, amongst other things, that her risk of harm to anyone in an intimate relationship with her is considerably higher than her treating team believe. You recommend a restricted hospital or hybrid order.[11]

Her treating team recommend an unrestricted hospital order, and understandably, her solicitor does not want to submit your report to the court. You are concerned that her treating team will therefore be unaware of Lara's pre-existing thoughts of poisoning her girlfriend, and of your risk assessment, which you consider relevant to the court's sentencing decision.

Questions

1. Will you disclose the report to the treating team?
2. Will you disclose the report to the court?
3. What other clinical, legal, clinico-legal, and ethical issues arise in the case?

---

[11] In E&W or NI; the alternative recommendation is required by the *Vowles* and *Edwards* judgments (see ethical case 18). In Scotland, you would recommend a restricted compulsion order or a hospital direction. In RoI you would simply recommend committal for treatment.

Clinical

A lot of weight may be attached to your assessment of the risks arising from Lara's bipolar disorder and lack of problem-solving skills. Your assessment will need to have been done to a high standard, as it will be tested under cross-examination.

Legal

A similar situation arose in *Egdell*,[12] in which an independent psychiatrist gained information from clinical interview suggesting that a patient who could shortly have been transferred out of a high-security hospital still posed an unacceptably high risk of harm to others. Dr Egdell disclosed his report to the treating team and urged it to be passed on to the Home Secretary.[13] The patient sued for negligence by breach of confidence, but the Court of Appeal dismissed his case, stating that Dr Egdell's actions were justified because there was 'a significant risk of serious harm to the public'.

Disclosure to the court was considered in *Crozier*.[14] A psychiatrist instructed by the defence diagnosed a personality disorder and recommended admission to a high-security hospital. The defence solicitor did not use the report, and the court sentenced Mr Crozier to nine-years' imprisonment for attempted murder (he had attacked his sister with an axe). The psychiatrist disclosed his report to the prosecution, who successfully applied to vary the sentence to a hospital order with restrictions. Mr Crozier appealed, citing the breach of confidence, but the court ruled that the public interest overrode the doctor's duty of confidentiality.

Clinico-legal

Egdell clearly provides legal authority (at least in E&W) for you to disclose your report to the treating team in this case, if that is the only way for the risk of harm to others to be properly managed.

An alternative approach would be to employ the power under the Data Protection Act[15] to make a limited disclosure of information to an appropriate body such as the hospital or the court, for the purpose of preventing future offences.

Neither legal basis infers a *duty* to disclose, merely the *right* to do so. If you chose not to disclose the information, and were later sued by a victim, as the law stands,[16] you would be unlikely to be found negligent unless the victim was very clearly identifiable and the harm to them reasonably foreseeable (in contrast to the Tarasoff judgment[17] in the USA).

Ethical

The information in your report is Lara's confidential medical information, and any decision to disclose it should in general be made by her, given that she has the capacity to decide. Disclosing it against her express wishes would amount to a breach of confidentiality. Moreover, the report was commissioned on her behalf by her solicitor, not by the court or prosecution, so it was not completed under the terms of any prior agreement with her that would have allowed it to be disclosed to the court or prosecution. Breaching confidentiality in a way that results in harm to the patient (e.g. the longer period of detention that would result from the treating team or court becoming aware of your conclusions) would be ethically wrong, unless the facts fall within one of the exceptions to the general duty of confidentiality in professional ethics (as codified in guidance from the GMC/IMC and the Royal College of Psychiatrists). In this case, they clearly do.

---

[12] [1990] 1 AllER 835.
[13] At the time the relevant Minister; now in E&W it would be the Ministry of Justice.
[14] *R v Crozier* [1991] CrimLR 138.
[15] DPA2018 in the UK, and in RoI.
[16] *Palmer (administratrix of the estate of Palmer) v Tees Health Authority* [1999] AllER 722; *Surrey County Council v McManus and others* [2001] EWCA 691; *K v Secretary of State for the Home Department* [2002] EWCA Civ 775.
[17] *Tarasoff v Regents of the University of California* 17 Cal 3d 425.

3

Personal injury by 'nervous shock'—PTSD

Themes: *PTSD (p.96), malingering (p.118), and use of psychological tests (p.130) [C]; reasonably foreseeable damage and causation (p.548) and nervous shock (p.640) [L]; distinguishing normal grief reaction (p.98) [CL]; and reporting versus treating (p.678) [E]*

Case description

Jeremy attends a solicitor, seeking compensation. He says that nine months ago he was walking along a bridge in central London with his wife, when he witnessed a drunken man drive a van onto the pavement in front of him, killing his wife and another pedestrian, and injuring three others. He knelt with his wife as she died at the roadside. He said he had not feared for his own safety as he had been some metres back from the van. The police accept Jeremy's witness statement at the time as truthful. The driver was charged with causing death by dangerous driving, and Jeremy has now been called to the trial as a witness, as well as to the inquest into his wife and the other pedestrian's deaths.

Jeremy has had nightmares ever since, cannot sleep, is constantly anxious, and is on long-term sick leave because he cannot function at work as a bus driver. He misses his wife terribly and thinks he will never get over her death. He says his employer's occupational health department has advised him to consider retirement on medical grounds. However, Jeremy says he cannot afford this, and asks whether he can claim compensation from the driver's insurance company.

The solicitor instructs you to prepare a report on whether Jeremy has PTSD, or any other mental disorder, and if so, whether it was caused by his being present at the incident, and to advise on treatment and prognosis. The solicitor says that Jeremy's GP has written a brief report already, stating that Jeremy suffers from PTSD. Shortly afterwards, the GP refers Jeremy to you for assessment and treatment of PTSD.

Questions

1. What are the clinical, legal, clinico-legal, and ethical issues in the case?

Clinical

Assessment of PTSD in the context of compensation claims can be difficult: the assessment relies heavily on claimants' own accounts of their symptoms, which they may have an interest in exaggerating or even feigning. There may also be a conflict of interest for you between treating the claimant in the interest of his welfare, and producing a court report in the interest of justice: so you should explain carefully which role you have agreed to take on and its implications, and offer him advice on colleagues who might be able to help with the other role.

The essence of PTSD is involuntary re-experiencing of elements of a life-threatening or otherwise severely traumatic event, with symptoms of hyperarousal, avoidance, and emotional blunting.

Symptoms usually arise within six months, with impairment of social, occupational, or other areas of functioning. The risk of developing PTSD after trauma is 8%–13% for men, and 20%–30% for women. Factors such as low education and lower social class increase vulnerability, as do low self-esteem, neurotic traits, previous or family history of mental disorder (especially mood and anxiety disorders), and previous childhood or adult trauma. Protective factors include higher IQ, higher social class, male gender, and psychopathic traits.

Your assessment and report should explicitly consider the possibility of malingering (see criminal law case 26 for details of such an assessment).

Take a full and detailed psychiatric history from Jeremy; do not just focus on his claimed posttraumatic symptoms. Read his GP records from before and after the incident, along with records from any other clinician treating him, his employer's occupational health records, plus the police report of the incident and Jeremy's witness statement. Speak to informants who know him well about his behaviour before and since. Then perform a detailed mental state examination, looking, for example, for a change in mental state when discussing the incident, or observable hyperarousal in response to unexpected noises from outside the consulting room. Posttraumatic avoidance can extend to cancelling appointments despite the potential legal or financial disadvantage, because he knows he will have to discuss the incident with you; ask the solicitor and police, if you can, about similar behaviour.

You may also wish to administer standardised test questionnaires for PTSD, anxiety disorder, depression, or malingering,[18] either yourself if you possess the relevant training, or via a clinical psychology colleague.

Legal

Where a person witnesses traumatic events occurring to others 'with whom he has close ties of love and affection', the law allows a claim for any adverse psychological impact, which it terms 'nervous shock'. The term has been described as inaccurate and misleading, but it continues as a useful abbreviation for a complex concept.

In law,[19] a nervous shock is a psychiatric illness or injury inflicted upon a person by the intentional or negligent actions or omissions of another. The shock must be 'a sudden assault on the nervous system': not, for instance, years spent caring for a negligently injured spouse or dealing with a negligently brain-damaged child's challenging behaviour or bereavement alone.[20] The shock must result in a diagnosed mental disorder (not just 'mental distress').

The courts have laid down additional strict requirements of proximity and foreseeability:

- The claimant must perceive a shocking event with their own unaided senses: for example as an eyewitness or hearing it in person or viewing its 'immediate aftermath' (e.g. seeing your spouse gravely injured in hospital straight after the incident). This requires close physical proximity to the event or its immediate aftermath, and would usually exclude events witnessed by television, or reported by a third party.
- If the nervous shock was caused by witnessing the death or injury of another person, the claimant must show a 'close tie of love and affection'.
- There must be no supervening event that occurred between the trauma and the onset of the mental disorder that could have caused it.
- It must have been reasonably foreseeable to the defendant that a person of 'normal fortitude' in the claimant's position would suffer mental disorder. If so, the defendant is liable for whatever degree of injury the victim suffers, even if this is exacerbated by a vulnerability that could not reasonably have been foreseen.[21]

The 'quantum' of compensation is determined by the nature and degree of the distress and disability arising from the mental disorder, the employment implications, and the cost of its treatment, taking into account the duration of treatment and its prognosis.

---

[18] For example the Impact of Events Scale Revised (IES-R), Beck Anxiety Inventory (BAI), Beck Depression Inventory version 2 (BDI2), or the Structured Inventory of Reported Symptoms (SIRS), respectively.

[19] Essentially the same legal principles apply in E&W, Scotland, NI, and RoI in this area of law.

[20] While recognising the claimant's plight, the courts have ruled in each such case that on public policy grounds defendants cannot be held liable for such gradual, long-term consequences.

[21] This is known as the 'eggshell skull rule', and is analogous to the subjective elements of the criteria for diminished responsibility, loss of control (provocation), and duress.

Clinico-legal

In assessing Jeremy for PTSD, or any other mental disorder arising from the trauma, you must exclude any pre-existing condition (as opposed to any mental vulnerability not amounting to a mental disorder); this can be difficult to achieve, especially if the GP and other records suggest some measure of mental dysfunction, but without any formal diagnosis having been made. You must also attempt to distinguish between mental disorder arising from witnessing the event and arising from bereavement, particularly if Jeremy's wife had died some time later, and his symptoms had only arisen after that date.

If you do, even provisionally, make a diagnosis of PTSD or other mental disorder, then it would be wise to advise early treatment, for Jeremy's wellbeing and to confirm the diagnosis through successful treatment. It will also assist his case if he can demonstrate that he has taken reasonable steps to limit the damage arising from the incident that he is claiming for.

Ethical

The GP asked you to assess and treat Jeremy. However, the risk of bias, or at least the external perception of bias, where a doctor both treats and reports for legal proceedings on a patient who is a litigant is obvious, in terms of the likely impact upon assessment for legal proceedings where there is also a therapeutic relationship. So you should not both 'treat' and 'report'.

Otherwise, all the usual requirements apply of maintaining a professionally disinterested stance in a case where you are reporting into legal proceedings.

4 Battery and negligence—treatment in prison

Themes: *personality disorder (p.78) and side-effects of depot antipsychotic (p.201) [C];*
battery (p.416) and clinical negligence (p.550) [L]; safe system of work (p.552) and preparing
for disciplinary and professional proceedings (pp.557, 642) [CL]; and making apologies
(p.642) [E]

Case description

You are a prison psychiatrist. You see Zak, a forty-two-year-old man with antisocial and
borderline PD. He expresses labile mood, irritability, impulsivity, and brief psychotic episodes. He often cuts himself, occasionally assaults others, and complains about being
poorly treated. He is unpopular with prison staff and other inmates.

You hope to engage Zak in an MBT programme, but he refuses to consider psychological treatment (and very little is available in the prison in any case). You therefore offer
a combination of a low-dose antipsychotic, zuclopenthixol, and a mood stabiliser to help
reduce his lability and impulsivity; you tell him about common side-effects of zuclopenthixol such as sleepiness, akathisia, and hypersalivation. Over several months, he takes
these drugs only occasionally. After a further discussion, he agrees to monthly depot
zuclopenthixol instead.

Zak accepts the first dose the next day without issue. However, the following month he
tells prison officers he doesn't want it, but then goes to the healthcare centre with them
anyway. He says again to the staff there that he does not want to be injected as he 'feels
odd in his head', but he does not repeat this when the nurse arrives with the depot, and
meekly allows it to be administered.

A few days later he begins to experience neck movements which are later diagnosed
as a retrocollis caused by the zuclopenthixol. You stop the prescription, but the torticollis
persists for several months; it is ameliorated by injections of botulinum toxin into his
sternocleidomastoid muscle.

Soon afterwards, you receive a letter from Zak's solicitor claiming damages for battery
and trespass to the person through administration of an injection without consent, and for
negligently prescribing a drug without informing him of the risk of a painful side-effect
that he went on to experience. The letter adds that you have been referred to the GMC/IMC
for investigation of your fitness to practice.

Questions

1. What immediate actions should you take?
2. Did the administration of the second dose of zuclopenthixol amount to battery?
3. If so, are you responsible for it?
4. Was your prescription of zuclopenthixol negligent?

5. What would you do differently in the future?
6. What other clinical, legal, clinico-legal, and ethical issues in the case?

Clinical

You should refresh your memory of events by referring to the patient's medical records, but must not make any retrospective changes. You may wish to make your own copy of relevant records if you will lose access to them (e.g. if they are held in a paper file, which will be retained by prison management); ensure that you have permission to do so and that you comply with data protection law.

Legal

Ultimately, the question of whether Zak was the victim of battery depends upon whether he consented to the injection at the point it was given. Any case will turn on the detailed evidence of the interaction between him and the person administering the depot injection.[22]

The legal question of negligence rests on whether you had a duty of care to Zak (i.e. he was sufficiently 'proximate' to you); whether you breached that duty; whether that breach caused harm; and whether harm was reasonably foreseeable.

You undoubtedly owed him a duty of care as he was your patient, and side-effects such as dystonic reactions, including torticollis, are reasonably foreseeable consequences of taking antipsychotics. The prescription of the drug (and thus its administration in accordance with your prescription) directly caused the harm that he suffered. So the question comes down to whether your prescription amounted to a breach of your duty, which in such cases incorporates three tests:

- Was your practice accepted as proper by a responsible body of medical opinion?[23]
- Did it have a logical basis?[24]
- If consent was required, did you inform the patient of everything a reasonable person in their position would have wanted to know, or that you should have known the patient would have wanted to know?[25]

Clinico-legal

The administration of low-dose antipsychotics, including by depot injection, for symptom control in patients suffering from severe personality disorder is a practice accepted as proper by a responsible body of medical opinion, and it is logical to use a low-dose antipsychotic to reduce arousal and impulsivity and to protect against transient psychotic symptoms. However, you did not mention the possibility of dystonia in general or torticollis in particular. A court would therefore have to decide whether torticollis was 'a material risk', in that a reasonable person in the patient's position would have attached significance to the risk, or was there evidence that you should reasonably have been aware that the patient himself would have attached significance to the risk? If it concluded that it was a material risk, it could find you negligent for not referring to it.

Even if the court did not find you negligent for the reasons above, you might be liable if the court found the depot to have been given without consent. Zak's statements and behaviour were inconsistent (saying twice that he did not want it, but not saying this to the administering nurse, attending the healthcare centre for his depot, and accepting it without refusal or resistance). Were the question to be settled in court, it would come down to determining what the evidence on balance was and/or whose account of events was found more believable.

---

[22] This was the key issue in *Freeman v Home Office No.2* [1984] 1 QB 524, which also concerned the administration of depot antipsychotic to a prisoner allegedly without his consent; the claimant claimed, unsuccessfully, that he 'could not' consent to medication because of his essentially vulnerable coerced relationship with prison staff, including healthcare staff.
[23] *Bolam v Friern Hospital Management Committee* [1957] 1 WLR 583.
[24] *Bolitho v Hackney Health Authority* [1998] AC 232.
[25] *Montgomery v Lanarkshire Health Board* [2015] UKSC 11.

Whether you are responsible for any treatment without consent would depend upon what system of work you had established as the clinical leader of the team. If your routine practice clearly involved the seeking of consent, you discussed issues of consent with other staff, you made clear that you expected staff to seek consent themselves before performing any procedure, you shared guidelines from other bodies about consent, and you took part in arrangements to ensure compliance with them, then this would demonstrate that you had done everything you reasonably could to ensure a system of work that sought informed consent in all cases, and the nurse was liable for any failure to conform to that system. If there was no evidence of you doing any of these things, it would be possible for you to be held responsible in negligence and in professional conduct proceedings.

The nurse should have made a point of confirming and recording the patient's consent to the injection before administering it. As a clinical leader of a team that includes nurses administering depots, you should ensure that this is part of their system of work and is covered in their supervision sessions; you should also consider arranging for patients' notes to be audited to see whether and how often consent is recorded explicitly in this way. (In practice, in most such teams you would work alongside a team manager and others who ensure a safe system of work is followed, but you should still check that they are doing this.)

You should also change your practice to as to inform patients of potential risks more carefully. A simple way of doing this would be always to supply them with a copy of a patient information sheet about side-effects of specific drugs, and, after mentioning the most frequent effects, to check whether there is anything rare that would have particular significance for them.

You should show the claim you have received to your employer and your medical defence organisation straight away. Although addressed to you, elements of the claim also affect other staff (e.g. the nurse who administered the injection and prison officers who were witnesses) and your employer, who may be vicariously liable.

Ethical

If you have not done so already, you should also consider acknowledging the harm the patient has suffered, explaining openly and honestly how it occurred, and apologising for it; this does not amount to an admission of legal liability.[26]

---

[26] If you are employed by the NHS, your employing organisation will be required to ensure you or someone else does this, under the 2015 'Duty of Candour'.

5

Capacity to make a will–depressive illness

Themes: *depression (p.94) [C]; testamentary capacity (p.540) [L]; mapping mental state onto the legal test (p.358) [CL]; and irrelevance of apparent 'fairness' to expert opinion (p.674) [E]*

Case description

Albert, a deceased unmarried retired teacher, was perfectionistic and obsessional. He had an episode of moderately severe depression in his forties from which he recovered fully. He made a will when he was forty-five, in which he left all his assets to his brother and sister, with whom he had occasional friendly but not close contact.

When he was sixty, he became severely depressed because of work stress. Although he improved somewhat on antidepressants, he retired on medical grounds, and thereafter only did voluntary work. He became lonely and isolated, until this was reduced slightly when an old friend resumed contact with him, and he became close to her and her teenage son. Nevertheless, his medical records suggest his mental health never fully recovered, and that he ruminated obsessionally upon his loneliness and upon whether he had behaved inappropriately to his friend's son or to past pupils.

Last year, aged sixty-five, he made a new will in which he disinherited his brother and sister, and left all his assets to the friend's son. He then died, aged sixty-six.

Albert's first will is accepted as valid, but his siblings dispute the validity of his allegedly supervening second will. Their solicitors instruct you to give an opinion on whether Albert had testamentary capacity when he made the second will.

Questions

1. Did Albert have testamentary capacity when he made his new will?
2. What other clinical, legal, clinico-legal, and ethical issues are there in this case?

> **Clinical**
>
> You will need access all of Albert's medical records, as well as needing to read any relevant witness statements, in order to determine his most likely mental state at the time that he made the second will. You should also speak to, or read a statement by, the solicitor who assisted him with the second will: ask whether she or he noticed anything odd about Albert at the time (solicitors have a duty themselves to be alert to possible lack of testamentary capacity[27]).

---

[27] *Key v Key* [2010] EWHC 408 (Ch).

Legal

The test of testamentary capacity is laid down in the leading case[28] as follows:

- understanding the nature and effects of making a will;
- understanding the extent of the property disposed of in the will;
- comprehending and appreciating the claims others might have that the will should give effect to; and
- having no mental disorder 'that shall poison his affections, pervert his sense of right, or prevent the exercise of his natural faculties; that is, no insane delusion shall influence his will in disposing of his property and bring about a disposal of it which, if the mind had been sound, would not have been made'.

The test was recently confirmed in *Walker v Badmin*,[29] which determined that the test of mental capacity set out in the Mental Capacity Act 2005 was not directly relevant.[30] However, a person might have the capacity to 'comprehend' in terms of the first three aspects of the test, but 'without having the mental energy to make any decisions of his own about whom to benefit', thus allowing an 'affective disorder' as capable of negating testamentary capacity.[31] The burden of proof is initially upon the party seeking to overturn the will to show some real doubt about its validity; after which the burden shifts to the party wishing the will to be upheld.

Clinico-legal

You will need to 'map' Albert's likely mental state at the time he made the second will onto each of the elements of the test above. Unless Albert was deluded at the time he made the will, and deluded in ways that related to any of the elements of the legal test, then it is very unlikely that his depression and ruminations could have caused him to have been unable to understand the nature of the will and its effects, the extent of his property, and others' possible claims. The only element of the test that *might* apply is the final limb.

So what is likely to matter is whether, on the balance of probabilities, Albert held deluded beliefs that 'poisoned his affections': for example, a delusional belief that he had behaved inappropriately to the friend's son and so wanted to make up for this in some way by bequeathing assets to him. Merely suffering a neurotic depressive illness, feeling lonely, fearing becoming even more depressed as a result, plus ruminating about inappropriate behaviour, and therefore favouring the young man in his will, would not likely be sufficient to pass this test, even if these factors substantially affected his judgment.

In summary, as best you can, you will have to give an opinion on whether Albert's depression, and any obsessional ruminations about inappropriate behaviour, could be said, on the balance of probabilities, to have 'poisoned' his affections (against his family) or 'perverted his sense of right'. Any information showing how he chose between the potential beneficiaries will also be relevant. Simply concluding that, had he not suffered from depression, he would probably not have made the dispositions that he did make, would not likely overturn the presumption of his testamentary capacity.

Ethical

Retrospective reconstruction of a testator's mental state at a particular time in the past, and mapping of that onto the test of testamentary capacity, may offer some limited latitude in judgment. It is important therefore not to take any view of the disputed will in terms of what seems to you to be 'fair'.

---

[28] *Banks v Goodfellow* (1869-70) LR 5 QB 549. This is a direct precedent in E&W, and has repeatedly been cited with approval by Scottish and Irish courts.

[29] *Walker v Badmin* [2015] WTLR 493.

[30] The public policy reason is that the common law sets a lower threshold for testamentary capacity than the MCA principles would do, reducing the number of elderly people with declining cognitive function who are prevented from making a will, and (it is hoped) reducing the numbers of successful challenges to revised wills from unhappy would-be beneficiaries.

[31] *Key v Key* [2010] EWHC 408 (Ch).

6

'Fitness to parent' and risk of harm to a child

Themes: *puerperal psychosis (p.153) [C]; family law principles (p.554) [L]; avoiding making findings of fact (p.654) [CL]; and intrusion of personal values (p.674) [E]*

Case description

You have been appointed as a single joint expert in care proceedings involving baby Lisa, aged three months. Lisa is in interim foster care; the Local Authority have indicated that they intend to put Lisa up for adoption.

Lisa's parents are Kelly, aged forty-one, and Kyle, thirty-one. Kyle was released from prison eighteen months ago, having served a ten-year tariff for murdering Kelly's two-year-old son Teddy while Kelly was at work and her older daughter, then aged eight, was at school. Teddy died from blows to the stomach and head; forensic evidence led to Kyle's conviction. Kyle has always denied killing Teddy, but has acknowledged that he failed to protect him, and that therefore his death 'must be my fault'.

Kyle's only prior convictions were common assault (drunken fights with other young men), drunk driving, and theft. He had never before been in prison. He had worked since leaving school in a variety of jobs, none for very long. His 'stormy' relationship with Kelly was his first serious relationship.

The prison and probation reports are positive about Kyle. He attended courses on anger management and domestic violence, and his behaviour was exemplary. He was assessed as posing a low risk of harm to others. He would have been released on parole considerably earlier had he admitted to killing Teddy.

Kelly maintained her relationship with Kyle throughout. Social services were involved as soon as she became pregnant, and warned her that they would seek to take the baby into care if she stayed with Kyle, but she refused to separate from him. Now that Lisa has been taken temporarily into care, Kyle has agreed to move out and live with his elderly mother, if that means Lisa can come home.

You are asked to carry out a psychiatric assessment on both Kelly and Kyle, and give an opinion about the risk that each may pose to baby Lisa, including whether Kelly is at risk of getting into future violent relationships if she leaves Kyle. Kelly refuses to meet you, but Kyle is entirely cooperative during the interview. He says he wants to show everyone that he is safe, and that he and Kelly will be good parents. He says Kelly is fed up with questions: she has looked after babies successfully in the past and does not see the need to talk to a psychiatrist.

Kelly was treated by her GP for mild postnatal depression after Teddy's birth; otherwise, neither she nor Kyle has any psychiatric history. Kyle takes over-the-counter remedies for anxiety and insomnia; he tells you he has nightmares about prison. You find no mental disorder in Kyle, and cannot comment on Kelly.

Questions

1. What clinical, legal, clinico-legal, and ethical issues arise in this case?

Clinical

This is a good example of the complexity of cases that come before the family court, and the lack of good-quality evidence about relevant issues. Kyle had no psychiatric defence when he killed Teddy; although from a psychological perspective one might wonder about his youth, and his capacity to tolerate the stress of caring for a toddler. The family court may hope that your psychiatric assessment will offer some explanation of why Kyle killed Teddy, and whether the same risk pertains to Lisa.

Actuarial risk factors that indicate lower risk to Lisa are that Kyle is now older; he has an enduring supportive relationship with Kelly; and he has no risk factors for violence other than his past offending. The absence of major mental illness may also be protective. The risk to Lisa also will decrease as she gets older, since babies younger than a year old are at the highest risk of fatal assaults by their carers. Finally, child abuse may be committed by parents who suffer a range of mental disorders, but the majority of child abusers have no formal diagnosis.

Clinically it might be helpful for you to recommend a parenting assessment of both parents, which could be in a residential placement. Parenting assessments can only be carried out by clinicians who are trained to undertake them; few psychiatrists are trained to do so. However, there are some national parenting centres with psychiatric expertise (usually CAMHS). In this case, Kyle's history may make it difficult to find a parenting assessment centre that will accept referral.

The presence or absence of mental disorder is less important than how any disorder, or personality disorder, and related psychological patterns falling short of disorder, may impact the relationship that Kelly and Kyle have with Lisa, and how they respond to her vulnerability and neediness. One of the concerns may be that Kelly has an avoidant attachment style; she can do practical care of babies but struggles to be emotionally close. This is the kind of psychological issue that might emerge during an extended parenting assessment.

Legal

There is no specific legal test of fitness to parent. Rather, there are the key principles that the welfare of the child is paramount, and that parents have responsibilities to, rather than rights over, their children.

Clinico-legal

Since there is no test of 'fitness to parent', so there is no 'mapping' exercise per se to conduct. And your assessment should not aim to assess parenting 'fitness' directly, as it is both an issue for the court, and an issue that in some respects goes beyond your expertise as a psychiatrist. Instead, you should address whether there is any evidence of mental disorder, or of other psychological factors, which could, or would be likely to, impair Kelly or Kyle's ability to act safely as a parent. The evidence base does not greatly assist, because all mental disorders *may* impact parenting, at least for brief periods. Some parents manage to provide good care despite their mental conditions; others struggle to parent with quite minor levels of disorder. The only obvious exception to this is puerperal psychosis, which can lead to sudden increased risk to children: and this could be relevant to Kelly, who is only three-months postnatal and has a history of such illness.

Generally, the question is best addressed by a direct parenting assessment, rather than by attempting to draw inferences about the nature of any effect upon parenting arising from symptoms of a given mental disorder (except perhaps in relation very serious mental illness or learning disability, but even here this should not be definitive). Most experts concur that a parenting assessment cannot be based solely on a psychiatric interview, but needs repeated assessments that include observation of the interactions between the baby and both parents, by experts who have clinical experience of treating families and of parent-infant psychotherapy.

Your report belongs to the family court and cannot be disclosed without the court's permission. As with all evaluations, you need to advise Kyle and Kelly of the limits of confidentiality in relation to what they say at interview. You must also be careful that you do not rely on 'facts' that are disputed and subject to court finding, and that you do not advise until you have seen a transcript of any judgement of the fact-finding hearing.

You may be asked to provide some comment on Kelly's refusal to see you. However, you should be careful about what inferences can properly be drawn from this, and you should not make any comment upon psychiatric diagnosis beyond what is in the GP notes.

The two main issues in this case are, first, whether your psychiatric assessment of Kyle can have anything to say about his likely parenting, and second, how his risk of harm is to be assessed many years after a serious and unusual act of violence.

With regard to Kyle's risk to Lisa, it is not surprising that his risk-assessment score was low. The absence of most criminogenic risk factors is a positive factor, but Kyle's reluctance to admit his role in Teddy's death is harder to interpret. And, although denial of offending may be unattractive, it is not empirically associated with higher risk of reoffending, especially in unusual offences like child homicide.

Ethical

The ethical issue in the case relates to the emotions that may be stirred up by it, including the common sense of disgust towards someone who has killed a child, especially one for whom they were responsible. Psychiatric evidence may have an important role in putting risk in its proper perspective and helping other professionals to appreciate the protective factors as well as the risk factors. However, you too may struggle with a negative emotional response to parents such as Kyle and Kelly, having a sense of unease that cannot be supported by clinical evidence.

The expert needs to remind themselves that they are assisting the court in its deliberations, and their duty is to provide the court with the best quality report that is possible in terms of evidence, and to make use of professional and personal methods of managing their own understandable feelings, such as mentoring and personal support.

7

Rules of evidence in family proceedings—disputed and established facts

Themes: *factitious disorder (p.118) [C]; rules of fact and opinion evidence (p.382) [L]; not giving opinion before facts are confirmed (p.654) [CL]; truth, honesty, and justice in emotive cases (p.674) [E]*

Case description

You are asked by the family court to provide an expert psychiatric assessment on Anna, a thirty-two-year-old woman whose children are subject to care proceedings brought by the Local Authority. Care proceedings have been started because Anna is suspected of inducing illness in her youngest child, a six-month-old baby. Key facts are disputed: the Local Authority argues that Anna has abused her children by repeatedly exaggerating and fabricating accounts of their illnesses over the last three years, which she denies.

Your instructions include questions about the risk that Anna poses to her children, including a question about whether she has any mental disorder that might lead her to pose a risk to her children. You are provided with extensive medical records of Anna and all her children, including the GP notes. You also have police records, with no convictions recorded, and the transcript of Anna's recent police interview, during which she answered 'no comment' to all questions.

In your interview with her, Anna denies all of the allegations, and talks in enormous detail about her children's illnesses, and her role as a carer. She also says that she herself suffers from a range of chronic disorders, which have never responded to any medical treatment. She is pleasant enough but becomes slightly hostile when you ask more personal questions about her childhood history and background, saying that she had a perfect childhood, excellent parents, and doesn't believe in seeing 'shrinks'. At the end of the interview, she demands to know your diagnosis of her, saying that 'everything depends upon your view of whether I'm mad or not'. You respond by saying that you can't comment at this stage until you have seen all the materials, and that, as far as you know, your report is only one part of the evidence before the judge.

In her notes provided there is evidence that Anna has a long and well-documented history of signs and symptoms that both her GP and local physicians think are functional somatic disorders, without an organic basis. She often attends out-of-hours health services and A&E departments, usually presenting at least once a month. However, she tends only to present to her GP to ask for sick notes, and has refused any referral to psychological therapies or a trial of antidepressants. You also note that factitious and induced illness was raised as a potential issue with both her first two children by local paediatricians, but never investigated further.

Questions

1. What will you do next?
2. What risk of harm to others do you perceive there to be?
3. What other clinical, legal, clinico-legal, and ethical issues does the case raise?

Clinical

This appears to be a *prima facie* case of abnormal illness behaviour in a parent, and in theory, you could provide the court with a summary of what is known about such behaviour generally. And there is a clinical evidence base, summarised in Royal College guidelines[32] which contains information about incidence, mortality, and morbidity and how the diagnosis is made. However, the guidelines state that factitious and induced illness (FII) is a diagnosis of *children* made *by paediatricians*. Its causes (only one of which is parental mental disorder) are a secondary issue.

But the facts of this case have yet to be established by the family court. The Local Authority have alleged that Anna has done a variety of things that have caused the children significant harm, but Anna disputes this. And the factual question of whether there has been exaggerated, fabricated, or induced illness in the children will be addressed by paediatric, not psychiatric, evidence.

If you assess Anna further before the fact-finding judgment, you can answer questions about whether she has a mental disorder (although this may be challenged in cross-examination), but you cannot address questions about abnormal illness behaviour and risk because whether this has happened at all is yet to be determined. In addition, there is no known functional link between any mental disorder and abnormal illness behaviour by parents.

You must not go beyond your expertise and comment on matters that are paediatric. And the details of the paediatric evidence are unlikely to assist you (what will assist the court in such cases is the independent paediatric review, which will offer an independent opinion on whether the clinical picture is best explained by abnormal illness behaviour by the parent).

Legal

In cases of child protection, to avoid delay, cases are often heard urgently in the family court, and children removed temporarily on interim care or protection orders.[33] The family court will then hold a fact-finding hearing, in which the Local Authority will set out its evidence that harm has been caused to the children in question. The finding will be determined upon the civil standard of proof (the balance of probabilities), not a criminal standard. The welfare of the child is legally central.

Clinico-legal

The Royal College of Psychiatrists guidance on FII and its management states that psychiatrists should not provide expert assessments of adults like Anna until after fact-finding hearings. The guidance also suggests not reporting until an independent paediatric review has been completed, ideally as part of the fact-finding process. If the paediatric evidence supports a finding of harmful parental behaviour, then subsequent psychiatric evidence may then help the court to understand the mechanism and meaning of the behaviour for the parent, the potential for future risk, and the potential for therapy to reduce the risk.

[32] Royal College of Paediatrics and Child Health (2009) *Fabricated or Induced Illness by Carers (FII): A Practical Guide for Paediatricians*. RCPCH.

[33] An order that gives the local authority temporary parental responsibility and allows it to take the child(ren) concerned into its care during proceedings. The legal frameworks differ between jurisdictions, but this could be an interim care order under s38 of the Children Act 1989 in E&W, an interim compulsory supervision order under s86 Children's Hearings (Scotland) Act 2011, an interim care order under s57 of the Children (Northern Ireland) Order 1995, or an interim care order under s17 of the Child Care Act 1991 in RoI.

So any formulation that you might consider of Anna's history and presentation must wait until the facts are resolved by the family court. Just as in the criminal court, if the subject of the allegations is denying them, then it is crucial that the psychiatrist does not usurp the role of the court with (unreliable) claims that there is a psychiatric history that explains the disputed 'facts'.

This is especially important in child protection cases because the CPS often wait for the family court to make findings before deciding whether or not to proceed to criminal charges, where the burden of proof is higher. If they do proceed, they should have access to all the family court bundle, but you may not disclose your report to anyone (including the police) without court permission or a court order.

Because the burden of proof is higher in the criminal court, it is not unusual for facts to be established at the family court that are not then proven in the criminal court. Defendants may be pleased by this, not realising that the family courts' findings are unaffected by criminal court (negative) findings, and that the harm to their child remains an established fact for child protection purposes.

Sometimes, despite one's best efforts, the court insists on having psychiatric evidence at the fact-finding stage. It is vital that, in your opinion, you emphasise that there are questions that you cannot answer because to do so involves addressing facts that are disputed. The main source of the difficulty is that many local authorities, solicitors, and courts still believe that a disorder exists called 'Munchausen's syndrome by proxy' that has *probative value* in terms of causation of behaviour. So it is often helpful to explain to the court that the varied terminologies in the psychiatric literature[34] are no more than descriptions of those same behaviours that the court needs to rule on factually.

Once the facts are established, they do then contribute to your risk assessment. In a case like this, if the court finds that Anna has induced illness in her child, then this finding provides evidence of past risk behaviour, which can be analysed alongside the presence or absence of other risk and protective factors. It is at this stage that an interview with Anna will be helpful in terms of her insight, her level of denial, and her willingness to consider what the court has found.

So you should not prepare a report without having considered the judgement in any fact-finding hearing, and stating that you have done so. The judgement will be the 'facts' of risk that you have to work with in coming to your view. It is not uncommon for the parents in the case to disagree with the judgement: this is understandable but does not count as 'fact'.

Ethical

No matter how obvious it seems to you that a person has done what they are accused of, it is vital that you do not comment upon disputed facts. The most ethically testing scenario is where someone 'confesses' in their interview with you to the disputed facts. If this happens, then you may need to stop the interview in order to discuss further with the lead solicitor who instructs you; and you may need to remind the person that your report is not confidential, and that you have a duty to the family court, and therefore the welfare of the children; which means that concerns about risk need to be shared. In practice, this scenario is very rare; and people are often politely uncooperative at interview, on the advice of their lawyers: another reason for recommending that clinical assessment takes place after fact-finding is complete.

It is not uncommon for paediatric experts to give opinions that comment on areas of psychiatric expertise. It will be of assistance for you to politely point out to the court where this has happened. In one such case, a paediatrician provided an opinion which stated that the most likely explanation for a child's sickness was that her mother had poisoned her, based on the fact that the mother had taken overdoses in the past when she was a teenager. This case went to the Court of Appeal, and the paediatrician apologised after psychiatric evidence was admitted effectively to rebut the paediatric opinion.

---

[34] The terms currently favoured include *Fabricated or induced illness* and *Factitious disorder imposed on another*.

8

Evidence at the Medical Practitioners Tribunal Service

Themes: *depression (p.94) and sexual boundary violation (p.302) [C]; professional conduct proceedings and principles (p.552) [L]; fitness to practise (p.642) [CL]; professional boundary violations (p.302) and balance of power in clinical relationships (p.302) [E]*

Case description

You are instructed by solicitors representing Amanda, a fifty-seven-year-old female consultant psychiatrist facing the allegation that she had had an inappropriate sexual relationship with a male patient. Amanda does not deny the relationship with the patient, who was referred by his GP with depression following his wife's death.

Amanda claims her judgement was affected by being depressed herself at the start of the relationship. Her mother had died suddenly of a heart attack, and her husband had left her. She had then taken several months' sick leave whilst being treated with antidepressants and CBT. When she returned to work, she discovered that her hospital had been reconfigured and her role had changed. She was asked to work in the elderly care service, where she met the patient in question.

Amanda says that when she realised her relationship with the patient had become more intimate, she transferred his care to another consultant. The relationship continued for five years, ending by mutual consent when the patient moved away to be near his adult daughters. He then told one of his daughters about the relationship, who reported Amanda to the GMC, alleging that Amanda had exploited and abused her father sexually when he was vulnerable.

You examine Amanda and find no evidence of depression. However, you are provided with good contemporaneous evidence that she did have a major depression at the relevant time, in addition to having a previous history of postnatal depression and anxiety (and, as a medical student, she had had to resit several exams because of this).

Her manager says there have been no other concerns about her behaviour, although there had been occasional comments that she seemed over-involved with some elderly patients, spending more time with them than other consultants did.

The patient in question declines to appear at any GMC hearing, but provides a statement in which he supports Amanda's account of events. You are asked by Amanda's solicitor to provide an opinion on her fitness to practice.

Question

1. How would you proceed, given these instructions?
2. What other clinical, legal, clinico-legal, and ethical issues arise in the case?

Clinical

Inappropriate sexual relationships represent a breach of professional boundaries, and they are commonest in those medical specialties where relationships can build up over time, such as general practice and psychiatry. There is an extensive literature on doctors who engage in sexual boundary violations, and any psychopathology that makes this behaviour more likely. Generally, the presentation resembles the scenario in this case, and only a minority of perpetrators deliberately groom and sexually assault their victims. Most doctors who appear at the MPTS on such charges have insight and admit wrongdoing. They usually argue in mitigation that the relationship was consensual; that they were under stress of some sort; and that they had tried to ensure that they stopped having a clinical relationship with the patient. It is not at all unusual for the relationship only to come to light after it ends, often after several years.

Although your duty as an expert is to the MPTS process, you may want also to consider Amanda's future mental health if she is censured, or even erased from the register, or how she might be rehabilitated if she is suspended. If she does have ongoing mental health needs, then she may benefit from being referred to one of the services that are dedicated to supporting doctors with mental health problems, such as the Practitioner Health Programme, or DocHealth.

Legal

The MPTS[35] deals with cases of misconduct that might impair a doctor's fitness to practise. It hears cases referred by the GMC after investigation by a case examiner. Cases of inappropriate sexual relationships are nearly always referred to the MPTS, and the GMC usually seek suspension or erasure from the medical register if the charges are proven. The burden of proof is on the GMC, but it only has to meet the civil standard of proof (the balance of probabilities).

The MPTS makes findings of fact, and then determines whether these facts demonstrate that fitness to practise is impaired. If fitness to practice is impaired on the grounds of misconduct, then the MPTS has a range of sanctions that they can consider, including no action. However, in cases of inappropriate sexual relationships, the tribunal must consider erasure and suspension.

The GMC's case is usually that such an abuse of trust damages public confidence in the medical profession, as well as causing harm and distress to patients or their families. In this case, the fact that the patient has not complained will be discounted by the GMC, and they are likely to press for the most severe sanctions if impaired fitness to practise is proved by reason of sexual misconduct.

Although you are instructed by the defence, your duty as an expert witness is to the tribunal. You may have to give evidence in person, and expect to be cross-examined as in any court. The standard expected of your assessment and report is exactly the same as for any other court.

Clinico-legal

Studies of the effects of sexual boundary violations find that patients feel betrayed when the relationships end, and that they are harmed because their treatment course is often halted or disorganised when their treating doctor becomes their partner. And people who have already experienced sexual exploitation may be particularly at risk of becoming involved in such relationships. Whilst studies of perpetrators indicate that there is a small number of sexually predatory doctors who prey on patients. The total number of cases is small: nineteen in one study, or about 20% of all cases referred to the MPTS (there are over 300,000 registered medical practitioners in the UK).

One challenge with psychiatric evidence at the MPTS is the lack of an evidence base from which to comment. Even within the domain of occupational health, there is very little in the way of empirical evidence about the relationship between common mental disorders and conduct that indicates impaired fitness to practice. And doctors are unusual offenders in forensic psychiatric terms: in that they rarely have histories or presentations that include the established risk factors for offending and rule breaking (e.g. antisocial attitudes, previous criminality, substance abuse, or childhood adversity).

---

[35] In the UK. In RoI, the IMC fulfils the investigatory and prosecutorial role of the GMC, and the trial role of the MPTS.

It is also rare for overt mental illness to lead to conduct concerns; although it may lead to performance problems. Personality dysfunction occurs in a minority of practitioners, usually at the level of dysfunctional traits rather than personality disorder, and Cluster A and C rather than Cluster B. Antisocial PD is rare in doctors, although narcissistic traits can sometimes be a contributory factor to professional misconduct. Most subjects of MPTS proceedings are male, aged older than forty-nine years, and qualified overseas.[36]

A key clinical factor is the issue of insight into misconduct, acceptance of responsibility, and willingness to engage in remediation. Lack of insight or regret, and denial of need for remediation is usually seen as both further evidence of misconduct as well as a risk-factor for future misconduct.

Your clinical opinion is likely to be used in mitigation, and in this case, you will be asked your view as to whether clinical depression could have given rise to Amanda's inappropriate behaviour. You will also be asked about the role of treatment in reducing the risk of the behaviour recurring in future, and you may be asked your view about Amanda's insight and whether she constitutes a risk of sexually inappropriate behaviour with other vulnerable patients. The GMC narrative will discount any 'relational' quality to what occurred, and will tend to present Amanda as a potential 'sexual offender'. Your evidence may be important in helping the MPTS understand what is known about sexual boundary violations by doctors, and setting out the risk and protective factors in Amanda's case.

Ethical

Since the Hippocratic era, it has been an ethical principle that doctors should never have sexual relationships with patients because of the disparity of power between doctor and patient and the potential for sexual exploitation.

Cases like Amanda's may generate a range of counter-transferential feelings in experts. An assessing expert may feel that Amanda is not a sexual predator, that there is no evidence that she did any harm to the man she had a relationship with, and that she does not pose a future risk of harm to vulnerable patients. The GMC's case will reflect the anger of the complainant, and it is important that the expert pay proper attention to this, and try to maintain an impartial and objective stance. A wrong has been done, and cases like this do harm the professional reputation of doctors in general, and psychiatrists in particular. Doctors have an ethical duty to uphold public confidence in the profession.

---

[36] Harris H and Slater K (2015) *Analysis of Cases Resulting in Doctors Being Erased or Suspended from the Medical Register.* DJS Research.

B.5

Mental capacity and mental health law cases

Mental capacity and mental health law—refusal of Caesarean section

Themes: *depression (p.94), adjustment disorder (p.98), and coercing treatment (p.186) [C]; mental capacity law (p.522) and advance decisions (p.536) [L]; determining mental capacity (p.523) [CL]; respect for autonomy (p.331); and refusal of treatment (pp.332–337) [E]*

Case description

You are asked for an urgent psychiatric assessment of Eleanor, who is thirty-nine weeks pregnant and has pre-eclampsia. The obstetricians have recommended an emergency Caesarean section to protect her and her baby's lives. Eleanor has refused, saying she is a vegan and opposed to any 'unnatural' form of childbirth. She has been verbally abusive to obstetric staff and has threatened to leave hospital if a Caesarean section is suggested again.

Eleanor has an extensive psychiatric history, starting with an eating disorder in her teens. She has harmed herself when stressed, and has other symptoms of borderline personality disorder. She has graduated from university, has a good work record, and has good support from local friends. She has no relationship with her family of origin, whom she claims abused and neglected her as a child. She says her baby was conceived during a one-night stand when she was drunk. She considers herself to have been raped, but says did not report it to police because the rapist had left the country. She was referred to perinatal mental health services, but declined the support they offered.

When you meet Eleanor, you are struck by how physically unwell she looks and how anxious she seems. She speaks rapidly and loudly, with intermittent tears. Although initially hostile, she becomes more open and explains she is frightened of having a Caesarean section because she does not want chemicals injected into her veins. She understands the obstetricians' recommendation plus reasoning, and she believes they are sincere in their advice. However, she insists she can give birth naturally and wants to take the chance, even if it is risky for her and the child. She tells you that she has been told that there is a more than 10% chance of her or her baby dying (or both), but thinks she will be fortunate 'because I'm a strong person'.

The obstetricians want to operate without delay and are sure that what they see as Eleanor's 'foolish' wishes indicate that she lacks the capacity to refuse. They ask you about the significance of her past psychiatric and perinatal history, and suggest that her mental health will suffer if she survives, and the baby dies.

Questions

1. How will you assess Eleanor and her situation?
2. What advice will you give?
3. What other clinical, legal, clinico-legal, and ethical issues arise in the case?

Clinical

You must conduct a thorough assessment, including reviewing her past notes, interviewing Eleanor herself, speaking to her treating team, and corroborating some information by speaking (with her permission) to her closest friend.

Assume that you note symptoms of anxiety, agitation, tearfulness, and lability of mood, exacerbated by the profound headache caused by the hypertension of pre-eclampsia. Further assume that you then conclude, on balance, that Eleanor's symptoms do not indicate a new mental disorder, but that if they do, it is probably an adjustment disorder, to which she is predisposed by her personality disorder, or possibly an emerging depressive episode.

Legal

The test of mental capacity is set out in statute,[1] with some minor variation between the four jurisdictions. The essential elements of the tests are:

- understanding information relevant to the decision to be made;
- remembering information long enough to make a decision;
- using[2] the information ('weighing it in the balance') so as to come to a decision; and
- communicating the decision by some means.

A person can be said to lack mental capacity if they are unable to do one or more of the above; in RoI for any reason; and in the UK by reason of 'an impairment or disturbance in the functioning of their mind or brain'.[3]

A number of cases have addressed the issue of capacity to refuse life-saving treatment. The landmark case was *Re C*:[4] a man with an active psychotic illness refused recommended amputation of a gangrenous foot. It was this case that set out the test of mental capacity that then was formalised in the above-mentioned statutory mental capacity schemes several years later.

The key point is that the law accepts that a decision to refuse life-saving treatment can be legally enforceable if it is made according to certain criteria, and that the exercise of autonomy includes a right to make decisions with dire consequences for oneself, even if they appear irrational or foolish to others. In other words, a person's mental capacity to make even the gravest decisions depends upon their mental functioning, not upon their status as mentally disordered or upon the outcome of their decision-making process.

Cases involving pregnant women have been particularly fraught, as the courts have sought to balance in some way the life of an unborn child against the undoubted rights of a competent adult (given that the foetus has no rights in law). There have been several cases in which a Caesarean section has been performed on a pregnant woman against her wishes in order to save her and/or her baby's life, in which the definition of mental capacity has arguably been stretched, even distorted. For example, in *Re MB*,[5] a woman refused a life-saving Caesarean section because of a needle phobia (although she

---

[1] The AWISA 2000 in Scotland, followed by the MCA 2005 in E&W, the ADMCA 2015 in RoI and the MCANI 2016 in NI.

[2] This includes believing in the information (and not discarding it because it conflicts with a delusion e.g.), and 'appreciating' the information (i.e. recognising how it could apply to oneself—which is made explicit in the MCANI but not the other statutes).

[3] Scottish law uses the phrase 'mental disorder, or inability to communicate because of physical disability'.

[4] *Re C (Adult, refusal of treatment)* [1994] 1 All ER 819.

[5] *Re MB (Adult, medical treatment)* [1997] 38 BMLR 175 CA.

later agreed to it), and the court found that the phobia impaired her capacity to decide on that specific treatment at that specific time, and ordered the operation could go ahead.

The case of *St George's v S*[6] was very similar, on its facts, to Eleanor's. Ms S had refused a Caesarean section despite severe pre-eclampsia threatening her life and that of her baby, on the ground that she wanted a natural birth. She was diagnosed with depression and admitted to a neighbouring psychiatric hospital for assessment under mental health law. Despite stating in writing that she refused 'any medical or surgical intervention', that same night she was transferred, while still detained, to St George's Hospital, where a Caesarean section was performed the next day despite her refusal of consent.[7]

Ms S later sued the hospital successfully, and the Court of Appeal reaffirmed the right of competent adults (as they found she had been) to refuse even life-saving treatment for themselves and their unborn children, and it reaffirmed that neither mental health nor mental capacity law could allow enforced treatment (other than for mental disorder) 'merely because her thinking process was unusual, bizarre, or irrational, and thus contrary to the overwhelming majority of the community at large'. It also ruled, in essence, that such emergency declarations could not be made without the involvement of the patients or their legal representative.

In some cases of people with mental disorder, the courts have authorised a Caesarean section under *mental health* law, under very particular circumstances. For example, in *Tameside*,[8] a forty-one-year-old pregnant woman with a history of paranoid schizophrenia refused an induction and possible Caesarean section to safeguard the life of her baby because of a delusional belief that the obstetricians actually wanted to harm her baby. The court held, bizarrely, that the induction and Caesarean section amounted to *treatment for her mental disorder* because continued pregnancy was expected to cause her mental state to deteriorate further, while simultaneously preventing effective treatment for it (as an effective antipsychotic dose could harm the baby), and because the death of her baby in the womb would further harm her mental health. Such an approach utilising the earlier nonobstetric decision in *Re B* that 'treatment for mental disorder' included 'treatment of the consequences of mental disorder'.[9] However, it is not recommended to rely on this precedent without obtaining legal advice and perhaps a High Court declaration.

Clinico-legal

You will have to consider whether Eleanor can understand the treatment she is refusing and the consequences of refusal, despite her fear and agitation. Consider in particular whether the pre-eclampsia is affecting her cognitive function, including her memory of what is said to her, or whether her PD traits are impairing her ability to use information that is emotionally charged. In the UK, you must also determine whether there is a mental or neurological disorder, as otherwise she cannot be found to lack mental capacity.

If your opinion is that she has the capacity to refuse treatment, then you must advise the obstetricians that they can do no more than encourage Eleanor to change her mind, perhaps utilising any psychological understanding of her you have developed through your assessment.

If you conclude that she currently suffers from mental disorder, you should make clear that, even if it warrants detention for treatment under mental health law, this cannot authorise any obstetric procedure in the absence of a court order.

---

[6] *St George's Healthcare NHS Trust v S; R v Collins and others, ex parte S* [1998] 44 BMLR 160.

[7] She had contacted a solicitor who advised her and the hospital that she had the right to refuse the Caesarean section despite her detention under mental health law. The hospital obtained an emergency declaration from a judge in chambers authorising the treatment on the basis that 'her capacity to consent … may be affected by her current mental state'. The hospital's solicitor had told the judge that it was 'a life and death situation with minutes to spare' and that S had been in labour for twenty-four hours, which was untrue—she had not begun labour. Moreover, the hospital did not inform the judge that S had instructed solicitors. The hospital trust was very severely criticised on both points in the subsequent litigation, which found that the application to the judge (and therefore the authorisation of surgery) had been unlawful, as had been the transfer from the psychiatric hospital. S returned to the psychiatric hospital three days later after recovering from the surgery, whereupon she was reviewed by a consultant psychiatrist and immediately discharged from detention because there was no evidence of mental disorder under the MHA.

[8] *Tameside and Glossop Acute Services Trust v CH* [1996] 1 FLR 762. She was thirty-one-weeks pregnant; her baby had intrauterine growth retardation and was expected to die if not delivered urgently.

[9] *Re B (Adult: Refusal of treatment)* [2002] 2 FCR 1.

If your view is that she lacks mental capacity, the obstetricians could then decide to operate if they were satisfied it was in her best interests (not those of her baby)—provided she had not previously made a valid applicable advance decision against a Caesarean section in any circumstance.[10] Even if she *had* made such an advance decision, the clinical timing of events would be such that the obstetric team might take the view that they had to save her life by carrying out the section, and they might be reasonably concerned that a mother's advance directive would not be a defence in a clinical negligence case if the baby suffered injury during delivery.

In practice in such cases, there are usually good grounds for questioning whether the women in question have capacity to make a decision of this gravity. What they need is support and reassurance that they will be helped and cared for after the baby is delivered; and that they will feel much better once the labour is over.

Similar clinical anxieties arise when people with eating disorders refuse life-saving treatment. In *Re E*,[11] the judge supported forced feeding to keep E alive, but a key point was that she was found to have lost mental capacity. Conversely, in *Re W*,[12] the judge agreed with the hospital that, although W had lost capacity, forced treatment (feeding) was not in her best interests, and in *Re X*,[13] the court agreed with the hospital that, although X had lost capacity, she should not be forced to accept even life-saving treatment. In certain circumstances,[14,15] but not others,[16] refeeding can be a treatment authorised under mental health law itself.

The narrowing of the grounds appears to have resulted from direct application in the UK of Article 8 (the right to private and family life) of the European Convention on Human Rights, and reflection on whether the severity of the intrusion on a person that force feeding represents is proportionate to the severity of their mental disorder and risk to their life.

Ethical

These are cases about autonomy and respect for the principle that people should be able to control what happens to their own body without intrusion from the State, even if their decisions have dangerous or fatal outcomes for them or their offspring. *St George's v S* emphasised how unjust it can be to force someone into undergoing surgery because of the negative consequences of not doing so.

Medical professionals typically find it very difficult to tolerate the anxiety caused when refusal of treatment will put a person's life at risk, especially that of a healthy baby. The frustration and anxiety for the obstetricians is that a perfectly viable baby is minutes and inches away from life without injury

---

[10] The law on advance decisions in the UK and RoI is complex. In brief, to be enforceable in E&W and RoI, such a decision would have to specify clearly that Eleanor did not want a Caesarean section, even if she would die without one, would have to be in writing, signed, and witnessed (in RoI by two witnesses, and a designated healthcare representative) and not have been subsequently withdrawn, explicitly or implicitly. Advance decisions cannot be enforced in Scotland or Northern Ireland; they are often taken into account by doctors but would probably not be accepted as grounds to withhold life-saving treatment. Another option would be for her to arrange, before she loses capacity, for someone else to refuse treatment on her behalf, under a relevant power of attorney where available, or following a court judgment.

[11] *A Local Authority v E (by her litigation friend, the Official Solicitor)* [2012] EWHC 1639 (COP).

[12] *Re W (medical treatment: anorexia)* [2016] EWCOP 13.

[13] *Re X* [2014] EWCOP 35.

[14] *B v Croydon Health Authority* [1995] Fam 133. B suffered from BPD and PTSD. Nasogastric tube feeding was held to be ancillary to the core treatment alleviating the symptoms of her disorder.

[15] *R v Collins, ex parte Brady* [2000] Lloyd's Rep Med 355. Brady suffered from psychopathy and narcissistic personality disorder, and his hunger strike was deemed to be a manifestation of his mental disorder. The judge ruled that force feeding was a lawful treatment under s63 MHA, but also lawful under common law (this was before the MCA) because Brady lacked mental capacity at the time to decide not to accept food.

[16] *An NHS Trust v A* [2014] Fam 161. A suffered from delusional disorder and paranoia, possibly paranoid personality disorder. He expressed suicidal ideation, refused food, and made a number of political statements about the failure of his applications for asylum in the UK. The court found that he lacked capacity, that force feeding could not be authorised under the MCA in circumstances in which a deprivation of liberty was not permitted, but that despite the MCA the court retained inherent jurisdiction to authorise treatment for incapacitated adults involving such a deprivation in their best interests even if the DoLS criteria had not been met. It added that the meaning 'medical treatment' under the MHA should not be extended to include treatment involving a deprivation of liberty greater than that 'beyond what is properly within the ambit of' the MHA without first applying to the High Court for a declaration.

or disability, and from having full rights to protection in law. If the baby were born alive, Eleanor would be open to criminal charges if she subsequently put her baby's life at risk, but she can refuse treatment to save the baby's life before birth if she is deemed to have capacity. There is also an ethical and legal inconsistency with regard to Eleanor's autonomy in relation to termination; any attempt by Eleanor to have an abortion at this stage would be a criminal offence.

As human interactions, discussions about refusal of life-saving treatment are often suffused with high levels of emotion, especially if disability or death are possible outcomes. And many of the nonobstetric legal cases described above represent yet more examples of the importance of communication skills in ethical discourse, and of how important it is that discussions reflect exploration of different value positions and perspectives.

However, it does seem that wherever there is uncertainty over evidence of relevant mental disorder, the courts are likely to support an unborn baby's life over their mother's autonomy, until it is demonstrated unequivocally that the mother did indeed make a clear, capacitous decision to take a course of action that threatened her life and the life of her baby.

It would also be intriguing to speculate on the role of child protection services in the life of the child if they survived their mother's high-risk autonomous decision.

2

'Appropriate treatment' test–personality disorder

Themes: *personality disorder (p.78), psychological treatment (p.204), and offender treatment programmes (p.220) [C]; treatability (p.471) [L]; appropriate treatment (p.IV.107) [CL]; and what counts as treatment (p.340), and harm caused by loss of liberty (p.324) [E]*

Case description

Daniel is a thirty-year-old man who was sentenced to ten-years' imprisonment for the manslaughter of his partner; his earliest date of release is in nine-months' time. He has three prior convictions for minor violence. He was a victim of childhood physical and sexual abuse. He has diagnoses of paranoid, antisocial, and borderline PD, and a history of drug use.

He was transferred to hospital six months ago and is currently detained in a medium secure PD service under your care. He has intermittently withdrawn from treatment and occasionally self-harms. He is unpopular on the ward.

Recently, Daniel stopped attending therapy sessions, and then stopped speaking to staff at all. He said he would continue until returned to prison. Based upon his progress before stopping, the treating psychologist has estimated that, even if Daniel engaged fully, there is only a 40% chance that psychological treatment would significantly reduce the risk of violence arising from his severe PD.

A majority of the team believe there is no purpose to Daniel being in hospital, and his bed should be used for someone willing to engage in treatment. Some team members think that this is a stage that must be worked through before treatment can succeed.

Daniel has applied to the tribunal for discharge; you are preparing the medical report for the hearing.

1. Should you recommend continued detention?
2. What other clinical, legal, clinico-legal, and ethical issues arise in this case?

Clinical

Your report will need to state the team's view on what treatment, if any, is recommended. It may be difficult to plan more than for the short term, given the difficulties with engagement, but a key question is whether any treatment can be provided now, or only at a later stage, after a change in attitude. If possible, Daniel should be involved in the discussion. If he will not engage in this then provide him with information, such as in the form of written summaries. Attempting to include him in your discussions is both clinically advisable and ethically desirable.

Legal

All jurisdictions require the purpose of detention under mental health law to be treatment. The strongest test is in Scotland, where proposed treatment must be 'likely to prevent the mental disorder worsening; [to] or alleviate any of the symptoms, or effects, of the disorder'. By contrast, in RoI, treatment only has to be 'intended for the purposes of ameliorating a mental disorder', and in E&W, it need only be treatment 'the purpose of which is to alleviate, or prevent a worsening of, the disorder or one or more of its symptoms or manifestations.'[17]

The difference between the first pair and the second pair may appear subtle, but the latter can allow detention for a treatment with a very low probability of success (indeed no legal requirement of probability per se) and which the patient refuses to accept, whereas the former cannot.

'Treatment' is also very broadly defined, and includes medical, nursing, and other interventions and care, though not simply detaining someone, even in a hospital.[18] Treatment need not address every aspect of Daniel's disorder, so that it may still be 'appropriate treatment' even if it focuses only on violence to others. Finally, it does not need to be the best or most appropriate treatment.

There is no treatability test at the time of writing in NI; when the MCANI comes into effect, there will be a 'best interests and prevention of serious harm' test which covers similar ground.[19]

Clinico-legal

If you are treating Daniel in Scotland, you will have no choice but to recommend remission to prison because continued psychological treatment would not be 'likely' to improve his condition. However, in the other three jurisdictions, the weaker tests mean that you can detain him for further attempts at treatment, (assuming the other criteria for detention are met) even if he refuses to engage in the treatment.[20]

You may recommend continuing attempts to engage Daniel. His unwillingness does not itself make the treatment inappropriate in law, especially if your opinion is that of the minority in your team, that after going through this stage he would engage meaningfully.

Any opinions you give in relation to the treatment and its likely effect must be directed towards both Daniel and about PD in general. The same treatment could be appropriate for one patient, but inappropriate for another.

Ethical

The treatability tests described above are all that prevents mental health law being used to control dangerous individuals without prospect of improvement[21]; nevertheless, in E&W and RoI, they are arguably too weak to ensure that patients are not detained for purposes other than their own likely health benefit.[22,23]

---

[17] Until 2008, the definition in E&W was the same as that in NI.

[18] The precise definitions in each jurisdiction are explored in ethical case 16.

[19] At the time of writing, this is scheduled for 2021 or later. Simplifying slightly, the tests, under schedule 1 paragraph 9, are that it would be in the patient's best interests to have the treatment, and that (unless there is no objection) failure to provide the treatment would create a risk of serious harm to the patient or others, and the treatment is a proportionate response to the likelihood and seriousness of the harm.

[20] This is the case in RoI only because Daniel has been transferred from prison. Treatment for PD alone is excluded under the civil sections of the MHA and from inpatient treatment sentences under the CLIA.

[21] In NI, the lack of such a test means such 'administrative detention' is theoretically possible until the MCANI comes fully into effect.

[22] See for instance *R (W) v Rampton Hospital Authority* [2001] EWHC Admin 134; *MD v Nottinghamshire Health Care NHS Trust* [2010] UKUT 59 (AAC), in both of which detention was upheld despite explicit acknowledgement of there being very little prospect of successful treatment.

[23] The government's own recent review of the E&W Act has advised 'Detention criteria concerning treatment and risk should be strengthened to require that: (a) treatment is available which would benefit the patient, and not just serve public protection, which cannot be delivered without detention; and (b) there is a substantial likelihood of significant harm to the health, safety or welfare of the person, or the safety of any other person without treatment' (*Modernising the Mental Health Act—Final Report of The Independent Review of the Mental Health Act*, 2018).

Some PDs are clearly associated with an enhanced risk of harm to the public, and evidence-based treatments do exist for people with certain types of PD. However, arguably the legal criteria allowing detention for treatment in hospital should reflect psychiatric reality, and the prospect of real therapeutic benefit: meaning that without likely therapeutic benefit from being in hospital, antisocial behaviour in convicted offenders should be addressed within the criminal justice system. Indeed, one of the principles of the UK government's 'offender personality disorder strategy' is now that services be predominantly based in the criminal justice system.

The issue goes to the heart of the ethical practice of psychiatry, since current legislation diminishes the right to liberty, can result in harm to the patient,[24] and alienates psychiatry from the rest of medicine by permitting enforced treatment without significant prospect of success, which is not possible for other medical conditions under mental capacity law.

Moreover, as a responsible doctor you should only recommend treatment you consider likely to be effective, whatever legal power might exist and despite the risk of harm to others, and not engage in 'psycho-legal gymnastics' aimed at 'detention come what may'. Patients who drop out of treatment sometimes do worse than those who never engaged, and the longer-term harm of detaining someone without prospect of benefit may create a state of grievance which, rather than preparing them for treatment (by encouraging engagement), creates an obstacle to future treatment.

[24] In *MD v Notts* above, it was accepted that continued detention would worsen the manifestations of the patient's profound narcissistic PD.

3

Choosing between mental health and capacity law— autism, mild LD

Themes: *autism (p.104) and mild intellectual disability (p.110) [C]; detention under mental health law (p.466) and under mental capacity law (p.522), and deprivation of liberty (p.532) [L]; and determining mental capacity (p.523), the least restrictive principle (p.190) [CL], and what it is right to treat (p.338) [E]*

Case description

Michael is twenty-eight years old and has autism and mild intellectual disability. He usually lives in a care home but has become increasingly distressed, banging his head and trying to stick forks in his arm. There is no clear reason for this, but care home staff say they can no longer manage him safely and want him admitted to hospital. The regime in the care home does not amount to a 'deprivation of liberty'.

When assessed, he is very distressed. You establish that he wants to leave the care home and will continue to hurt himself until he does. However, he is unable to explain why. He communicates with the assistance of a speech and language therapist who knows him well; she is also unsure why he is so distressed. He is not in any physical pain; there have been no significant changes in his care or carers and no recent events that could explain his unhappiness.

He is assessed as lacking capacity to decide where he lives because of an inability to weigh or use the information relating to the decision. However, he is able to communicate that he wants to leave the care home, and does not object to going to hospital. You and he agree that he should be assessed in hospital, on a ward with a locked door but no special security.

Questions

1. How should do you decide which legal route to use?
2. What other clinical, legal, and ethical issues arise in this case?

> **Clinical**
>
> Review the past diagnostic records and reconsider his diagnoses. Consider any formulation of his problems, and therefore his treatment needs (if any). Then consider his care and treatment in the care home and what may have happened to precipitate the deterioration.

Legal

Deprivation of liberty is a legal term, perhaps most clearly defined in the landmark case *Cheshire West*.[25] The test turns on whether the person is 'under continuous supervision and control' and 'whether they are free to leave'. Almost every person admitted to any psychiatric hospital ward would be considered to be deprived of their liberty, especially if the ward is locked. Any deprivation of liberty must be lawfully authorised, and in this context that means under either mental health or mental capacity legislation.[26] (Sometimes the same provision will also authorise treatment, and sometimes a separate authorisation is needed.)

Mental capacity law only applies to patients who lack capacity, and can only be used to detain someone if special safeguards are met.[27] If in such circumstances the patient also has mental disorder, then they could also be detained under mental health law. Where both regimes apply, you should proceed with whichever would be less restrictive for the patient in their particular situation.

Scottish mental health law[28] includes a test of 'significantly impaired decision-making ability' before detention is lawful—a lower threshold than under Scottish mental capacity law.[29]

Clinico-legal

If it is assumed that there has been full exploration of different explanations of Michael's apparent deterioration in mental health using appropriate means, and on more than one occasion, then the main issue will be whether detention is indicated, and if so, under which legal regime.

You should consider whether Michael has the capacity to consent to the deprivation of liberty associated with his admission to hospital. If he does, detention would not be required. However, in this case it is assumed that he lacks capacity.

Some think that mental capacity law is by default less restrictive, although this appears to be based upon the idea that being 'sectioned' under mental health law is more stigmatising. You should consider the likelihood that Michael will not be compliant in future, or his capacity could fluctuate, in which case detention under mental health law would be less restrictive, as fewer delays and reassessments would then be likely.

Ethical

The fact that care, or treatment, amounts to 'deprivation of liberty' does not mean that it is inappropriate. It means only that it reaches a certain threshold such that statutory authorisation is required. Identifying and authorising a deprivation of liberty should not be a substitute for, or impede the delivery of, the highest quality of care. The focus of decision-making must remain Michael's expressed interests (or best interest if appropriate). Nothing in either law is intended to prevent timely and appropriate medical treatment.

---

[25] *Cheshire West and Chester Council v P* [2014] UKSC 19, [2014] MHLO 16.
[26] Or in exceptionally rare cases, the inherent jurisdiction of the High Court.
[27] The Deprivation of Liberty Safeguards or (from later in 2020) Liberty Protection Safeguards in E&W; the MCANI authorisation procedure; a decision-making order or agreement in RoI; or an intervention or guardianship order in Scotland.
[28] Mental Health (Care and Treatment) (Scotland) Act 2003; Mental Health (Scotland) Act 2015.
[29] Adults with Incapacity (Scotland) Act 2000.

4 Assessment at the police station–psychosis and murder charge

Themes: *schizoaffective disorder (p.73), ASPD (p.82), assessing level of security (p.190), and diversion from custody (p.268) [C]; advance statement (p.536), police bail (p.398), and remand to hospital (p.498) [L]; fitness to be interviewed (p.573) [CL]; and balancing welfare and justice (p.314) [E]*

Case description

You work in a Criminal Justice Liaison Service. A police liaison nurse calls you about Malcolm, a thirty-nine-year-old man arrested on suspicion of attempted murder and arson with intent. He allegedly set a fire under his mother-in-law's bed while she slept. The nurse, and the Forensic Medical Examiner who has also assessed him, think him psychotic and that he lacks capacity: he ignores everyone most of the time and appears to talk to an invisible figure, although he told the FME he was not unwell, and certainly did not need medical treatment.

You consult Malcolm's medical records and note that he is known to a local CMHT, that he has well-established diagnoses of schizoaffective disorder and ASPD, and that his team have been trying to track him down since staff at his hostel reported last week that he had stopped taking his oral antipsychotic medication. You also see that, during a hospital admission two years ago, after he had recovered from a psychotic episode, he made an 'advance statement' in his collaborative crisis plan that, if he relapsed again, he wanted to be treated with oral medication in the community, and if necessary, be admitted to a particular open ward at his local hospital, where he had a good experience in the past.

The nurse thinks Malcolm should be detained and diverted to hospital immediately, but the custody sergeant, while not doubting he needs medical treatment, will not bail him because of the seriousness of the alleged offences. The nurse asks you to step in and speak to the custody sergeant.

Questions

1. What is the relevance of Malcolm's advance statement?
2. Assuming you agree with the nurse and FME's assessments, what will you say to the custody sergeant?
3. What additional steps do you need to take, whichever route to admission is adopted?
4. What other clinical, legal, clinico-legal, and ethical issues arise in this case?

Clinical

The immediate clinical concern is to ensure he receives treatment in a suitable place, where he and others will be safe. However, any clinical recommendation you make under mental law could be 'trumped' by criminal justice law and procedure, and you should take this into account.

Legal

There are several legal provisions which may be relevant, including safeguards for mentally disordered people in custody (e.g. the presence of an appropriate adult), the criminal law itself, and law allowing transfer to hospital. Transfers could be under civil provisions of mental health law, or on the order of a court.

Treatment can be started at the police station if Malcolm changes his mind and assents to it, or if he is at such risk of immediately harming himself or others that the treatment is justified, immediately necessary, and proportionate to the likelihood and seriousness of harm[30]; or potentially under mental capacity law. Mental health law does not allow treatment to be coerced outside hospital settings.[31]

In certain circumstances, advance decisions to refuse treatment can be binding on professionals.[32] Even if not binding (as Malcom's request for certain treatments would not be in the UK), relevant advance statements of wishes should be taken into account when patients lack capacity. However, mental health law can override even binding advance decisions.

Clinico-legal

Police officers tend to be reluctant to allow treatment in custody unless a member of healthcare staff will remain indefinitely after it has been given (because of concern about failing to spot, or being unable to deal with, any side-effects, or other consequences, of the treatment). At present, Malcom is refusing treatment, and the risk to him and others does not make it immediately necessary.

In discussing Malcolm with the custody sergeant, you should acknowledge and respect the rules with which the sergeant must comply, and the legitimacy of seeking to prosecute Malcolm. But you should ensure the sergeant understands and records that Malcolm appears to be suffering from an acute psychotic episode, and requires urgent treatment in hospital. You could discuss what safeguards might enable police bail to hospital pending further investigation to be agreed (e.g. admission under civil mental health law to a secure ward with an undertaking from the treating team not to release Malcolm without prior discussion with the police). However, given the gravity of the charge, this is unlikely. In any event, you are not in a position to undertake a sufficiently robust risk assessment, including data from witness statements, in order to determine what level of secure care Malcolm needs.

Assuming Malcolm remains in police custody until brought before the court later that day or the following morning, you should arrange to recommend to the court that he be remanded to hospital by the court,[33] with a backup plan of liaison with the local prison inreach psychiatric team were the court to remand him to prison instead.

If Malcolm is likely to have done what is alleged, this would dramatically alter your assessment of the risk of harm he might pose to others, including staff and other patients in a hospital. At this stage,

[30] The precise wording varies between jurisdictions, and the proportionality requirement does not apply in Scotland.

[31] An exception would arise if Malcolm were already subject to a Community Treatment Order in E&W, or a Compulsory Treatment Order covering community treatment in Scotland, or had been conditionally discharged under a restricted hospital order or compulsion order, in which case he could in principle be required to take treatment while at the police station, on pain of otherwise being readmitted to hospital, but no force could be used to compel him without first recalling him to hospital.

[32] In E&W and RoI, if the patient lacks capacity, the advance decision clearly covers the treatment and its circumstances (and has not been withdrawn, superseded or resiled from), and certain formalities are met. In RoI, requests for certain treatment, as well as refusals, can be binding. The law in Scotland does not yet make such decisions binding; the common law in NI may do.

[33] This would involve liaison with the psychiatric diversion team covering that court, and forwarding to them your recommendation for remand to hospital, under s35 MHA in E&W, s52A CPSA in Scotland, Art42 MHNIO, or s4(6) CLIA in RoI.

in the absence of a comprehensive risk assessment, you must assume he might have done it, and therefore arrange for admission to a to a unit with sufficient physical, procedural, and relational security. This is likely to mean a medium secure forensic psychiatric ward.

Separately, you should assess whether he is unfit to be interviewed at present, and even if he is fit, highlight to the custody sergeant that he is a vulnerable detainee.

Ethical

This case raises two relevant ethical principles: ensuring prompt treatment for someone who is severely unwell, and prosecuting someone alleged to have committed a very serious offence, in the interests of justice and public protection. Neither principle can properly 'trump' the other: a balance must be struck between them.

At the same time, as a psychiatrist you cannot be neutral with respect to these two principles. Since you are the clinical leader of a liaison team assessing him, Malcolm is your patient, and you owe him a duty of care (whilst to the custody sergeant he is a detained suspect). Your primary duty is therefore to ensure that he receives as full an assessment as necessary, and urgent treatment as quickly as possible, through negotiation with the criminal justice system.

It is important that any emotional response to your advice being discounted by the custody sergeant does not interfere with your subsequent decision-making, and has no detrimental impact on Malcolm.

If charges against Malcolm are authorised and he is remanded into custody, your duty of care does not end there, and you should ensure proper follow-up throughout the criminal justice process.

5 Residual common law powers–delay in emergency situations

> **Themes:** *schizophrenia (p.73), organic personality change (p.116), risk of impulsive aggression (p.168) [C], detention by police under mental health law (p.494), false imprisonment (p.436), and residual common law powers (p.476) [L]; processes for authorising detention in emergency (p.476) [CL]; and conflict between duty to patient and the law (p.298) [E]*

Case description

You have been Joe's community psychiatrist for two years, following discharge from hospital. He had been convicted of common assault and received an unrestricted hospital order. He has schizophrenia, and organic personality change resulting from a serious head injury with a hammer when he was aged seventeen years.

He had eight convictions prior to the head injury, all for common assault. His risk of impulsive aggression remains high; his behaviour has been difficult to predict, although his aggression is usually triggered by delusions or hallucinations. Joe is prescribed clozapine and sodium valproate, which he accepts voluntarily. He lives in a mental health care home. He does not use drugs or alcohol.

The police have detained Joe today, for throwing bricks at a shop. When the police arrived, he shouted that there was a bear in the shop; he had scratched a symbol into his forehead. He was first taken to A&E, where his injuries were found to be superficial and to require no treatment, and then to a place of safety in a psychiatric hospital.[34]

On arrival, Joe was very agitated, muttering about animals possessing people. He kept following staff out of the room. He refuses to allow you to speak to him, and swears at you when you try. You think that, on balance, he has capacity to refuse admission, and he certainly objects to the idea of treatment. Together with the relevant professionals[35] you agree that he meets the criteria for civil detention for assessment. However, with one hour of the legal detention period left, no bed is available.

Questions

1. What would you advise should happen next?
2. What other clinical, legal, clinico-legal, and ethical issues arise in this case?

---

[34] Under s136 MHA in E&W, art130 MHNIO, s297 MHCTA in Scotland, and s12 MHA in RoI.
[35] An Approved Mental Health Practitioner (AMHP) in E&W, Mental Health Officer in Scotland or Approved Social Worker in NI, plus in E&W or NI a second doctor. In RoI another suitable adult must be involved.

> **Clinical**
> The clinical imperative is to ensure that Joe receives appropriate treatment without delay.

> **Legal**
> Mental health law in the UK sets strict limits[36] on how long a patient can be detained because of presumed mental ill-health on the order of a police officer. And where it allows for the period to be extended, this is only for a single additional twelve-hour period, and only because the patient's condition (e.g. intoxication) prevents assessment: not because of delays in the arrival of staff, or in obtaining a bed. After this time, Joe must either be released or detained under an alternative legal provision; otherwise detention will be unlawful 'false imprisonment', for which he can claim compensation.
>
> Had you believed that Joe lacked capacity, there might be scope to detain and treat him under mental capacity law; although in such situations, where the criteria of mental health law also apply, you should attempt to use mental health law first. (If he did lack capacity, in order to detain and treat him against his will, you would need to satisfy yourself that the treatment, and any force or threatened force, were necessary to prevent harm, and proportionate to the likelihood and seriousness of that harm.[37])
>
> As he retains capacity, the legal question becomes whether any residual common law power exists to allow you to continue to detain Joe until a bed becomes available and you can implement the assessment order under mental health law.
>
> There was from 2005, at least in E&W, case law that any person, including staff in a mental hospital, can take reasonable and proportionate action to prevent immediate significant harm to others.[38] However, a subsequent English case,[39] amplifying an earlier Scottish one,[40] left the law unclear in relation to the powers of mental health staff: it stated on the one hand that there is no common law power to detain (under the doctrine of 'necessity', for instance) in a situation in which the Mental Health Act applied, but also that 'it is unlikely … that there will be a false imprisonment … if there is no undue delay during the processing of an application for admission under sections 2 or 4 … '; which appears to mean that the courts will allow brief periods of detention beyond a time limit as long as there is no 'undue delay' in applying for a section.
>
> Until either Parliament or the courts rectify this unsatisfactory legal situation, clinicians and their employers are left to decide, in situations like Joe's, whether to risk being held to have detained patients without lawful authority, or to risk being found to have negligently released persons who then harm themselves or others. The only option may be to base this difficult decision on the likelihood and severity of harm that would result if the patient were not detained.

> **Clinico-legal**
> Your dilemma is whether to authorise detaining Joe for longer, in the absence of a statutory power, until he is admitted or to risk harm being done if you release him. Your hospital should have issued you with guidance for this situation, which you should follow.

[36] Twenty-four hours in E&W, or thirty-six if extended because of the patient's condition; twenty-four hours in Scotland; forty-eight hours in NI, reducing to twenty-four when the MCANI comes into effect. There is no time limit in RoI.
[37] This is the simplified wording from the MCA in E&W, the MCANI, and the ADMCA in RoI. The AWIA in Scotland refers to force being 'immediately necessary'.
[38] *R (Munjaz) v Ashworth Hospital Authority* [2005] UKHL 58.
[39] *R (Sessay) v South London & Maudsley NHSFT and another* [2011] EWHC 2617. In this case, Ms Sessay had been removed unlawfully from her home by police who believed they had the power to take her under s5 of the MCA. She remained unlawfully detained in the hospital's s136 suite for a further period of time (the hospital staff wrongly believing that she had been detained by police under s136) until she was lawfully detained under s2. The hospital had taken thirteen hours to complete detention under s2, which was held to represent an unnecessary delay. Ms Sessay was compensated for false imprisonment by the police and (for the thirteen hours) by the hospital trust.
[40] *Black v Forsey* 1988 SLT 572, HL(Sc). The House of Lords held that the MHCTA was a complete code and there was no common law power to detain in Scotland when mental health law applied, and detention of the patient after the expiry of the time limit for renewal was unlawful.

Your decision-making will, in part, depend upon your analysis of the patient's treatment needs, and the risks and benefits of different options. You should consider the risks to Joe and the risks to others from Joe, as well as your assessment of how likely it is that, if you continue to detain him, it will be possible to admit him without 'undue delay'.

Whatever your decision, you should not implement it without taking into account the views of colleagues, and escalating the decision through your employer's management hierarchy (e.g. informing your Clinical Director or Medical Director before acting).

Ethical

Your duty is to make the care of your patient your first concern; yet this may conflict with your obligation to act within the law (if the common law does not permit Joe's continued detention, which is unclear). If so, acting within the law may result in harm to your patient's health, and potentially to other people. You may wish to discuss the situation and your planned action with your medical indemnity organisation.

You also have a duty to make decisions in consultation with patients; although, in this situation, your patient has made his opinion clear and now refuses to talk to you. You should try to explain whatever decision you make, nevertheless.

Critiquing decisions

In Part A we outlined ways in which we all make decisions, both the apparently rational processes that we may fool ourselves into thinking dominate our decision-making and the nonrational processes, with attendant heuristics and bias, that actually influence the vast bulk of our day-to-day decision-making, including describing ways in which our values influence and guide both. That is, we addressed what might be termed *internal fine-grain decision-making*. And we then invited you, the reader, both to make decisions in each of the cases in Part B of the book, and then to reflect upon how you came to those decisions, including viewing your processes through the prism of the theory presented in Part A and in relation to some practical NHS decision-making guidelines. Finally, in regard to 'real-world' practice, we suggest not only that past decisions might be critiqued in this way but also that any decision 'taken but yet to be implemented' might similarly be subjected to personal critique *before* their implementation.

We turn now, in Part C, to offer a brief description of the wide range of paradigms that are utilised in *external* critiquing of decisions implemented (i.e. critiquing by someone, or body, other than the original decision-maker), recognising that they vary in the extent to which each is capable of approaching, or will be likely to approach, the methods and standard of fine-grain internal critiquing described in Part A. That is, against the standard of what should be high-quality internal self-critiquing of decisions.

Perhaps understandably, the reader may immediately assume that Part C is about critiquing decisions that 'went wrong': that is, where there was a bad outcome. This is most acutely observed within forensic psychiatry in the inquiry literature, particularly inquiries into homicides committed by mentally disordered individuals. However, what makes a decision 'good' or 'bad' should not be the outcome, but the *process* by which the decision was reached. And this leads to the key practice advice 'show your workings': that is, show how you reached the decision and upon what information it was based. Since having to reflect upon and then write down your thinking (even if only in brief notes) will encourage both rigour and insight in regard to the decision process being applied. Also, only by doing so will there be, *ex post*, some record of how a decision came to be made, as well as what alternative decisions were rejected, and why.[1] And it is in this vein that we would offer the further advice to self-critique all your past major decisions (whether the outcome was 'bad' or 'good'), and thereby learn by reflecting.

Further, outcomes are not properly singular,[2] although they tend to be viewed as such when looked at in retrospect after some bad outcome has occurred. For example, giving community leave to a patient (e.g. as in clinical case 16), followed by an assault by the patient upon another whilst on leave, will tend to be viewed solely in terms of the outcome of having given leave, and even solely in terms of the assault having occurred—but proper outcome assessment should be comprehensive, so as to take account also (in this example) of what might have been the likely negative outcomes of *not* granting a programme of leave, for example, in terms of failed or delayed rehabilitation, and lost liberty, or even of a frustrated patient committing a more serious assault on the ward—an example of WYSIATI and the narrative fallacy (see Part A). That is, it is important to guard against

---

[1] Reconstructing retrospectively a decision process without the aid of contemporaneous notes is highly likely to be heavily distorted by knowledge of what was the outcome of the decision: that is, it is likely to layer 'hindsight bias' upon any previous 'decision bias'.

[2] See Cohen A and Eastman N L G (1997) Needs assessment for mentally disordered offenders and others requiring similar services: Theoretical issues and a methodological framework, *British Journal of Psychiatry* 171: 412–416; and Cohen A and Eastman N (2000) *Assessing Forensic Mental Health Need: Policy, Theory and Research*, Gaskell, which both elaborate on 'perspectives' on need and 'outcome' measures in forensic mental health care.

observed (usually bad) outcomes being viewed without consideration of other outcomes that properly should reflect a *range* of objectives of treatment.

Moreover, stakeholders are usually multiple, with each bringing their own approach to decision-making and, often crucially, different values (see Values-based decision-making in Part A).

Having come to a decision, including one taken but not yet implemented, it is good practice to unpick that decision critically, in terms of the types of decision processes outlined in Part A. Asking, for example, How did I come to this (proposed) decision?; also How did I come to reject the alternative decisions I could have made? As suggested, we might call this 'fine-grain' critiquing: really getting into reflective detail of our previous individual internal decision processes, including recognising the role that our (often conflicting) values played, as well as considering what were any group processes of the team within which we work (again often expressing conflicting values). And here the reader might like to read again the table of ease, bias and heuristics in Part A that offered some common forensic practice examples of heuristics and bias, plus some suggested means to counteract them.

Understandably we may, in real practice, often come to engage in this 'fine-grain' process, particularly when there has indeed been a single bad outcome or at least a near miss,[3] and if the outcome, or near miss, is bad enough, we may do so unhelpfully by way of nonconstructive obsessive rumination, rather than via structured and informed self-reflection. But we should be routinely critiquing *all* our major decisions, irrespective of their outcomes.

However, these processes are all *internal*, usually to the individual clinician or to their team. Yet critiquing decisions made is often also undertaken, almost always when there has been a particularly bad outcome, by way of a range of methodologies and bodies that are *external* to the individual decision-taker (and here we include e.g. 'internal service inquiry', since this also is external to the individual clinician or team). And this will risk *not* being 'fine-grain', in the terms of Part A, and/or the method adopted may vary from being analysis that is grounded in clinical reality (and thereby be potentially flawed by that route). In summary, therefore, although any critique paradigm *should* take note of all of theory presented in Part A, different paradigms will tend to do so, or be capable of doing so, to differing degrees and in differing ways.

In essence, what we are interested in therefore in this Part C is the extent to which different external critique methods are capable of taking note of, and applying, or will tend to take note of, the theory of decision-making described in Part A in coming to their conclusions, as well as considering what data and processes their particular methodologies privilege, downplay, or ignore.

---

[3] Although critiquing near miss events is still, at least in the NHS, rare, arising only perhaps in the context of audit across cases in the aggregate or within honestly pursued individual clinician appraisal.

C.1
The critique matrix

We can perhaps most easily address external critiquing of decisions by considering a 'matrix' with two dimensions (see civil law case 1 as an example). First, is the level of critique: that is, is the subject matter an individual case, a case type, or a whole area of practice? Second, is the method of critique: for example, clinical, legal, professional regulatory, internal service inquiry, external inquiry, or peer review. Various methods can be applied to the different levels of critique; albeit some methods do not fit some levels (e.g. the clinical method of audit only operates on case types or areas of practice, not individual cases).

We propose to elaborate on the varying methods by describing the nature and limitations of each, and by recognising therefore how each may be inadequate and/or biased when set against the standards of 'fine-grain' theory described in Part A.[1] Such inadequacy or bias may be inferred, first, by virtue of restrictions arising from its formal process, perhaps most obviously in the law[2]; and secondly, by virtue of the fact that all external methods are, as with individual or team cognitive decision-making, potentially influenced by many of the same factors described in Part A. Any investigation itself involves making decisions, and is undertaken by human beings, who will unavoidably bring their own heuristics, biases, and values, and their group interaction with their colleagues.

The origins of the *in*validity, or at least restricted validity, of a critique method will lie most profoundly in the method failing adequately to investigate what were the contemporaneous heuristics, biases, and values that can be identified as having been active at the time clinical or other decisions were made, and/or then substituting the external critiques' *own* heuristics, biases and values for those previously identified heuristics and biases, without adequate justification for such substitution.[3] These biases and heuristics may include, for example, a critique forum unconsciously substituting an easier question for what was, in fact, a difficult one; applying a causal model to a situation requiring statistical inference (leading to 'hindsight bias'); basing confidence on narrative coherence rather than statistical probability; selecting answers based on narrative familiarity and cognitive

---

[1] Here we intend by *bias* to refer to *inherent* aspects of a method of critiquing that tend to influence the outcome, rather than referring to that method being used in a biased fashion (e.g. because of prejudice on the part of one or more of the individuals involved).

[2] For example, the rules on admissibility of evidence which exclude evidence of risk of harm that would have been taken into account in a clinical risk assessment.

[3] Consider, perhaps, the recent controversial prosecution of a retired senior police officer for failings in the series of events that led to the deaths of ninety-six people at Hillsborough Stadium in 1989. It can be argued that one of the values applied by many police officers in 1989 was that of solidarity amongst police officers in the face of any perceived attack. It can also be argued that one of the values being applied in contemporary public debate and the subsequent legal proceedings is that justice must be done, meaning that the families of those who died must be able to see someone being held to account for the deaths of their loved ones. Both of these are understandable values—but both are potentially in conflict with the value of revealing the truth.

ease; representing categories of choices in terms of prototypes or exemplars; overweighting unlikely but associatively coherent events and underweighting likely but dissonant ones; as well as inappropriately applying the anchoring, availability, and affect heuristics.

Instead, a valid critique should seek out (amongst other things) what were the heuristics, biases, and values that underpinned the decision process and then express a view as to whether, at the time and in the circumstances of the decision-making, those aspects were justifiable, even if they were not what the external reviewer would have applied.

In summary, therefore, there is a range of external critique paradigms, and the paradigm within which a critique is conducted will very likely influence the conclusions reached—to the extent that different paradigms applied to the same 'bad outcome' may come to differing conclusions, even when they purport to ask the same, or at least nearly the same question.[4] An illustration of this is offered by comparing the possible conclusions of an internal NHS inquiry and legal proceedings for negligence: the latter is constructed to address a series of very specific legally defined questions, with rules as to what evidence is admissible, and in what manner it is considered, and where there are strict rules concerning the location of the burden and standard of proof, whereas the former can be set up in any one of a number of ways, usually with far less attention to any required rules of procedure, fact finding, or blame attribution. So that, for example, a healthcare professional may be subject to managerial sanction arising from the internal NHS inquiry, and/or be sanctioned by their professional regulator, and yet be found not to be legally liable for the bad outcome that ensued.

---

[4] As will become apparent, different critiquing methods often do address *different* questions, albeit arising from the same 'bad outcome', and are designed to do so. However, even where the forum chosen is specific for only one purpose, or group of purposes, the outcome of its deliberations can sometimes influence, even 'contaminate', either formally or informally, conclusions that should properly arise from a different forum (see Case Study below).

C.2
Legal critiquing in general

Legal critique is, for clinicians, perhaps the most feared critique paradigm. Not merely by virtue of the potential for legal sanction but also because it is in this context that they are most likely to feel in an alien world, subject to language and rules that are not of their clinical world.

The two 'territories' of medicine and law[1] are profoundly different in their purposes and methods, as is evident from the difficulties often experienced in clinico-legal practice, and will have been observed within many of the cases in Part B, of 'mapping' a medically defined mental state onto any given, or a number of different legal definitions or tests. Although some legal domains are more reflexive than others in being able to incorporate the constructs and methods of medicine,[2] whatever legal domain one is in will contain profound differences of method and process from clinical practice because law tends ultimately towards being a closed or 'autopoietic'[3] intellectual system.

Most fundamentally and practically, whereas medicine is investigative by method, and admits all potentially relevant data in order to determine truth, law in common law jurisdictions is mainly adversarial, and thereby restricts data to that which, in fairness, is 'admissible' and to process that is similarly fair. So as to come to truth, the finding of which is constrained by its pursuit of justice.

All the specific legal domains potentially relevant to critiquing clinical or clinico-legal decisions are laid out in Parts IV and V of the handbook. However detailed consideration of the following case study of alleged clinical negligence, and the various legal contexts and fora within which that case was considered, will serve to introduce the contrast between legally based critiquing, across a range of contexts and fora, with 'fine-grain' clinically based critiquing.

---

[1] The concepts of medicine and law as 'territories' or 'lands' is explored in the opening chapter of Part IV of the handbook.

[2] See King M and Piper C (1995) *How the Law Thinks about Children*, 2nd ed. Arena, who describe family law being more reflexive than other legal domains, particularly criminal law.

[3] See Teubner G (1993) *Law as an Autopoietic System*. Blackwell, who describes law as ultimately capable only of 'creating from within itself'; that is being nonreflexive in its response to evidence from other disciplines. Albeit different domains of law are *variously* nonreflexive: for example family law is much less so than criminal law (again see King M and Piper C (1995) *How the Law Thinks about Children*, second edition. Arena).

C.3

A case study of critiquing clinical decision-making within multiple paradigms

The well-known case of a higher trainee paediatrician Dr Bawa-Garba, who was convicted of manslaughter as a result of her role in the death of a young boy with Down's syndrome, illustrates the differences of process and outcome between prosecution for gross negligence manslaughter, civil legal negligence, professional regulatory proceedings, and internal service inquiries.

All the material given in the description that follows is in the public domain, released by the inquiries concerned.

The clinical case

Dr Bawa-Garba was a higher trainee in paediatrics who reportedly had an impeccable training record before she went on maternity leave in 2010. She returned to clinical work in 2011, and was placed almost immediately in an acute paediatric setting, one she had had no recent experience of before she had gone on leave.[1]

---

[1] We have chosen a case of a paediatrician because of its wide notoriety. However, there are examples in psychiatry, as well, such as that of general psychiatrist who was sanctioned by the GMC for having 'failed to disclose that he had no previous experience of acting as an expert witness in a homicide case; and … [being] reckless in a number of respects in his work as an expert for his failure of acquaintance with criminal expert witness practice.' The sanction was upheld by the High Court: *Kumar v GMC* [2012] EWHC 2688 (Admin).

The details of the clinical story are important, and are as follows.[2] 'On 18th February 2011 Jack Adcock (a young boy with Down's syndrome) was admitted to Leicester Royal Infirmary with a history of severe gastroenteritis. He had previously had an AVSD [atrio-ventricular septal defect, a "hole in the heart"] repair, doing well on enalapril. He had a temperature of 37.7 degrees centigrade, dehydration and shock. A blood gas showed a pH of 7.0, a base deficit of -14, lactate 11mmol. He was prescribed a fluid bolus and maintenance fluids. Blood tests, including CRP, were undertaken and a chest X-ray ordered. There was a delay of two and a half hours in reviewing the chest X-ray, during which time Jack showed some recovery ... (with) improvement in blood gas, to pH 7.24. Jack was moved off the Children's Assessment Unit (CAU) to the wards, where an un-prescribed dose of enalapril was administered [by his mother]. Approximately one hour later he suffered a collapse from which he was very sadly unable to be resuscitated.'

The account continues, 'the registrar that day was Dr Hadiza Bawa-Garba, a high-flying doctor, with an unblemished record ... who had ... just returned from 13 months' maternity leave. Her last general paediatric post, ST4, commenced four years earlier in a DGH, outside Leicester. She had received no Trust induction. When she came to work that day she found that the registrar covering CAU was on training, away from the wards. Dr Bawa-Garba was requested to cover CAU as well as her own ward duties. Working under her were a foundation doctor and SHO. Both had only rotated to paediatrics that month. The consultant covering CAU was teaching outside the city. ...

Provision of care was dogged by the breakdown in IT facilities for the whole hospital, meaning that the team were constantly phoning to try to get results. Even when back online, the flag system for abnormal results was down. The nursing staff were hard pressed, with staffing and equipment shortages logged. Jack was looked after by an agency nurse with a certificate in adult nursing. ...'

As regards the aftermath, the account reads, 'It is not clear what de-brief for the staff involved was undertaken after the tragic events of that day, but Dr Bawa-Garba met with her consultant in the hospital canteen, where she felt under pressure to fill in areas of a trainee encounter form.'

The account adds, 'She continued to work without problem and indeed with plaudits.'

Almost finally, 'a serious untoward incident inquiry was undertaken following the patient's death, which was completed on 24th August 2012. A 14-person investigation team concluded that a single root cause for the death[3] was unable to be identified. Numerous parts of the clinical process were identified as needing change. The report highlighted 23 recommendations and 79 actions that were undertaken by Leicester Royal Infirmary as a result of the organisational learning.'

The legal cases

Dr Bawa-Garba was arrested and questioned on 17 December 2014 and later charged with manslaughter on the grounds of gross negligence. She was convicted on 4 November 2015, after twenty-five-hours' deliberation by the jury, on a majority verdict of ten to two. On 8 December 2016, she was denied leave to appeal, and on 13 June 2017, she was suspended for a year by the Medical Practitioners Tribunal Service [MPTS]. The GMC then

---

[2] Summary taken directly from *Position of University Hospitals of Leicester NHS Trust in Relation to Dr Hadiza Bawa-Garba*, April 2018.
[3] See below concerning 'root cause analysis'.

successfully appealed to the High Court to overturn the MPTS suspension, and instead erase Dr Bawa-Garba from the Medical Register. Health Education England withdrew her training number.

The Position Statement of the hospital notes, 'on 7th December 2017, considering the arguments surrounding the GMC case for erasure, the judge asked to know what was different about ... the day of the tragic events surrounding Jack's death. This may presuppose that all works smoothly on other days, although we do not know the level of incidents, recorded or unrecorded error, near miss, death or disability from care on other days.'

On 12 February 2018 the Court of Appeal reinstated Dr Bawa-Garba on the Medical Register (subject to the originally imposed suspension).

In criminal law there is an initial four-stage test for gross negligence manslaughter that includes: 'a breach of the doctor's duty of care which ... causes (or significantly contributes to) the death; and the breach should be characterised as gross negligence, and therefore a crime.' [4] This is then further elaborated: 'the death was reasonably foreseeable; where the conduct of the defendant was *so bad* in *all the circumstances* as to go beyond the requirement of compensation and to amount to a criminal act or omission; ... and *so reprehensible* as to justify ... that it amounted to gross negligence and requires *criminal* sanction[5,6] ... an obvious risk is a present risk which is clear and unambiguous, not one which might become apparent on further investigation'[7] (emphases added). That is, within legal critiquing, a distinction is drawn between criminal and (lesser) civil negligence.

Thus, having been found guilty in the criminal court, Dr Bawa-Garba was initially only suspended for one year by the MPTS (see civil law case 8 as an example of an MPTS case), which decision was then successfully appealed by the GMC to the High Court, specifically on the basis that the MPTS had wrongly 'gone behind' (reconsidered the reasoning lying behind) the doctor's criminal conviction, for the decision then to be replaced by erasure from the Medical Register. That decision was in turn reversed by the Court of Appeal in favour of the original MPTS decision, effectively on the basis that the purpose, and legal role, of the MPTS was entirely different from that of a criminal court, in that its focus was not criminal negligence but fitness to practice, which required particular and careful consideration of *all the circumstances* in which the doctor had been placed when she made her erroneous clinical decisions, and also of her training record overall.[8]

The case is of particular note for our purposes in that Dr Bawa-Garba's decision-making was critiqued by way of criminal law, professional regulation, legal appeal, and then further legal appeal, as well as by way of a coroner's inquest, and by an internal NHS inquiry using 'root cause analysis' (see below). She was first found guilty of gross negligence manslaughter in a criminal court; second, subject to criticism for her actions in an (adjourned, incomplete) coroner's inquest; third, deemed sufficiently clinically competent as merely to be suspended for a period from practice and offered further support and training at an MPTS hearing; fourth, deemed so clinically incompetent as to justify erasure from

---

[4] *R v Adomako* (1994) 3 WLR 288.

[5] *R v Rose* [2017] EWCA Crim 11681.

[6] Notably, as critiqued by some lawyers (e.g. Sir Robert Francis QC, in his evidence to the relevant Parliamentary Select Committee), the definition is effectively for the jury to determine, since there is no clear legal test per se.

[7] Inquiries conducted after adverse incidents may not fully hold, in practice, to this latter caveat in the law of criminal negligence; thus expressing 'hindsight bias'.

[8] The GMC argued, in both the High Court and Court of Appeal, that the jury must have taken account of these factors in finding her guilty, given that the definition of the criminal offence *requires* consideration of 'all the circumstances'. However, the forum and manner of consideration of such matters is profoundly different within an MPTS hearing compared with a criminal trial, in front of a jury.

the Medical Register as a result of criminal conviction of gross negligence manslaughter in a criminal court; then deemed sufficiently competent to be reinstated in the Court of Appeal; and finally, an internal NHS inquiry failed to find her to be worthy of sanction, identifying numerous parts of the clinical process as needing change, rather than focusing on the doctor's causal role.

Dr Bawa-Garba has not, at least to date, also had to face civil negligence proceedings, although she could have done.[9] All doctors can potentially be sued in civil negligence in regard to their role in a clinical misadventure; albeit the negligence need not cross the high threshold required for criminal negligence. Here she would have been judged against the *Bolam* standard of whether what she did was within the practice of a responsible body of medical practitioners at her level of experience, properly supervised,[10] so long as the practice considered 'was capable of withstanding logical analysis'.[11]

The internal NHS inquiry[12] referred to above concluded, having of course taken account of 'all the circumstances', that there had been 'failure of medical staff to understand the significance of, and to communicate abnormal blood test results; failure of nursing staff to recognize the significance of abnormal observations and record and monitor according to clinical need; ambiguity of the observation and investigation tools used in the hospital; poor communication of the clinical condition between staff because of the absence of effective systems of handover (medical and nursing); failure to appreciate the child's over-all clinical picture and underlying medical history due to a failure to engage a timely cardiology review; failure to follow guidelines (Leicester Medicines Code) for non-prescribed medication because of a custom and practice for administering non prescribed regular medication.' In other words, there were indeed myriad 'circumstances' entirely beyond the practice of Dr Bawa-Garba that clearly contributed to the patient's death. And yet it seems clear that, although the criminal court, High Court, Appeal Court, MPTS, and Trust inquiry all addressed such 'circumstances', and rendered them significant, they did so in differing ways and concluded them to be of differing relevance, indeed crucially different relevance.

Finally, there seems little evidence that any of the fora, even the NHS inquiry, adequately addressed Dr Bawa-Garba's 'fine-grain' decision-making in terms of the types of rational or heuristic theories presented in Part A. And, almost certainly, that is because doing so does not 'fit', or cannot be accommodated within, the particular forum. Rather, self-reflection (perhaps guided within supervision) seems most likely to be capable of facilitating this. And it is to this that we now turn in regard to her case.

In her reflective notes Dr Bawa-Garba did indeed reflect in a 'fine-grain' fashion on how she had come to make the decisions she made, some of which had contributed to the Jack Adcock's death. And, of note, in the government-sponsored independent inquiry into the operation of gross negligence medical manslaughter chaired by Professor Sir Norman Williams,[13] one of the key recommendations was that notes of such self-reflection should not be accessible to any disciplinary or professional practice body, on the basis that the risk

---

[9] In practice, the decision on whether to take out civil negligence proceedings often turns on other factors, such as whether there is a living victim with unfunded care and support needs, and whether the amount of damages that might be awarded in a successful negligence action (which could then pay for that care), and the likelihood of proving negligence, are sufficient to warrant the costs of the legal proceedings.

[10] *Bolam v Friern Hospital Management Committee* [1957] 1 WLR 583.

[11] *Bolitho v Hackney Health Authority* [1998] AC 232.

[12] University of Leicester Hospitals Group NHS Trust, Final Report, Unexpected Death, Initial Report Form Reference W65737.

[13] www.nationalarchives.gov.uk/doc/open-government-licence/.

of future disclosure with adverse consequences would be such as to *inhibit* self-critique and learning. This perhaps emphasises that self-critique is usually likely to offer a crucial route to learning, and to avoiding future harms, with blame being the enemy of learning.[14]

So, in summary, the forum is all. And there is always some risk of 'contamination' across fora, either or both by way of factual matters determined in one context being used unthinkingly, without regard to the prescribed purposes of that context, in another, or by interpretation of data in one context being adopted inappropriately by another (see also below). Very obviously, contamination applied in Dr Bawa-Garba's case, when the GMC argued, initially successfully in the High Court, that the MPTS should not have 'gone behind' her criminal conviction in determining that, once past suspension for a year, she would remain fit to practise.[15]

[14] Successive Secretaries of State for Health have seemed to accept this, and yet no significant inroads into the blame culture of the NHS have been achieved. Perhaps suggesting that there is a systems- based inherent resistance to avoidance of blame, perhaps for fear that if blame does not alight upon individuals in respect of an individual case it may alight upon the particular NHS organisation, or even upon the culture of the NHS as a whole.

[15] There are some criminal convictions that do automatically result in erasure from the Medical Register, notably murder and rape.

C.4

Other specific critique paradigms

Civil negligence

Whereas the purpose of criminal negligence is to punish for criminal wrongdoing, the purpose of civil negligence is to compensate victims for the effects of negligent clinical practice and to 'police' practice against (i.e. discourage) such negligent practice (see e.g. civil law case 4).

So, turning to the example of patient suicide (as in civil law case 2), here, there can be, and often is, critiquing of clinical practice in the civil courts, in terms of negligence, and in the Coroners Court (see below). Where counsel for a bereaved family may, for example, in the latter aim both to collect evidence and to achieve a finding that will assist in a negligence action, as wells as using critiquing within an MPTS hearing to similar intended effect (aside from also using any nonlegal internal hospital or external inquiry). And again, all these legal fora apply differing processes and critically appraise the case against differing criteria. Yet, although they are addressing apparently different questions, again there is much room for 'cross-over' between fora, including by data and findings originating within one forum being used within another.

Of course, a given legal process may *properly* include as evidence nonlegally based investigation of adverse outcomes; hence, for example, a court addressing alleged negligence, or breach of health and safety law or regulations, may receive evidence from an internal hospital, or external inquiry. So that information and conclusions from one form of investigation then becomes evidence within another. We will turn in a moment to address inquiries in more detail.

Coroner's inquests

Where a patient dies within medical care, and the criteria for a coroner's inquest are met,[1] this leads to another form of legal critique of clinical care. And, as indicated above, the evidence presented, and sometimes the verdict of the inquest, can then be used in subsequent civil litigation in negligence.

---

[1] These amount to reason to suspect that the deceased died a violent or unnatural death; the cause of the death is unknown; or the deceased died while in custody or state detention.

Examples of when a death must be reported to a coroner of a patient in medical care include where there is a question of negligence or misadventure about the treatment of the person who died. And there must also be an inquest held in relation to any death in custody (of particular relevance to clinical forensic psychiatric practice). So quite clearly there is 'cross-over' with potential civil or even criminal negligence.

The coroner will decide on the scope of an inquest and determine the nature of enquiries to be undertaken. And once he or she is in receipt of all reports and statements, which may include hospital internal inquiry reports, these will be shared with the 'interested persons', and then a decision will be made as to which witnesses are required to attend the inquest hearing to give evidence in person, and whose evidence can be read into the record in their absence.

The coroner may also, as part of the inquest process, instruct for him- or herself independent experts to advise on possible negligent care, and both the family of the deceased and the health care provider can also do so, through their instructed counsel.

When recording the cause of death, the coroner or jury may give a verdict that includes accident or misadventure, unlawful killing, natural causes, open verdict, suicide, and may include 'aggravation of cause by lack of care'. Also, there may be offered a brief 'narrative', setting out the facts surrounding the death in more detail and explaining the reasons for the decision.

The process of the hearing is not adversarial but inquisitorial. So that the method of critique does not suffer the constraints imposed upon fact finding and conclusions often attendant other forms of (adversarial) legal hearing. And it might be thought therefore that inquests are less incongruous with 'fine-grain' clinically based critique methodology than some other legal processes. However, counsel for 'opposing' sides in an inquest hearing can encourage an adversarial climate, albeit the coroner may attempt to inhibit this.

Inquiries

Across all of the legal fora lurks inhibition of finding '*the* truth' by way of restricted data and methods of inferring from data, in favour therefore of finding '*a* truth' (see above). So that, by comparison with 'nonlegal' inquiry, there are constraints. However, criticism of nonlegal fora is often that they too may not be 'fair', by virtue of not applying legal tests and process, or clear burdens and standards of proof; albeit any inquiry can be subjected to judicial review in regard the process it applied if that process was fundamentally flawed.

Inquiries vary greatly in character, process, and type, and represent a huge topic; and one that has been the subject of, often highly critical, commentary. However, the claim for them, especially nonstatutory inquiries, is that—unconstrained by legal procedure and rules—they can more comprehensively and openly investigate what occurred and why[2] than can legal process. That is, they are capable of walking closer to 'clinical reality', by being unconstrained by legal process.

There is, in regard to NHS services, a hierarchy of inquiries, including those internal to the hospital Trust or Board; those that are internal but with led by an impartial external chair (some being legally qualified); those that are external and fully independent[3]; and

---

[2] That is, they address 'the truth ... what happened; how did it happen; and who, if anyone, was responsible, culpably or otherwise, for it having happened?' (Blom-Cooper L (1993) Public inquiries, in Freeman M and Happle B (eds) *Current Legal Problems, 46 Part II, Collected Papers*. Oxford University Press, pp. 204–220.

[3] At least, of the hospital or Trust concerned. As the external body is another part of the NHS, the independence of such inquires has been called into question.

those that are public and judicially led. The latter, for example, may utilise, or take into account, the findings of one of the lower-level inquiries (if more than one level is applied to the case). And the tool that is applied by internal inquiries at least is usually root cause analysis (RCA, see below).

In essence, there is an inherent and necessary trade-off between 'fairness' and seeking the truth in comparing inquiries with legal process. Albeit, apparently paradoxically, legal process itself places restrictions on data inclusion and the process of consideration also for reasons of 'fairness', so that (un)fairness operates in two directions. And in psychiatry the starkest example of this may well again be homicide inquiries. In that nonstatutory inquiries have variable terms of reference (sometimes in regard to apparently similar cases); offer no procedural or prescriptive legal rights or safeguards[4]; make no presumption of 'innocence'; can, if they wish, deliberate in private; and have no prescribed and known rules of procedure.[5] There is also no entitlement to cross examination or a right of appeal to any court to challenge the inquiry's findings (albeit their process can, rarely, be open to judicial review if it is deemed to have been clearly flawed and/or unfair, or can be overturned through the decision being deemed *Wednesbury* unreasonable[6]). And, of course, the findings can sometimes potentially be used in subsequent separate, usually civil negligence, legal proceedings (see above and below).

Some argue that lack of legal procedure combined with privacy optimises the pursuit of truth[7]; but such aspects inherently offer lesser protection to witnesses who are professionally at risk and yet are required to attend.[8] Nonstatutory inquiries also depend inconveniently upon the patient's consent for access to medical records.[9] Finally, inquiries can be biased by way of serving public catharsis.[10]

So, as a result of these features, and despite their alleged efficiency, whether inquiries do find *the* truth may be sometimes open to doubt. And certainly it seems unlikely that they will subject their own process to 'fine-grain' *self*-critiquing of their critiquing of others; in that the quasi-judicial (but not judicial) nature of their proceedings, driven by them often being legally chaired, hardly lends itself to investigation of 'fine-grain decision-making' by actors in the drama (compare such inquiries e.g. with self-reflective practice, see above and below). Indeed, for a witness to expose themselves to such fine-grain self-analysis in front of others, even if not in public, would seem unwise.[11] So that effective inquiry and truth-finding can be heavily inhibited by any inquiry process that could, somehow, result

---

[4] With the exception of so called 'Salmon letters', which give attendees forewarning that they may be open to criticism within the hearing.

[5] Boardman, Lord (1994), House of Lords; Hansard 552 (41) at Col. 208-10, 16 February.

[6] *Associated Provincial Picture Houses Ltd v Wednesbury Corporation* [1948] 1 KB 223

[7] Clothier Sir C (1996) Ruminations on inquiries, in Peay J (ed) *Inquiries after Homicide*. Duckworth, pp. 50–56.

[8] Eastman N L G (1996) Towards an audit of inquiries: Enquiry not inquiries, in Peay J (ed) *Inquiries after Homicide*. Duckworth, pp. 147–172.; Eastman N L G (1996) Inquiries into homicides by psychiatric patients: Systematic audit should replace mandatory inquiries, *British Medical Journal* 7064(313): 1069–1071.

[9] Thorold O and Trotter J (1996) Inquiries into homicide: A legal perspective, in Peay J (ed) *Inquiries after Homicide*. Duckworth, pp. 39–49.

[10] Reder P and Duncan S (1996) Reflections on child abuse inquiries, in Peay J (ed) *Inquiries after homicide*. Duckworth, pp. 93–98.

[11] One of NE's clinical supervisors in forensic psychiatry was subjected to a homicide inquiry in respect of one of his patients and wished, for himself, to understand how he had come to make any decisions that might have contributed to the killing, and so told his QC of his intention to be completely open with the inquiry panel in reflecting self-critically in front of the inquiry panel; to be told in the strongest terms by the QC that he was to do no such thing, being assured effectively that that was not within the 'model' of inquiries (personal communication).

in sanctioning of the witnesses.[12] As well as being at risk of clinical invalidity by way of substitution of its own heuristics and bias, and/or of substituting, often crucially, its own 'values balance' (see above).

Finally, homicide inquiries are similar to the homicides into which they enquire. Both are 'events'. By contrast, delivery of mental health care is a process, and, throughout medicine, it is generally agreed that a clinical process is most effectively investigated and improved by cycles of audit.[13]

By contrast, with the previously mandatory[14] requirement of an external inquiry after a psychiatric homicide, other psychiatric deaths (from suicide), and other medical and surgical deaths are much more commonly solely the subject of local or national audit, or of adjudication by the NHS Ombudsman. Hence, a wholly different government approach has usually been adopted to psychiatric homicides from that which is adopted in relation to the far more numerous suicides, or surgical and medical deaths. And this is likely to be driven by different public perception both of mental illness,[15] compared with other illness, and of the nature and acceptability of psychiatric risk compared to surgical or other medical risk.

At the aggregate rather than individual case level there is however the National Confidential Inquiry into Suicides and Homicides by People with Mental Illness, which collects data across cases, and does seek not to apportion responsibility but to encourage service improvement. It therefore progresses by collection and correlation of individual case data, with the aim of 'service learning'.

In summary, it seems inevitable that many of the biases in rational, and also nonrational, methods of decision-making that are applied to clinical decision-making will be mirrored in any inquiry there may be into a decision previously made, perhaps especially since such inquiries occur, of course, after there is known to have been a bad outcome (with the obvious risk therefore of hindsight bias). Hence, that bad outcome can, likely will, taint or bias inquiry into the service that experienced it, especially if not constrained by legal process.

Root cause analysis

This form of critique aims to address the risk of clinical invalidity that may attend other forms of inquiry, whether legal or other.

The former National Patient Safety Agency (NPSA) adopted, and adapted for health services, RCA, which has become the standard method within the NHS of investigation of untoward incidents. It holds to a number of general standards in terms of asking:

- Was the investigation process conducted with the appropriate level of *independence*?
- Was the investigation process *proportionate* to the incident and any associated risks?

[12] Within procedural rules of inquiries is provision for 'Salmon letters', which are sent to advise a witness that they may be subject to particular criticisms within the inquiry.
[13] See Eastman N L G (1996) Inquiries into homicides by psychiatric patients: Systematic audit should replace mandatory inquiries, *British Medical Journal* 7064(313): 1069–1071.
[14] Homicide inquiries ceased to be mandatory in 2013, so that now NHS England determines whether one should be held on the basis of whether there are likely to be lessons to be learned, given how many have been held. Though this would seem to decide whether to hold one depending upon conclusions that could only be reached by doing so.
[15] Pescosolido B A, Monahan J, Link B G, Stueve A, and Kikuzawa S (1999) The public's view of competence, dangerousness and the need for legal coercion of persons with mental health problems. *American Journal of Public Health* 89(9): 1339–1345; Link B G, Phelan J C, Bresnahan M, Stueve A, and Pescosolido B A (1999) Public conceptions of mental illness: Labels, causes, dangerousness and social distance. *American Journal of Public Health* 89(9): 1328–1333; Pearson G (1999) Madness and moral panics, in Eastman N and Peay J (eds), *Law without Enforcement: Integrating Mental Health and Justice*. Hart Publications, pp. 159–172.

- Did the investigation begin and end in a *timely* manner?
- Was the investigation process *open and transparent*?
- Did the investigation team *keep relevant parties appropriately informed*?
- Was the investigation *based on evidence*?

And crucially:

- Did the investigation *look for improvements* and *not to apportion blame*?

However, none of these criteria, or other aspects of RCA, necessarily require or encourage 'fine-grain' analysis of decision-making in the terms of theory presented in Part A, so that it is likely to be serendipitous whether such fine-grain analysis occurs.

RCA does seek to avoid specifically *hindsight bias*, that is, 'the tendency for people with the "benefit of hindsight" to falsely believe, once all the facts become clear, that the actions that should have been taken to prevent an incident seem obvious, or that they could have predicted the outcome of an event'. However, the NPSA notes 'although considered a serious pitfall in investigation terms, hindsight bias has been documented as a potentially *useful* mechanism in terms of the specific focus of learning from incidents[16]... in that it is a by-product of an adaptive mechanism that can make human memory more efficient. So that the basic idea of this "RAFT" model (Reconstruction After Feedback with Take the Best) is that any feedback or correct information received (in this case in the form of a now known, but previously unpredicted, incident outcome) is used to automatically update a person's knowledge base; although it is important to remember that failure to recognise hindsight bias in incident investigation can result in misinterpretation of findings and may ultimately mask the real lessons to be learned'.

The NPSA also cautions against *'outcome bias'*; that is, 'the tendency to judge a past decision or action by its success or failure, instead of being based on the quality of the decision made at the time. No decision maker knows for sure whether or not the future will turn out for the best following any decision they make. Yet individuals whose judgements are influenced by outcome bias can hold decision makers responsible for events beyond their control. Similarly, if an incident leads to death it is often considered very differently, and critically, compared to an incident that results in no harm, even where the incident or error is exactly the same. And when people are judged one way when the outcome is good, and another when the outcome is bad, accountability levels become inconsistent and unfair. So that, to avoid the influence of outcome bias, one should evaluate the decision or action taken at the time it was taken, and given what was known or going on at that time, irrespective of the success or failure of the outcome'.

In summary, the essence of the RCA method is addressing 'the 5 Whys[17]', so that by repeatedly asking 'the question', it is hoped that it will be possible successively to peel away the layers of 'symptoms', which can then lead to identifying the 'root cause' of a problem. However, this 5 Whys method has some inherent limitations.[18] 'First, using 5

---

[16] Although this may be cold comfort to any clinician who is coincidentally criticized and/or sanctioned by way of such hindsight bias.

[17] The idea that, given enough (up to five) layers of abstraction from the initial description of the problem, the questioner can identify a reason why the process being followed failed. 'Whys' in this sense must be focussed on things potentially under control, and exclude *ex machina* responses such as there not being enough resources (e.g. time, money, and staff), even though these may also be true.

[18] Anderson S, Root cause analysis: Addressing some limitations of the 5 Whys, in *Quality Digest*, 17 December 2009. https://www.qualitydigest.com/inside/lean-article/root-cause-analysis-addressing-some-limitations-5-whys-121709.html.

Whys does not always lead to root cause identification when the cause is unknown (i.e. if the cause is unknown to the person doing the problem solving), so using 5 Whys may not lead to any meaningful answers. Second, an assumption underlying 5 Whys is that each presenting symptom has only one sufficient cause. Yet this is not always the case, and 5 Whys analysis may not reveal "jointly sufficient" causes that explain a symptom. Third, the success of 5 Whys is to some degree contingent upon the skill with which the method is applied, and if even one Why attracts a bad or meaningless answer, the whole procedure can be thrown off. Finally, the method is not necessarily repeatable; and three different people applying 5 Whys to the same problem may come up with three totally different answers. Other drawbacks to 5 Whys have also been cited, including the method's inability to distinguish between causal factors and root causes, and the lack of rigour where users are not required to test for causal sufficiency.

As regards the level of investigation (see also above), there may be single RCA, or RCA aggregation with multi-incident investigation. Whilst the process of investigation should include determining 'the key points of the mapped chronology ... so that the reader of the report can gain a clear understanding of the events leading up to the incident'.

Clearly the agenda of RCA is to reduce, so far as possible, causes of bias in the investigation process. However, it tends to focus on identifying sequences of events. And, although this is surely a prerequisite for a further stage of interpreting how individual decisions within those events were made, whether it can consistently address cognitive heuristics and bias to the level described in Part A is perhaps doubtful. That said, it may well be superior in regard to bias to some other forms of inquiry, and certainly, the advantage of RCA is that it reduces or eliminates *some* of the heuristics and biases (as set out in Part A) that can impair unstructured inquiry processes.[19] However gaining its benefits may well depend upon the matter under investigation.

Finally, the conclusions should distinguish between 'root causes' and 'contributory factors'. And, as we noted in the above case study, in that case a single root cause for the death was unable to be identified.

Audit

An audit (by definition) investigates aspects of a service, or part of a service across defined cases. That is, it is an aggregate exercise, pursuing a cycle of improvement of both clinical process and outcome. Of course, how an audit is set up can be influenced, or biased, by the particular process adopted, or, in a different sense, by way of choice of the variables that it seeks to measure and improve. And, given its 'microscope up' approach, including concentration on outcomes, it is very unlikely naturally to be 'fine-grain' in its method.

Appraisal

Appraisal occurs across a clinician's practice, even if it does include addressing particular untoward events that have occurred since the last appraisal, and includes also using self-reflection (see above). It is potentially extremely 'broad brush' in its character, unless

---

[19] See for example *The Independent Inquiry into the Care and Treatment of John Barrett*, NHS London, November 2006, whose conclusions were wholly different in regard to critiquing the consultant forensic psychiatrist responsible for the patient's care from the findings in regard to her (non-) culpability found within the subsequent Court of Appeal case.

decisions are taken explicitly to include detailed and fine-grain self-reflection (although it does require collection of a great deal of detailed data about the person's practice). And, even if there is much detail, the analysis of such data is often largely impressionistic, whilst the data collected is effectively chosen by the doctor (unless there is a known unto-ward incident). So, perhaps contrary to what the GMC or NHS, for example, might hope, it is generally not an effective fine-grain tool; albeit collection of large amounts of data might suggest otherwise.

Yet reflection surely should be the method most open to self-critique within the models described in Part A (see below), and therefore of high validity. And almost certainly the clinician is *potentially* a better guardian of their own practice than is appraisal. Finally, appraisal of specifically clinico-legal practice can be subject to formal process through a feedback system: for example, the Royal College of Psychiatrists' Centre for Quality Improvement feedback system designed specifically for expert psychiatric witnesses.[20]

Peer review

Peer review is inherent to medical appraisal, and revalidation, in that it is a required aspect of the former, and feeds into the latter. However, it has not, until recently, been required to include specifically clinico-legal practice. Although the expert witness practice of psychiatrists is now under increasing scrutiny by the courts and the GMC, including within appraisal of a doctor's overall practice.

Appraisal of expert witness practice must address not only technical competence, including evidence of a real understanding of the interface between medicine and law, but also ethical probity, which is the more challenging appraisal focus. And, although within *all* psychiatry there is much room for the influence of values, in the expression of expert opinion, this is enhanced by the fact that the questions to which medical knowledge is ultimately put are not clinical questions but legal and ultimately *moral* questions (by way of 'clinico-legal mapping'). Hence, for example, an expert witness may, perhaps even without realising they are doing so, have a view of what the outcome of a legal case should be, and then accordingly (even unconsciously) amend either their clinical opinion about mental state or the mapping of that mental state onto the relevant legal test. And teasing this out within the legal process itself is not always reliably achieved.[21]

Bias can arise from sources 'within' experts, including as a reflection of their 'relation-ship' with the subject of assessment or their own values, or as an inherent reflection of the adversarial legal system. And routes to the expression of bias are numerous, throughout the method of assessment, report drafting, and giving of oral evidence.[22] And this empha-sises the importance of robust peer review.

The importance of peer review (*ex post*, not prereporting and giving oral evidence[23]) is illustrated by the requirement that, in order to be on 'the Home Office list', forensic

---

[20] *The Multi-Source Assessment Tool for Expert Psychiatric Witnesses*, originating in the work of Professor Keith Rix.

[21] The sudden infant death syndrome criminal cases in which Professor Sir Roy Meadow was eventually criticized for inaccurate use, or interpretation of mortality statistics within a single family, which appar-ently continued across a number of cases for some years, without the justice system rooting it out, may illustrate the point.

[22] See the handbook pages NNN.

[23] Since the opinion must be that of the expert; albeit they may validly seek advice on a specialist point from an expert colleague, though must make plain that they have done so.

pathologists must practice in groups, in order to minimise the chance of 'base-line drift'; the risk of such being enhanced where an expert operates in the absence of peer review.

Peer review, which usually is applied to single cases, can take a number of forms, which cannot be addressed here. However, clearly such review can vary in how 'fine'- or 'coarse'-grained is the review.

Self-critique

Finally, we return to self-critique, because it is *potentially* the most rigorous form of critique, if applied honestly and with rigour. No one can potentially know your mind better than you; albeit 'self-deception' is common in all of us. So that, at the heart of effective self-critique is 'self-inquiry'. And here we do come full circle back to Part A, in terms that self-critique is fully open potentially to the use of 'fine-grain' critiquing, *at all decision stages*. That is, as you prepare to make a decision, as you make it, as you decide to implement it after critiquing it, and as you peer into the recesses of your mind and look back critically on those stages, whether the outcome was 'bad' or even 'good'. Indeed, it may be as important to self-critique good-outcome decision processes as bad-outcome processes. And, although you may be encouraged by others, including employers, mainly or solely to seek to learn from bad-outcome decisions, you should press yourself to learn from all-outcome decision processes. Critiquing only what turned out to be bad decisions is a bad habit to acquire.

C.5
Conclusion
Self-critique as the gold standard

The destination we have arrived at after reviewing a range of critique paradigms is, perhaps in a somewhat self-serving fashion for the casebook, that individual self-reflection represents the gold standard. And that the very best guardian of good practice, be it clinical, clinico-legal or ethical, and potentially even the greatest safety from external critique, is via learning the habit of self-reflection: that is, awareness and constant vigilance throughout daily practice in regard to the thinking and values we apply to cases. We hope that addressing the cases in Part B of the casebook will assist colleagues in pursuit of such good practice.

POSTFACE

As we indicated in the *Preface*, this is a book aimed at learning by doing on paper. However, its ultimate aim is, of course, to enhance learning by doing in reality. Although we hope that we have done something to aid the latter for colleagues, readers will be only too aware of any disparities there may be between learning on paper and learning by doing. And we hope that, to the extent that there are failings in the cases we offer to represent reality, our readers will keep us informed of such. Similarly, if there are failings that readers observe, or improvements that could be made, in either of Parts A or C, we hope you will tell us. And if there are changes that might be made towards improving the 'companion' relationship between the casebook and the second edition of the handbook, again please tell us.

Finally, you are of course at liberty to use the cases of Part B within teaching exercises. However, we hope that, in doing so, you will credit their origins. And, if you alter the case scenarios, we hope that you will make plain the ways in this has been done, and to what purpose.

INDEX

For the benefit of digital users, indexed terms that span two pages (e.g., 52–53) may, on occasion, appear on only one of those pages.

Tables and boxes are indicated by *t* and *b* following the page number